P9-DMB-651

PREVENTION'S

Healing with Vitamins

The Most Effective Vitamin and Mineral Treatments for Everyday Health Problems and Serious Disease—From Allergies and Arthritis to Water Retention and Wrinkles

By the Editors of *Prevention* Magazine Health Books

Edited by Alice Feinstein

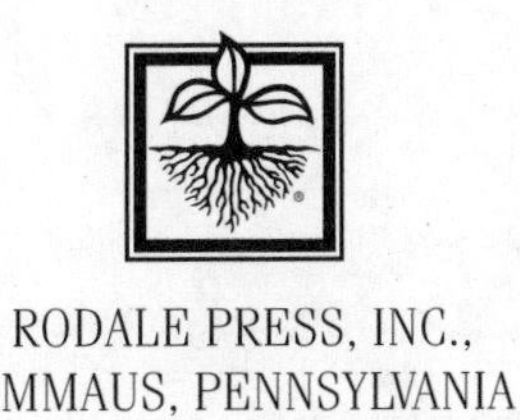

RODALE PRESS, INC.,
EMMAUS, PENNSYLVANIA

Notice

This book is intended as a reference volume only, not as a medical manual. The information given here is designed to help you make informed decisions about your health. While vitamins and minerals are nutrients that your body needs, in larger amounts they can have powerful druglike effects on your body. It is possible to overdose on certain vitamins and minerals, and it is possible to experience side effects. Vitamins and minerals can also interact with medications. For all of these reasons, you should always check with your physician when using doses above the Daily Values. This volume is not intended as a substitute for any treatment that may have been prescribed by your doctor. If you suspect that you have a medical problem, we urge you to seek competent medical help.

Printed in the United States of America on acid-free ♾, recycled paper ♻

Library of Congress Cataloging-in-Publication Data

Prevention's healing with vitamins: the most effective vitamin and mineral treatments for everyday health problems and serious disease—from allergies and arthritis to water retention and wrinkles / by the editors of Prevention Magazine health books; edited by Alice Feinstein.

p. cm.

Includes index.

ISBN 0–87596–292–0 hardcover

1. Vitamins—Therapeutic use. 2. Minerals—Therapeutic use. 3. Dietary supplements—Popular works. I. Feinstein, Alice. II. Prevention Magazine Health Books.

RM259.P74 1996

615'.328—dc20 96–10202

Distributed in the book trade by St. Martin's Press

2 4 6 8 10 9 7 5 3 1 hardcover

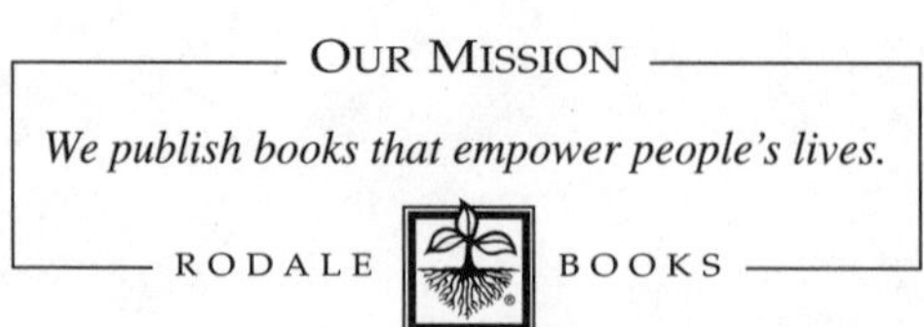

***Prevention's Healing with Vitamins* Editorial Staff**

Managing Editor: Alice Feinstein

Writers: Selene Y. Craig, Jennifer Haigh, Brian Paul Kaufman, Gale Maleskey, Ellen Michaud

Assistant Research Manager: Carol Svec

Book Researcher: Christine Dreisbach

Assistant Book Researcher: Carol J. Gilmore

Fact-Checkers: Susan E. Burdick, Carlotta Cuerdon, Valerie Edwards-Paulik, Jan Eickmeier, Karen Marmarus, Deborah Pedron, Kathryn Piff, Sally A. Reith, Sandra Salera-Lloyd, Anita Small, Bernadette Sukley, Michelle M. Szulborski, Margo Trott, John Waldron

Associate Art Director: Faith Hague

Cover and Interior Designer: Vic Mazurkiewicz

Studio Manager: Joe Golden

Technical Artist: William L. Allen

Layout Artist: Mary Brundage

Senior Copy Editors: Susan G. Berg, Jane Sherman

Production Manager: Helen Clogston

Manufacturing Coordinator: Patrick Smith

Office Staff: Roberta Mulliner, Julie Kehs, Bernadette Sauerwine, Mary Lou Stephen

Rodale Health and Fitness Books

Vice-President and Editorial Director: Debora T. Yost

Art Director: Jane Colby Knutila

Research Manager: Ann Gossy Yermish

Copy Manager: Lisa D. Andruscavage

Prevention Magazine Health Books Board of Advisers

Joanne Curran-Celentano, R.D., Ph.D.
Associate professor of nutritional sciences at the University of New Hampshire in Durham

Robert DiBianco, M.D.
Director of cardiology research, the Heart Failure Clinic and the Risk Factor Reduction Center, all at Washington Adventist Hospital in Takoma Park, Maryland, and associate clinical professor of medicine at Georgetown University School of Medicine in Washington, D.C.

Maria A. Fiatarone, M.D.
Assistant professor in the Division on Aging at Harvard Medical School, chief of the physiology laboratory at the Jean Mayer USDA Human Nutrition Research Center on Aging at Tufts University and attending physician in general medicine and geriatric medicine at Brigham and Women's Hospital, Beth Israel Hospital and West Roxbury Veterans Administration Medical Center, all in Boston

Mitchell Friedlaender, M.D.
Director of cornea and refractive surgery at Scripps Clinic and Research Foundation in La Jolla, California

Scott Haldeman, M.D., Ph.D., D.C.
Associate clinical professor in the Department of Neurology at the University of California, Irvine, and adjunct professor at the Los Angeles Chiropractic College

Arthur I. Jacknowitz, Pharm.D.
Professor and chairman of the Department of Clinical Pharmacy at West Virginia University in Morgantown

Mary Ann E. Keenan, M.D.
Chair of the Department of Orthopaedic Surgery at Albert Einstein Medical Center, orthopaedic director at Moss Rehabilitation Hospital and a full professor in orthopaedic surgery and physical medicine and rehabilitation at Temple University School of Medicine, all in Philadelphia

William J. Keller, Ph.D.
Professor and chair of the Department of Pharmaceutical Sciences in the School of Pharmacy at Samford University in Birmingham, Alabama

Robert D. Kerns, Ph.D.
Chief of the psychology service and director of the Comprehensive Pain Management Center at the VA Connecticut Health Care System in West Haven, Connecticut, and associate professor of psychiatry, neurology and psychology at Yale University

Charles P. Kimmelman, M.D.
Professor of otolaryngology at New York Medical College in Valhalla and a physician at Manhattan Eye, Ear and Throat Hospital

Albert M. Kligman, M.D., Ph.D.
Professor of dermatology at the University of Pennsylvania School of Medicine and an attending physician at the Hospital of the University of Pennsylvania, both in Philadelphia

Jeffrey Lisse, M.D.
Associate professor of medicine and director of the Division of Rheumatology at the University of Texas Medical Branch at Galveston

Jack W. McAninch, M.D.
Chief of urology at San Francisco General Hospital and professor and vice-chairman of the Department of Urology at the University of California, San Francisco

Morris B. Mellion, M.D.
Clinical associate professor of family practice and orthopaedic surgery at the University of Nebraska Medical Center and medical director of the Sports Medicine Center, both in Omaha

Thomas Platts-Mills, M.D., Ph.D.
Professor of medicine and head of the Division of Allergy and Immunology at the University of Virginia Medical Center in Charlottesville

David P. Rose, D.Sc., M.D., Ph.D.
Chief of the Division of Nutrition and Endocrinology at the Naylor Dana Institute of the American Health Foundation in Valhalla, New York, and an expert on nutrition and cancer for the National Cancer Institute in Rockville, Maryland, and the American Cancer Society

William B. Ruderman, M.D.
Practicing physician at Gastroenterology Associates of Central Florida in Orlando

Yvonne S. Thornton, M.D.
Visiting associate physician at Rockefeller University Hospital in New York City and director of the Perinatal Diagnostic Testing Center at Morristown Memorial Hospital in New Jersey

Lila A. Wallis, M.D.
Clinical professor of medicine and director of "Update Your Medicine," a series of continuing medical educational programs for physicians, at Cornell University Medical College in New York City

Andrew T. Weil, M.D.
Associate director of the Division of Social Perspectives in Medicine at the University of Arizona College of Medicine in Tucson

Richard J. Wood, Ph.D.
Associate professor in the School of Nutrition at Tufts University in Medford, Massachusetts, and chief of the mineral bioavailability laboratory at the Jean Mayer USDA Human Nutrition Research Center on Aging at Tufts University in Boston

Contents

Part One

Vitamins and Minerals for Health

Part Two

Therapeutic Prescriptions for Healing

Introduction

Tapping Into Nature's Vital Healing Power

Vitamins are not magic pills. But let's face it: It's really tempting to think of them that way. Anything that can help you live longer, look younger, stave off cancer and heart disease, enhance your immune system, fight off illness and boost your energy certainly sounds pretty miraculous or magical.

A few decades ago, when word started to spread about the healing potential of vitamins and minerals, the general public went wild for bottled nutrients. So did health writers and even some doctors. For a while, it was starting to sound like megadoses of vitamins could cure anything. Just take enough vitamins or the right combination of vitamins, and bingo! You were on your way to total health.

Well, that bubble burst soon enough. Of course, vitamins and minerals can't cure everything. But they can do a lot. Research breakthroughs over just the past few years are making interest in the topic heat up all over again. Some of the things that scientists have discovered about the healing power of these vital nutrients all but boggle the mind.

Let's take a brief look at just one study that didn't get all that much publicity. Researchers in London looked at 180 middle managers employed in the manufacturing industry in Britain. In a rigorous study, they gave one group a typical multivitamin/mineral supplement and another group a look-alike pill that did not contain nutrients. At the end of eight weeks, those receiving supplements revealed in tests that they perceived an improvement in their quality of life. The group not receiving supplements did not perceive a change. Researchers concluded that the supplements seemed to play a role in improving the managers' moods and reducing their stress levels. All of this from just a daily multivitamin pill . . . with hard scientific data confirming that it works.

As more and more rigorous scientific studies accumulate showing spectacular health benefits from vitamins and minerals, we're all back where we were a few decades ago: eager to take advantage of all of this healing potential—and thoroughly confused. While the reasons for taking vitamins and minerals are now based on solid science, shopping for nutrients is still nothing less than overwhelming.

You know what happens when you make a trip to your local pharmacy or supermarket to buy nutrients. You're faced with overwhelming choices. Shelf after shelf in aisle after aisle offers nothing but confusion. Letters and numbers, single nutrients and combinations, capsules and tablets, bottles in different sizes and colors from different companies, covered with enticing claims that compete for your attention and your precious consumer dollar.

What's a person who wants to take vitamins and minerals in a safe and responsible manner supposed to do? All you really want to know, after all, is what really works.

Well, search no more. That's what this book is all about.

Over the past year and a half, five writers on the staff of *Prevention* Magazine Health Books interviewed hundreds of the nation's top doctors and researchers, asking exactly those questions that you want answered: Which vitamins and minerals can you take to prevent, cure or ameliorate specific diseases? How much of the nutrients do you take? Are they safe? What kinds of results can you expect?

These writers also scanned computer databases and reviewed thousands of scientific studies to answer these questions. And in this fast-breaking, ever-changing, ever-expanding arena of nutritional therapy, they've put it all together in one easy-to-use volume. You're holding it in your hands right now. If you want to know which nutrients to take and in what amounts, simply look up the disease you want to know about.

Along with the scoop on how to use nutrients to fight disease, the writers made several important discoveries during the course of their research.

One is that supplements are not a substitute for good nutrition. It will come as no surprise to anyone who pays attention to natural healing and prevention that scientists can't beat nature when it comes to packaging healing therapies.

And that's why, so often in this book, you'll find doctors and researchers saying that you should get your healing vitamins and minerals from foods whenever you can. At the same time, doctors and researchers in this book often recommend taking supplements—at least a multivitamin for what they call insurance. Why is that?

It's often not practical to get adequate therapeutic amounts of vitamins and minerals from foods. That's right, therapeutic. Large doses of some nutrients have such powerful effects on the body that they act like drugs.

That brings us to the second important discovery that the writers made: Vitamin and mineral supplements should be treated with the same care and concern for safety that you reserve for prescription and over-the-counter medications.

Large doses of certain nutrients can be toxic. They can cause side effects.

They can interact with medications that you might be taking. So there are a few rules to follow when using this book.

Please take the Medical Alerts seriously. They are there for your safety. If you are under a doctor's care for a serious disease, you should talk to him about your interest in using nutrients as part of your treatment. With all of the scientific breakthroughs in this area, doctors are increasingly open to nutritional therapy. You may be pleasantly surprised to find your doctor willing to work with you to find the right dosages and monitor your progress.

And if you're pregnant or nursing a baby, make sure you mention any supplements you're taking, even a multivitamin, to your physician.

Finally, pay attention to the Daily Values of any vitamins and minerals you're taking. Daily Values are a relatively new system from the Food and Drug Administration designed to help you keep track of your body's nutritional requirements.

Many researchers and doctors feel that the Daily Values for certain nutrients—vitamin C, for example—should be set much higher. They've also found that the body's need for nutrients goes way, way up when it's fighting disease. That's why you'll find the recommendations in this book often go way beyond the Daily Values for many nutrients.

Here's wishing you all of the healing that nature's nutrients can supply.

Alice Feinstein
Managing Editor

Part One

Vitamins and Minerals for Health

Beta-Carotene

Daily Value: *None*

Good Food Sources: *Sweet potatoes, carrots, cantaloupe, spinach and other dark green, leafy vegetables*

Beta-carotene has frequently been portrayed as the blockbuster nutrient that will save the world from cancer, heart disease, aging, cataracts and a host of other ills.

And it may well be. Preliminary studies over the past few years have indicated that the more beta-carotene-rich fruits and vegetables people eat, the less likely they are to get cancer—particularly cancers of the lung, stomach, esophagus, mouth and, in women, the reproductive tract.

In the Physicians' Health Study at Harvard Medical School, for example, a preliminary report indicates that heart attack risk was cut 50 percent in a group of men between the ages of 40 and 84 who took 50 milligrams (83,000 international units) of beta-carotene every other day.

But in 1994, researchers began to question the therapeutic effects of beta-carotene. A study of 29,000 male Finnish smokers found that men who took 20 milligrams (about 33,000 international units) of beta-carotene a day actually had an increased incidence of both lung cancer and heart disease.

"It was an unexpected result," admits Norman Krinsky, Ph.D., professor of biochemistry in the Department of Biochemistry at Tufts University School of Medicine in Boston. "It does not coincide with what people had expected."

Some scientists suspect that the unexpected increase in heart disease and lung cancer among the Finns may have been caused by one or the other of two problems. First, the smokers had been puffing away on cigarettes for so many decades—three, to be exact—that the cancer process had been initiated even before researchers started handing out beta-carotene. Second, the heavy drinking in which the smokers also had apparently engaged—and which was not reported in the original study—may have influenced the effectiveness of the beta-carotene, according to Joanne Curran-Celentano, Ph.D., associate professor of nutritional sciences at the University of New Hampshire in Durham. Dr. Curran-Celentano cautions that the Finnish study is not suggesting that beta-carotene supplementation caused an increase in cancer or in heart disease. Poor diet and long-term heavy smoking and drinking may have put the men at high risk, she says.

Many researchers and physicians still recommend fruits and vegetables rich in carotenoids for disease, according to Dr. Krinsky. In light of the Finnish study, however, some researchers may be more cautious about recommending beta-carotene supplements.

Contributing to their reluctance and caution in recommending supplements are relatively new laboratory techniques that have revealed that most foods containing beta-carotene also contain other powerful disease-fighting members of the carotenoid family such as alpha-carotene, lycopene, zeaxanthin and lutein. In fact, says Dr. Krinsky, it may be these substances that have been doing most of the disease-preventive work, while beta-carotene has been garnering all of the credit.

Using Beta-Carotene Safely

People should be reaching for carotenoid-rich foods rather than supplements," says Dr. Krinsky. "But for those among us who do not take in five to nine servings of dark green, leafy vegetables and yellow fruits and vegetables a day, it might be wise to supplement the diet with a moderate dose of beta-carotene—maybe 5, 10 or 15 milligrams (between 8,000 and 25,000 international units) a day." With respect to the question about whether or not to supplement, there is no easy answer, he says.

Too much beta-carotene in the body can turn the skin orange. The discoloration fades as levels of the nutrient return to normal.

Biotin

Daily Value: *300 micrograms*

Good Food Sources: *Brewer's yeast, corn, barley, soybeans, walnuts, peanuts, molasses, cauliflower, milk, egg yolks, fortified cereals*

Your nails are a disaster. They've been clipped, filed and buffed, then coated with polish. And they still look thin, brittle and pathetic.

They will never appear in *Vogue*. But they do happen to be just about the first thing folks notice when you shake hands or pet their dogs. So what are you gonna do?

Well, you may want to take a tip—no pun intended—from some of the men and women who went to a nail doctor in New York City. In a study conducted by Columbia University College of Physicians and Surgeons in New York City and Thomas Jefferson University Hospital in Philadelphia, these people took an average of two milligrams (2,000 micrograms) a day of biotin, a B-complex vitamin that is necessary for your body to process the fat and protein that you eat.

Except for those of us who have brittle nails or a genetic inability to absorb biotin, most people really don't need to worry about whether or not they're getting enough. That's because unless you have a genetic defect that alters the way your body uses this nutrient, either you get enough of it through the eggs, milk and cereals in your diet or your body will manufacture what you need.

People with Type II (non-insulin-dependent) diabetes may prove to be a different story. When Japanese researchers studied the biotin and blood sugar levels of people with diabetes, they found that the higher someone's blood sugar, the lower his level of biotin. They also noted that people with diabetes have significantly lower biotin levels than people who don't have the disease.

Nobody knew quite what this meant, but the researchers wanted to see what would happen if they raised biotin levels in those with diabetes. So they gave nine milligrams (9,000 micrograms) of biotin to 18 people with diabetes every day for a month.

The result? After 30 days, the participants' blood sugar levels fell to nearly half of their original levels. For the full details on using nutrients to treat diabetes, see page 211.

Using Biotin Safely

Biotin may be one of the safest of all vitamins. There are no reports of toxicity, even when it's taken in high doses above the Daily Value of 300 micrograms.

Biotin is destroyed by certain food-processing techniques such as canning and heat curing. So it's always better to choose fresh fruits, vegetables and meats over canned or cured foods.

Calcium

◆

Daily Value: *1,000 milligrams*

Good Food Sources: *Skim milk, nonfat yogurt, cheeses, collard greens, mustard greens, kale, broccoli, canned salmon with bones, sardines with bones, corn tortillas processed with lime, calcium-fortified orange juice*

◆

By now, just about everyone knows that getting enough calcium helps prevent diseases such as osteoporosis. Less well known is just how calcium goes about doing this.

When you eat cheese or drink milk, the calcium in these foods is absorbed through your small intestine and into your blood. The amount of calcium in your blood is regulated by a substance called parathyroid hormone. When calcium intake is low, parathyroid hormone signals for bone to be broken down, releasing calcium into the bloodstream. "Diets with adequate calcium intake produce less parathyroid hormone, so we conserve more calcium and more bone," says John Anderson, Ph.D., professor of nutrition in the Schools of Public Health and Medicine at the University of North Carolina at Chapel Hill.

Calcium then combines with phosphorus to help form hard, crystal-like substances that create the latticework undergirding strong bones and teeth. In fact, 99 percent of the calcium in your body is stored in your skeleton. Researchers call this ongoing process of removing old bone and forming new bone remodeling.

You also need a stable level of blood calcium for normal heartbeat, nerve and muscle function and blood clotting. Living cells require calcium to act as a messenger and to help respond to hormones and neurotransmitters.

Even though calcium is vital for bone growth and maintenance in everyone, experts don't advise a one-size-fits-all intake. Here are daily intake levels as set by the Consensus Development Conference of the National Institutes of Health in Bethesda, Maryland.

- Infants, up to age 6 months: 400 milligrams
- Infants, ages 6 to 11 months: 600 milligrams
- Children, ages 1 to 10 years: 800 to 1,200 milligrams

- Adolescents and young adults, ages 11 to 24: 1,200 to 1,500 milligrams
- Men, ages 25 to 65: 1,000 milligrams
- Women, ages 25 to 50: 1,000 milligrams
- Pregnant and nursing women: 1,200 to 1,500 milligrams
- Women at menopause (ages 51 to 65) who are taking estrogen: 1,000 milligrams
- Women at menopause (ages 51 to 65) who are not taking estrogen: 1,500 milligrams
- Men and women over age 65: 1,500 milligrams

Using Calcium Safely

If you want your supplement to be rich in calcium but aren't crazy about eating aluminum or lead, steer clear of those made of natural calcium carbonate, says Richard Wood, Ph.D., associate professor in the School of Nutrition at Tufts University in Medford, Massachusetts, and chief of the mineral bioavailability laboratory at the Jean Mayer USDA Human Nutrition Research Center on Aging at Tufts University in Boston. "They can be contaminated by these other things that you don't want in your diet," he says. Even some forms of dolomite, a natural calcium-magnesium combination supplement, have been found to contain these metals.

On the other hand, pharmaceutical-grade calcium carbonate should be free of metals. Calcium gluconate, calcium lactate and calcium citrate are also metal-free, but each of these types contains less concentrated forms of calcium. Calcium carbonate is also found in several brands of antacid tablets, and many people use these antacids as sources of calcium. But some antacids also contain aluminum, a metal that can prevent adequate mineralization in bone. So be sure to choose tablets that are aluminum-free, such as Tums or Rolaids.

Calcium is best absorbed when it's taken with food and at a dose not exceeding 500 milligrams. This means that if you're taking supplements exceeding that amount, you should take them in divided doses throughout the day. Also, avoid taking calcium supplements with high-fiber wheat bran cereals, which can reduce absorption by 25 percent.

High calcium intake (more than 2,000 milligrams a day) may cause constipation and kidney stones and inhibit zinc and iron absorption. High blood levels of the mineral cause the body to excrete any excess, which in turn triggers a loss of magnesium.

Folic Acid

Daily Value: *400 micrograms*

Good Food Sources: *Fortified cereals, pinto beans, navy beans, asparagus, spinach, broccoli, okra, brussels sprouts*

Folic acid is a nutritional powerhouse that makes things happen within the body. It works with approximately 20 different enzymes to build DNA, the material that contains the genetic code for your body, and is essential for normal nerve function.

It also seems to prevent heart disease and stroke by reducing the body's levels of homocysteine, an artery-attacking chemical that accumulates in the blood of people who eat meats.

What's more, folic acid may help protect against cancers of the lung, colon and cervix. In a study at the University of Alabama in Birmingham, researchers found that women whose cervical cells were loaded with folate (the naturally occurring form of folic acid) were two to five times less likely than women with low folate levels to develop cervical dysplasia when exposed to various risk factors such as cigarette smoke, the human papillomavirus, contraceptives and childbirth. (Cervical dysplasia is a condition involving the development of abnormal cells in the cervix. This condition can progress to cancer in some women.)

Folic acid also protects a woman's fetus from life-threatening birth defects of the brain and spine. Unfortunately, a survey by the March of Dimes has found that 90 percent of women of reproductive age are unaware of this fact, and only 15 percent are aware that the federal government has recommended that all women capable of bearing children get 400 micrograms of folic acid every day. This amount of folic acid is available in a multivitamin/mineral supplement. Still, only 28 percent of the women surveyed take a vitamin containing folic acid every day.

Using Folic Acid Safely

Folic acid has virtually no side effects, even when taken in high amounts, although one study did find that people taking 15 milligrams (15,000 micrograms) a day complained of nausea, bloating, problems sleeping and irritability. Doses of more than 400 micrograms a day can mask symptoms of pernicious anemia, a potentially fatal vitamin B_{12}–deficiency disease.

"In general, 0.4 milligram (400 micrograms) of folate is a good amount to get in a day, and with careful planning that can be achieved," says Meir Stampfer, M.D., Dr.P.H., an investigator at the Harvard School of Public Health. A day's worth of folate could look like this: one cup of orange juice (110 micrograms) and one cup of folate-fortified cereal (160 micrograms) plus a cup of raw spinach in a lunch or dinner salad (130 micrograms). Although folate is available in these and many other foods, be aware that as much as 50 percent of the nutrient is destroyed during food processing, storage and household preparation. In general, much of the folate in foods is killed by heat and light.

Several substances can increase your need for the vitamin, including alcohol, tobacco, aspirin and other nonsteroidal anti-inflammatory drugs, oral contraceptives, pancreatic extracts, estrogen, antacids, arthritis drugs such as methotrexate and medications prescribed for convulsions, malaria and bacterial infections.

Iron

Daily Value: *18 milligrams*

Good Food Sources: *Beef, Cream of Wheat cereal, baked potatoes, soybeans, pumpkin seeds, clams*

There's no doubt that many of us can use more iron than we're getting. Roughly 20 percent of Americans are deficient in this mineral. The group most likely to be coming up short: women in their reproductive years.

"I would say that women need to be a little more thoughtful than men about iron, probably in the same way that women should be a little more cautious about calcium intake because of osteoporosis," says Adria Sherman, Ph.D., professor and chair of the Department of Nutritional Sciences at Rutgers University in New Brunswick, New Jersey.

Iron, which is absorbed in the intestines, comes in two forms: heme and nonheme. Found in meats, the heme form is well-absorbed. Men get about two-thirds of their iron needs met by heme iron; the amount varies for women. Nonheme iron is found in vegetables and isn't as well-absorbed.

Most of the iron you consume goes to form hemoglobin, the substance that helps your red blood cells transport oxygen from your lungs to the rest of your body. The rest is stored in the bone marrow, liver, spleen and other organs.

Because iron also plays a key role in helping to prepare your immune system's infection fighters for battle, a deficiency may lead to colds. Low iron levels can also cause fatigue, pallor and listlessness—hallmarks of anemia, says Dr. Sherman. In children, low iron levels can cause stunted growth and impaired learning. Other symptoms of iron deficiency include split nails, a sore tongue and cold hands and feet. An annoying condition called restless legs has also been linked to low iron.

Some experts even believe that vague gastrointestinal problems such as gas, belching, constipation and diarrhea may be rooted in iron deficiency. If you suspect that you may be deficient in iron, ask your family doctor or your gynecologist to test your blood at your yearly exam.

Using Iron Safely

Here's a fact about iron supplements that should encourage healthy respect: Researchers studying ten years of records at a large Winnipeg, Manitoba, hospital found that an average of five iron supplement poisonings occur each year.

Although accidental iron poisonings occur most often in children who ingest supplements containing iron that are formulated for adults, high levels of iron can also be toxic to adults. Therefore, most experts recommend that you don't take iron supplements unless your doctor confirms the need with a blood test.

A daily intake of 25 milligrams or more for an extended period of time may cause undesirable side effects. Symptoms of acute iron poisoning include pain, vomiting, diarrhea and shock. Still, doctors normally recommend iron supplementation for pregnant women and for infants.

Among the variety of iron supplements, experts say those made with ferrous salts are better absorbed. Among them, ferrous sulfate is considered best.

Slow-release and coated iron tablets may cause less diarrhea, nausea and abdominal pain, but since the site of maximum absorption is the beginning of the small intestine, delaying the time of release decreases the overall amount of iron absorbed by your body. Taking the tablets with a meal could go a long way in helping to reduce stomach upset, but then again, the food may interfere with the iron absorption. Therefore, since it is advantageous for absorption, experts recommend taking iron supplements between meals if you do not experience side effects or you can tolerate iron taken in this manner.

Magnesium

Daily Value: *400 milligrams*

Good Food Sources: *Brown rice, avocados, spinach, haddock, oatmeal, baked potatoes, navy beans, lima beans, broccoli, yogurt, bananas*

Imagine a product that not only may help prevent a heart attack but also may successfully ease premenstrual syndrome, high blood pressure, heart arrhythmia, asthma and kidney stones.

This single-source solution to some of our most vexing health problems doesn't come from the high-tech laboratory of some pharmaceutical company. It's magnesium. And the more studies researchers conduct, the more impressive this mineral looks.

"There's no question that magnesium is the most looked-at mineral in nutrition today," says Herbert C. Mansmann, Jr., M.D., professor of pediatrics and associate professor of medicine at Jefferson Medical College of Thomas Jefferson University in Philadelphia. "The research papers on this topic are increasing exponentially."

Investigators may be breaking new ground, but magnesium has a long healing history. Epsom salts—first discovered in Epsom, England, and essentially made of magnesium sulfate—has long been the key ingredient of soothing hot foot soaks. Magnesium in this form has the ability to draw water from inflamed muscles and tissues.

Inside your body, magnesium serves several crucial roles, including helping to turn food into energy and helping to transmit electrical impulses across nerves and muscles. These impulses generate what's called neuromuscular contraction, literally causing your muscles to flex. Take away magnesium, and muscles—even the smooth muscles that routinely squeeze blood vessels—will cramp.

Magnesium is also vital for making sure that calcium is used properly. Too much calcium, however, can cause you to lose magnesium in your urine.

Prescription asthma drugs, diuretics (water pills), digitalis and other cardiovascular medications, alcohol and caffeine are notorious for removing magnesium from your body. People with diabetes who have high blood sugar lose a lot of magnesium in the urine. Even stress can remove magnesium from your system.

"It's very easy to not get enough into the system or to lose what's in there. And that's rarely recognized until someone has advanced magnesium deficiency, with a low blood level of magnesium," says Dr. Mansmann. But this much is known: Up to 40 percent of the American population gets less than 75 percent of the Daily Value of magnesium, says Dr. Mansmann. Just how many suffer needlessly from magnesium deficiency–related health problems is anyone's guess.

Symptoms of magnesium deficiency include nausea, muscle weakness, irritability and electrical changes in the heart muscle.

Using Magnesium Safely

Picking a magnesium supplement may not seem like a decision worthy of intense study. But select the wrong one, and you may find yourself in the bathroom more frequently. Dose for dose, magnesium gluconate causes one-third of the amount of diarrhea of magnesium oxide and one-half of the frequency of diarrhea of magnesium chloride, according to Dr. Mansmann.

Other benefits of magnesium gluconate: It can be taken on an empty stomach, while the other two forms can cause stomach upset in some people. Magnesium gluconate is absorbed more quickly than other forms. And you don't have to take quite as much, since the amount of magnesium per capsule that your body can use is higher.

As a general rule, you need about six milligrams of magnesium for every kilogram (2.2 pounds) of body weight. That means that if you weigh 150 pounds, you should be getting about 400 milligrams a day. If you develop diarrhea, simply take your magnesium in divided doses throughout the day, or reduce the dose by 20 to 25 percent until normal soft bowel movements return, says Dr. Mansmann.

If you have kidney or heart problems, always check with your doctor before taking supplemental magnesium.

Niacin

Daily Value: *20 milligrams*

Good Food Sources: *Chicken breast, tuna, veal, fortified breads and cereals*

The niacin story is one of triumph and potential tragedy. The triumph: One form of niacin, nicotinic acid, dramatically lowers the risk of heart disease at a fraction of the cost of prescription drugs. The tragedy: Used improperly, slow-release niacin can cause severe side effects, including liver damage.

"In the right hands, it's a very useful medication. It lowers harmful cholesterol and raises good cholesterol better than any drug we have," says James McKenney, Pharm.D., professor in the School of Pharmacy at Virginia Commonwealth University Medical College of Virginia in Richmond. "But taken indiscriminately by an uninformed person without a professional monitoring his condition, it can be dangerous."

Although more research needs to be done, it's thought that niacin somehow limits the liver's ability to produce cholesterol.

A less controversial use of niacin has no less positive results. Niacin prevents pellagra, a now rare condition that often starts with skin inflammation, includes diarrhea and depression and ends in death. In the deep South at the turn of the century, this ailment afflicted over 100,000 people, largely because their diets consisted mainly of cornmeal.

Not only does corn contain a form of niacin that the body cannot readily use, but a diet consisting of nothing but corn can also create an amino acid imbalance, says Marvin Davis, Ph.D., chairman of the Department of Pharmacology at the University of Mississippi at Oxford.

Thanks to the fortification of flours and cereals with niacin, pellagra is rare in all but alcoholics and people suffering from severe gastrointestinal problems, says Dr. Davis.

Niacin supplements may also reduce the incidence of asthma-induced wheezing, perhaps because this nutrient prevents the release of histamine, a biochemical normally released during allergic reactions. Harvard University researchers found that people who got the most niacin in their diets were significantly less likely to have bronchitis or wheezing than people who got the least. Lower blood levels of niacin were also linked to increased wheezing.

Using Niacin Safely

It's virtually impossible to get too much niacin in your diet. But when you take niacin supplements in the doses needed to improve your cholesterol levels, you are likely to experience side effects ranging from flushing, itching and excessive nervousness to headaches, intestinal cramps, nausea and diarrhea. And high doses of niacin, especially the slow-release form, can cause liver damage. That's why this kind of therapy needs to be taken under medical supervision.

Niacinamide, a form of niacin that is included in multivitamin/mineral supplements, does not produce the side effects associated with niacin itself. It also does not reduce blood cholesterol levels.

Pantothenic Acid

Daily Value: *10 milligrams*

Good Food Sources: *Whole grains, mushrooms, salmon, peanuts*

In a world that pops painkillers for hangnails and spreads toxic chemicals on lawns to produce greener grass, pantothenic acid may mean the difference between life and death.

In an ongoing series of laboratory studies, Won O. Song, Ph.D., associate professor of nutrition at Michigan State University in East Lansing, has found that the body uses coenzyme A, a substance containing pantothenic acid, to detoxify many of the harmful man-made compounds found in herbicides, insecticides and drugs.

Until now, pantothenic acid—one of the B vitamins—has been taken for granted, says Dr. Song. "It is very important. It is involved in so many different metabolic pathways, including the conversion of food to energy, the synthesis of important hormones and the body's utilization of body fat and cholesterol," she explains.

Those most likely to be deficient in pantothenic acid are older folks, people with serious drinking problems and people who take cholesterol-lowering drugs, says Dr. Song.

Signs of deficiency, which rarely occurs except with severe B-complex vitamin malnutrition, include the sensation of burning feet, loss of appetite, depression, fatigue, insomnia, vomiting and muscular cramping or weakness.

Using Pantothenic Acid Safely

Pantothenic acid has been taken in a wide range of doses all the way up to 10,000 milligrams a day, with no ill effects reported except an occasional case of diarrhea. The amount of pantothenic acid required to detoxify all of the man-made chemicals to which people are exposed is unknown.

Up to 50 percent of pantothenic acid is destroyed by processing, canning or cooking. That's why the best sources are unprocessed whole grains, fortified or enriched cereals to which the nutrient has been added and multivitamin/mineral supplements.

Phosphorus

Daily Value: *1,000 milligrams*

Good Food Sources: *Halibut, nonfat yogurt, salmon, skim milk, chicken breast, oatmeal, extra-lean ground beef, broccoli, lima beans*

What do a Bengal tiger and a teenager have in common? Depending on their chow, they may both be getting too much phosphorus.

Years ago, after noticing that the big cats in some zoos simply lay in their cages all day, researchers found that the animals' feed was high in phosphorus and dangerously low in calcium. To be sure, a calcium-phosphorus imbalance has yet to be linked to teenage couch-potato syndrome. But some experts believe teens who drink too much soda may have a phosphorus imbalance that could lead to osteoporosis later in life.

The mineral phosphorus is needed for many of the chemical reactions in the body. Phosphorus compounds help regulate the release of energy that fuels our bodies. By combining with calcium, phosphorus also helps form hard, crystal-like substances that create the latticework undergirding strong bones and teeth. In fact, 85 percent of the body's phosphorus is located in bone.

That may be part of the problem. The mechanism regulating the body's balance of calcium and phosphorus is so finely calibrated that getting too much phosphorus actually causes calcium to be removed from your skeleton and sent to your blood. Long-term calcium loss has been found to cause osteoporosis, a weakening of the bones that can lead to tooth loss and fractures.

Eating natural forms of phosphorus, which is found in everything from chicken and broccoli to milk and fruits, isn't likely to give you too much of this mineral. But some experts are worried that drinking too much soda—such as cola, root beer, and even clear drinks—can tip your delicate calcium-phosphorus balance in the wrong direction. Moreover, by forsaking milk for soda, you're further reducing your calcium intake, says John Anderson, Ph.D., professor of nutrition in the Schools of Public Health and Medicine at the University of North Carolina at Chapel Hill.

"That's where you get hurt the worst. You are compounding the problem. You are getting low calcium and high phosphorus," says Dr. Anderson.

It seems soda and many processed foods contain either phosphoric acid or some form of phosphate, both of which are hefty sources of phosphorus.

"Phosphoric acid is used in cola soft drinks to give them an acid taste," says Dr. Anderson. "Added to foods, phosphates may act as preservatives or perhaps even help alter the physical quality."

In rare cases, people who use antacids containing aluminum hydroxide for long periods of time might suffer from weakness, loss of appetite, malaise and bone loss. This chemical apparently prevents phosphorus from being absorbed.

Using Phosphorus Safely

Experts say there's virtually no reason to ever take a phosphorus supplement. It's easy to get enough phosphorus from your diet.

Potassium

Daily Value: *3,500 milligrams*

Good Food Sources: *Dried apricots, baked potatoes, dried prunes, cantaloupe, bananas, spinach*

If monkeys eat as many bananas in the wild as they do on television, there is no way that any of them will ever suffer from high blood pressure.

That's because potassium—in humans, anyway—is a key factor in keeping blood pressure at the right level for maximum cardiovascular health.

How does potassium regulate blood pressure? Scientists believe it may have something to do with potassium's ability to pump sodium out of the body's cells and reduce body fluid. Potassium may also affect blood vessel tone, or resistance. Or it may be that potassium modifies the way blood vessels react to circulating hormones that affect blood pressure, such as vasopressin and norepinephrine.

In any case, potassium's ability to lower blood pressure is such that some scientists suspect low dietary levels of the mineral may actually trigger high blood pressure in certain people.

Aside from its miraculous effect on blood pressure, potassium is also necessary for good muscle contraction, healthy electrical activity in the heart and rapid transmission of nerve impulses throughout the body. This is why heartbeat irregularities are considered a classic sign of potassium deficiency. Other symptoms of deficiency can include muscle weakness, numbness and tingling in the lower extremities, nausea, vomiting, confusion and irritability.

Using Potassium Safely

Most of us get around 2,650 milligrams of potassium every day, reports the National Center for Health Statistics in Hyattsville, Maryland. That's not enough. And that's why you probably need to add at least three more servings of potassium-rich fruits and vegetables to your diet every day, says David McCarron, M.D., professor of medicine and head of the Division of Nephrology, Hypertension and Clinical Pharmacology at Oregon Health Sciences University in Portland.

Why not simply take a supplement? Dietary sources of potassium are better tolerated than pharmacologic preparations, experts agree, although potassium supplements—available over the counter or, in larger doses, by prescription—may be necessary for those who take diuretic medications. Diuretics help the body lose excess water but also deplete its potassium supply. (Digitalis, a heart medicine, can also cause you to excrete potassium.) If you use over-the-counter supplements, it is usually best, according to Dr. McCarron, to keep your total daily potassium intake from diet and supplements to 3,500 milligrams.

When a potassium supplement is required, talk to your doctor or pharmacist about which kind is best for you. Some doctors feel that potassium chloride is better absorbed than potassium bicarbonate, potassium citrate or potassium gluconate. Supplements containing more than 99 milligrams of potassium are available only by prescription.

Too much potassium (more than 5,000 milligrams a day) can upset the balance of minerals in your body and cause heart and kidney problems.

Other potential side effects include muscle weakness, tingling in the hands, feet or tongue and a slow or irregular pulse.

People with diabetes or kidney disease should consult their doctors before taking potassium supplements, as should people on certain medications, including nonsteroidal anti-inflammatory drugs, potassium-sparing diuretics, ACE inhibitors and heart medicines such as heparin.

Riboflavin

Daily Value: *1.7 milligrams*

Good Food Sources: *Poultry, fish, fortified grains and cereals, broccoli, turnip greens, asparagus, spinach, yogurt, milk, cheeses*

Riboflavin will probably never bathe in the nutritional spotlight like vitamin C, magnesium and vitamin E. But a smattering of experts say that it's about time we give this nutrient, also known as vitamin B_2, its due.

"It's not fashionable per se, but you're going to be hearing more about it," says Jack M. Cooperman, Ph.D., clinical professor of community and preventive medicine at New York Medical College in Valhalla.

Emerging research shows that riboflavin can act as an antioxidant, potentially helping to prevent cancer and control cholesterol buildup by helping to tame harmful free radicals. Free radicals are naturally occurring renegade molecules that damage your body's healthy molecules by stealing electrons to balance themselves. Antioxidants neutralize free radicals by offering their own electrons and thus protect the healthy molecules from harm.

Riboflavin assists a number of important chemical processes in the body. Folate and vitamin B_6, for example, need riboflavin to undergo the chemical changes that make them useful. Amino acids are transformed by riboflavin into what are called neurotransmitters, chemicals crucial for thinking and memory. A shortage of red blood cells, which causes symptoms such as anemia, has been linked in some cases to a lack of riboflavin. "The key concept to remember here is that riboflavin is one of the essential B vitamins necessary for all sorts of chemical processes inside the body, such as helping to turn food into energy," says Dr. Cooperman.

Riboflavin deficiency can affect your vision, causing your eyes to become light-sensitive and easily fatigued. Other symptoms of deficiency include blurred vision and itching, watering, sore or bloodshot eyes. Severe dermatitis is another hallmark of riboflavin deficiency.

Fortifying cereals and flours with riboflavin began during World War II, when meats and dairy products, among the best sources of the nutrient, were rationed. But folks who choose to limit their dairy and meat consumption may still be at risk for deficiency. "We've done a study that shows there is a correlation between low milk intake and riboflavin deficiency, particularly among African-American youths," says Dr. Cooperman.

People who exercise regularly may not be getting enough riboflavin, either, since activity seems to help speed the vitamin's removal from the body.

Using Riboflavin Safely

There's no need to worry about a riboflavin overdose. Any excess of this particular vitamin is excreted from your system. And unlike most other vitamins, this one quickly lets you know that you've reached your saturation point. Two hours after taking a supplement containing riboflavin, your urine will turn bright yellow, says Dr. Cooperman.

Huge amounts of riboflavin, 2,000 times the Daily Value, have been known to cause kidney stones, but there is no reason to take this much.

Both oral contraceptives and alcohol seem to reduce your body's ability to absorb riboflavin. So if you use either, you might want to consider taking a B-complex vitamin to cover all the bases, says Dr. Cooperman.

Selenium

Daily Value: *70 micrograms*

Good Food Sources: *Lobster, Brazil nuts, clams, crab, cooked oysters, whole grains*

Selenium may play a pivotal role in whether some viruses live harmlessly in the body or turn into rampaging pathogens that kill.

Laboratory studies at the University of North Carolina at Chapel Hill first suggested that selenium is the switch that triggers a Jekyll-and-Hyde personality in viruses. Subsequent studies at the University of Georgia in Athens indicated that selenium depletion in a cell may be what throws a switch on HIV, the virus that causes AIDS, and launches that particular viral terrorist on a cellular rampage that wipes out its human host. The irony is that the virus intends no harm. It is simply looking for more selenium.

If subsequent studies prove that selenium depletion is the trigger that shifts the AIDS virus into overdrive, the answer to keeping even this lethal virus in check may be as simple as making sure the body has adequate levels of selenium, says Will Taylor, Ph.D., an AIDS researcher at the University of Georgia, who led the Georgia study. For the full story on selenium and AIDS, see page 311.

Although its effect on viruses is probably selenium's most dramatic achievement, the mineral has other important roles in the body as well. It activates substances that protect the eyes from cataracts and the heart from muscle damage. It binds with toxic substances such as arsenic, cadmium and mercury to make them less harmful. It boosts several infection-fighting elements of your immune system.

And last but not least, selenium protects cells against damage from free radicals, naturally occurring maverick molecules that damage your body's healthy molecules by stealing electrons to balance themselves. Vitamin E has this same protective effect. In fact, selenium and vitamin E work so well together against free radicals that they frequently substitute for one another. That's why a deficiency of one of these nutrients can frequently lead to a deficiency of the other.

While there are no clear symptoms of selenium deficiency, some research has suggested that an insufficient level of the mineral may play a role in the development of heart disease.

Using Selenium Safely

As far back as the thirteenth century, Marco Polo noted that certain forages on which his animals grazed in western China caused the animals' hooves to drop off.

In subsequent centuries, scientists found that the cause was a toxic level of selenium in the plants that animals ate and that high levels of selenium in the diet could affect humans as well as horses. The only difference seems to be that humans lose hair and nails as opposed to hooves. Other side effects of excessive selenium intake include a persistent garlic odor on your breath and skin, a metallic taste in your mouth, dizziness and nausea for no apparent reason.

Today we know that the Daily Value is 70 micrograms. Some experts suggest that you look for a selenium supplement labeled "l-selenomethionine" and avoid those marked "sodium selenite" because l-selenomethionine is less likely to cause side effects and won't react with vitamin C to block selenium absorption.

To fight the AIDS virus, therapeutic doses of 200 to 400 micrograms have been suggested. But scientists caution that selenium supplements in excess of 100 micrograms per day should be taken only under medical supervision.

There is some debate over whether we need to take selenium supplements. Acid rain and the use of fossil fuels may be depleting the amount of selenium in the food chain. A further reduction in selenium intake can be linked to the many processed foods we eat. For these reasons, some experts have argued that the optimum amount of selenium may be much higher than the Daily Value suggests. The Brazil nut seems to be the richest source of selenium available. It takes only one or two nuts to meet the Daily Value.

If you are counting on the foods you eat as your primary source of selenium, here's something for you to think about. Plants get their selenium contents directly from the soil in which they grow. Generally, the soil in those states east of the Mississippi and west of the Rockies has a low selenium content. Crops that are grown in these areas will also have low selenium contents. Livestock is also affected, because the animals graze on plants grown in the same soil as our crops. Compounding this problem are the ions produced when we burn fossil fuels such as coal and oil. These ions acidify the soil, which hinders selenium uptake and reduces the amount of selenium found in the crops even more.

Sodium

Daily Value: *2,400 milligrams*

Good Food Sources: *Cheeses, including cottage cheese; most meats, especially ham and bacon; canned soups; canned vegetables; processed lunchmeats; shellfish; canned tuna; cereals; breads; baked goods; salad dressings; potato chips; pickles; sauces.* Note: *Although we all need a certain amount of sodium to survive, most people get too much rather than too little.*

Despite getting bad press, sodium is a mineral that your body needs as much as any other. It regulates the amount of fluid that your body contains, it facilitates nerve and muscle impulses, and together with potassium, it maintains the permeability of your cells' walls. This is a vitally necessary job if nutrients and other substances involved in cell maintenance are to be able to come and go as they're needed.

But scientists have also believed for decades that sodium has a direct effect on blood pressure—an effect that is proving to be highly controversial. The controversy is fueled by studies indicating that people with high blood pressure who reduce their consumption of sodium can lower their blood pressure readings by about five points. Lowering pressure just a few points cuts the risk of heart disease and stroke. By the same token, other studies indicate that low-salt diets do not lower blood pressure in about half of the people who try them.

Doctors have suspected for quite a while that low-salt diets won't help many people. Figuring that low-salt diets might help some and couldn't hurt others, however, they have continued to recommend that people with high blood pressure watch their salt intakes, says David McCarron, M.D., professor of medicine and head of the Division of Nephrology, Hypertension and Clinical Pharmacology at Oregon Health Sciences University in Portland.

That may be changing. Researchers at Cornell University Medical College and the Albert Einstein College of Medicine, both in New York City, decided to actually count the number of heart attacks among men with high blood pressure who consumed low amounts of sodium, then compare that figure with the number of heart attacks among men who had high blood pressure and higher sodium intakes.

The results? The men who ate the least sodium were four times more likely to have heart attacks than those who ate the most. And the less sodium they ingested, the higher their risk.

In effect, a low-sodium diet among people with high blood pressure was associated with the very problem it was designed to prevent. For more details on sodium and blood pressure, see page 297.

Using Sodium Safely

The amount of sodium your body needs to perform the nutrient's normal functions and keep your blood pressure on an even keel is a hot topic within the scientific community.

Some scientists feel you need no more than 500 milligrams a day of sodium chloride, the form in which sodium is usually found in foods or your saltshaker. Others say that your body is naturally constituted to readily handle 4,000 to 5,000 milligrams a day without a problem. And still others point out that the amount of sodium in your body at any given time is actually determined by aldosterone, a kidney hormone, anyway. So why worry about how much you're eating? Too much sodium in the body, and your kidneys will act to excrete the excess; too little, and they'll make sure enough sodium is retained in your body's fluid.

Clearly, more research is needed to sort out sodium's role in the body. But until that happens, how much sodium chloride should you allow in your diet?

Well, don't run out and start scarfing down salty chicken noodle soup, pickled herring or processed lunchmeats such as bologna laden with excess salt. You can still do well on 2,400 to 3,000 milligrams in your diet on a day-to-day basis, according to Dr. McCarron, who has spent the better part of 15 years researching the subject. One teaspoon of table salt contains about 2,000 milligrams of sodium.

Sulfur

Daily Value: *None*

Good Food Sources: *Meats, poultry, fish*

Most of us think of sulfur as a nostril-burning by-product of the combustion engine that pollutes urban air. But it is also a mineral that our bodies need to neutralize toxins.

Absorbed from protein-based foods, drinking water and even noxious air, the sulfur taken into our bodies combines with toxins to form harmless compounds that can then be escorted to the nearest exit.

Sulfur is also combined with the proteins that structure cartilage, tendons and bone in the body as well as with the proteins in our hair and nails.

Sulfur is not related to sulfa drugs or sulfites, which are sometimes added to foods.

Using Sulfur Safely

Sulfur is so widely available from foods, water and air that the National Research Council has established no Recommended Dietary Allowance. It also seems to be impossible to get the wrong amount of sulfur—either too much or too little.

Thiamin

Daily Value: *1.5 milligrams*

Good Food Sources: *Rice bran, pork, beef, fresh peas, beans, wheat germ, ham, oranges, enriched pastas, breads, oatmeal and other cereals*

It's tucked discreetly into baked goods and cereals. You probably wouldn't know you're getting thiamin unless you read about it on a food label. But thanks to this water-soluble B vitamin, you're able to turn the starches and sugars in your breakfast bowl into energy.

Unlike the United States, many parts of the world still don't fortify cereals with thiamin, also known as vitamin B_1.

Although rice and whole grains—dietary staples throughout the world—naturally contain thiamin, the process of refining them for consumption removes the nutrient. Folks living on little but devitalized rice and grains soon become thiamin-deficient and develop a disease called beriberi, with symptoms such as weakness, heart enlargement and limb swelling that make even walking difficult, says Howerde Sauberlich, Ph.D., professor in the Department of Nutritional Sciences at the University of Alabama in Birmingham. "I've seen cases of this myself where people were having difficulty walking, and almost miraculously, within a few hours after being given thiamin, they could walk," he says.

Thiamin's ability to make energy available for the body has ramifications for the brain. "If you dramatically reduce thiamin intake, you reduce the ability of the brain to use glucose. And if you reduce that, you have impaired mental function," says Gary E. Gibson, Ph.D., professor of neuroscience at Burke Medical Research Institute at Cornell University in White Plains, New York. A severe thiamin deficiency not only kills the brain cells responsible for memory but also may cause an increase in the protein that causes Alzheimer's disease, says Dr. Gibson.

Thiamin deficiencies have also been found to cause mood changes, vague feelings of uneasiness, fear, disorderly thinking and other signs of mental depression—symptoms that researchers say often affect memory.

Using Thiamin Safely

Although thiamin toxicity—its symptoms include itching, tingling and pain—has been caused by massive doses administered by injection, there has been no evidence of toxicity from oral thiamin, even when doses as high as 500 milligrams (333 times the Daily Value of 1.5 milligrams) were taken daily for a month. Experts say that excess thiamin is easily cleared by the kidneys.

Trace Minerals

Just because they're called trace minerals doesn't mean that copper, iodine and even molybdenum aren't as important as, say, calcium, a biggie that we all know about. It simply means that you require smaller daily amounts of these nutrients—in the case of some trace minerals, less than a milligram a day. Minerals taken in such tiny amounts are often measured in *micro*grams, or one-thousandth of a milligram.

Several trace minerals—copper, chromium, cobalt, manganese and molybdenum—are firmly established as essential to humans. That means that you can't live without them, at least not for very long. It means that these minerals are necessary for certain vital chemical reactions in the body to occur and that no other elements can take their places. It also means that the National Research Council has developed daily intake guidelines to help you make sure that you are getting enough.

The Estimated Safe and Adequate Daily Dietary Intakes were established for essential nutrients (including many trace minerals) that have some research to support an estimated range of requirements, but not enough to establish a Recommended Dietary Allowance or a Daily Value.

Luckily, trace minerals are found in a variety of foods and in water, so we usually get enough of every one of them to function normally, though we may not always get optimum amounts.

Several additional trace minerals, including boron, silicon and vanadium, have been proven essential to assorted bacteria, fungi and other microbes. And all plants need boron in order to grow. As technology improves and research deepens, these minerals may one day be shown to be essential to humans as well.

Many trace minerals act as coenzymes, so-called catalysts in chemical reactions. That means they function as spark plugs, getting chemical reactions going without actually being changed in the process. That's important, because our bodies are giant laboratories, where billions of chemical reactions are taking place all of the time.

Trace minerals play roles in your body's production of neurotransmitters, biochemicals that send messages through your nervous system; in the production of major hormones secreted by your thyroid and adrenal glands; and in your body's ability to burn carbohydrates and fat for energy and to weave molecules into the tissues that become your bones, blood vessels, skin and teeth. Along with other food components, trace minerals help you grow, reproduce and maintain your body over the years.

Getting enough trace minerals is a perfect reason to abide by one important bit of nutritional advice: Eat a varied diet that contains whole foods. Whole grains, nuts, seeds, beans, fresh fruits and vegetables, mushrooms, shellfish, herbs and spices are the richest sources of trace minerals. A few processed foods also contain high amounts: ham, canned pineapple juice, cocoa and beer, which contains trace minerals from the brewer's yeast used to concoct the stuff. Yes, chocolate and beer fit into a healthy diet—in moderation, of course. And you heard it here first!

If you're relying on supplements to make up for what is lacking in your diet, pick a good multivitamin/mineral supplement that supplies an array of trace minerals in the ranges recommended below. With very few exceptions, there's no reason to take supplements of individual trace minerals. That's because most trace minerals are toxic in high amounts. "The dose makes the poison," explains Curtiss Hunt, Ph.D., a research biologist with the U.S. Department of Agriculture Grand Forks Human Nutrition Research Center in North Dakota. Until more is known about these elements, especially how they interact with other nutrients, it's prudent to stick to amounts that researchers know are safe. And if you have health problems, get your doctor's okay before you begin taking any supplement.

Boron

Estimated Safe and Adequate Daily Dietary Intake: *None*

Good Food Sources: *Parsley, apples, cherries, grapes, leafy vegetables, nuts, beans*

If you've heard of boron at all, it may have been in regard to this trace mineral's apparent bone-building properties. In several studies, boron has been found to help people better absorb and use minerals such as calcium and magnesium.

"Boron also seems to play a role in the body's ability to generate energy, especially during exercise," says Dr. Hunt. He found that animals that were exercised and got adequate boron in their diets gained more weight and grew larger than animals that were exercised and fed a low-boron diet.

Boron may work by activating certain hormones, Dr. Hunt says. In postmenopausal women, adequate boron raised blood levels of both estrogen and testosterone. It also might help in converting vitamin D to its active form.

Bodybuilders who have used boron to jack up testosterone levels, however, have been disappointed. "Large amounts of this mineral don't affect hormone levels in people who are already getting adequate amounts," Dr. Hunt says.

Using Boron Safely

There is no Estimated Safe and Adequate Daily Dietary Intake for boron. So how much should you get? Probably about the amount you're getting now, if you're eating a well-balanced diet that contains at least five servings of fruits and vegetables a day. That's 1.5 to 3 milligrams of boron a day.

Supplements are not necessary or desirable, Dr. Hunt adds. "We don't yet know enough about boron to determine if amounts of more than three milligrams a day are safe," he says.

Chromium

Daily Value: *120 micrograms*

Good Food Sources: *Brewer's yeast, broccoli, ham, grape juice*

Think of it as the shovel that gets the fuel into the furnace. This trace mineral hooks up with insulin to help transport glucose (blood sugar) across cell membranes and into cells, where it can be burned for energy. People who don't get enough chromium may develop a condition called glucose intolerance; they have high blood sugar levels and often high insulin levels. The high blood sugar levels do not drop much when additional insulin is given, but they do go down when people get the chromium they need. Glucose intolerance can set the stage for Type II (non-insulin-dependent) diabetes.

Signs of chromium deficiency include diabetes-like symptoms of high blood cholesterol and problems with insulin levels.

"Most likely to benefit from chromium supplementation are people newly diagnosed with diabetes who have mild glucose intolerance and mildly elevated blood glucose," explains Richard Anderson, Ph.D., lead scientist in the nutrient requirements and functions laboratory at the U.S. Department of Agriculture Beltsville Human Nutrition Research Center in Maryland. Chromium has not proven as helpful for people with long-standing or severe diabetes.

Since chromium helps insulin work better, it may also raise blood sugar levels in people with low blood sugar, as shown in studies by researchers with the U.S. Department of Agriculture.

Chromium also seems to help raise HDL cholesterol, the "good" kind that helps escort bad cholesterol out of your body.

Sweet treats drain the body's supply of chromium. Complex carbohydrates such as pastas and potatoes help preserve chromium.

Using Chromium Safely

Even balanced diets designed by dietitians contain less than 50 micrograms of chromium and average about 15 micrograms per 1,000 calories, far less than the 120 micrograms that's recommended, according to an analysis by Dr. Anderson.

Trivalent chromium, the kind found in foods and supplements, is considered to be quite safe. "The safety of dosages of up to 200 micrograms a day is well-established, and ongoing studies using amounts of up to 1,000 micrograms a day have uncovered no toxic effects," Dr. Anderson says. "We have yet to establish an unsafe dose, because no amount we have given so far has proven to be toxic."

Still, it's best to get no more than 200 micrograms a day from supplements without medical supervision.

On the other hand, if you work around chromium-containing compounds, you'll want to steer clear of fumes and dust. Industrial chromium, a completely different form than that found in foods, is toxic.

People with diabetes who take chromium should be under medical supervision, since their insulin dosage may need to be reduced as blood sugar drops.

Many studies detailing chromium's benefits have used chromium picolinate, an easily absorbed form. Chromium nicotinate and amino acid forms of chromium are less easily absorbed than chromium picolinate but can supply adequate amounts of the mineral. The least absorbable form is chromium chloride, which is found in some multivitamin/mineral supplements. This type binds with other components in foods and becomes mostly unabsorbable.

Chromium is sometimes sold as glucose tolerance factor (GTF), a combination of chromium, nicotinic acid (a form of niacin) and amino acids. GTF may vary so much in composition that it is not a reliable source of chromium, Dr. Anderson says.

Cobalt

Estimated Safe and Adequate Daily Dietary Intake: *None*

Good Food Sources: *Dairy and other animal products*

Cobalt is at the core of every molecule of vitamin B_{12}, a nutrient that's essential for the body's formation of red blood cells. That function is vital, and it's the only known function of cobalt in humans.

Using Cobalt Safely

No Estimated Safe and Adequate Daily Dietary Intake has been set for cobalt; you get the amount you need from preformed vitamin B_{12}. Although B_{12} deficiency is not uncommon (some true vegetarians may develop B_{12} deficiency), cobalt deficiency has never been seen in people.

Copper

Daily Value: *2 milligrams*

Good Food Sources: *Shellfish (especially cooked oysters), nuts, seeds, cocoa powder, beans, whole grains, mushrooms*

Thanks to shiny new pennies, we all know that copper is a bright orange metal. Most of us don't know that need to consume a certain amount of copper in order to survive. Anyone who is concerned about heart disease or osteoporosis, and that's just about everyone, should be paying attention to copper.

Copper plays a role in the body's formation of strong, flexible connective tissue, in the production of neurochemicals in the brain and in the functioning of muscles, nerves and the immune system.

"One of copper's best-understood roles so far is its function in the cross-linkage of collagen and elastin," explains Leslie Klevay, M.D., Sc.D., of the Grand Forks Human Nutrition Research Center. "Copper helps knit together these two very important connective tissues, which are used throughout the body to build other tissues."

Copper-deficient animals have weakened hearts and blood vessels and may die from heart failure or a ruptured aorta, the main artery from the heart. They also have bone defects that are identical to osteoporosis. "Copper is essential for the network of connective tissue in bone on which minerals such as calcium are deposited," Dr. Klevay explains. Copper-deficient animals also develop cartilage breakdown similar to that which takes place in osteoarthritis.

Copper also interacts with iron, so copper deficiency eventually leads to anemia.

Copper deficiency may be more prevalent than we know. It may be more of a marginal condition than a true deficiency in people eating normal diets, Dr. Klevay says. Still, some experts suspect that many people are getting less than optimum amounts and may suffer from chronic illnesses such as heart disease and osteoporosis as a result. Lower blood levels of copper have been found in women with osteoporosis than in women with strong bones.

Using Copper Safely

Copper is often found in multivitamin/mineral supplements. If you want to get additional copper that way, look for a supplement that offers 1.5 to 3 milligrams of copper chloride or copper sulfate, Dr. Klevay says. "I prefer that people get their copper from foods," he adds.

Few people get more than 2 milligrams of copper a day from diet alone, and a fair number of people consume less than 1.5 milligrams a day, an amount that Dr. Klevay considers the bare minimum.

Copper is toxic in large amounts (it's most likely to cause vomiting), so there's simply no good reason to take more than three milligrams a day, Dr. Klevay says.

Zinc interferes with the body's ability to absorb copper, which is why experts who recommend zinc supplements often suggest extra copper as well, generally in a ratio of 1 milligram of copper to 10 milligrams of zinc. So if you're taking 15 milligrams of zinc (the Daily Value), you should be getting 1.5 milligrams of copper a day. And copper supplements are definitely off-limits to people with Wilson's disease, an inherited disorder that makes copper accumulate in the liver.

Fluoride

Estimated Safe and Adequate Daily Dietary Intake: *Adults, 1.5 to 4 milligrams. Children up to age 6 months, 0.1 to 0.5 milligram; ages 6 to 11 months, 0.2 to 1 milligram; ages 1 to 3 years, 0.5 to 1.5 milligrams; ages 4 to 6 years, 1 to 2.5 milligrams; ages 7 to 18 years, 1.5 to 2.5 milligrams.*

Good Food Sources: *Fluoridated water, tea, marine fish with bones, such as canned salmon and mackerel*

You might think that because fluoride is added to water and toothpaste, it's one of those nutrients that you just can't live without. That's not the case, although its potential for making visits to the dentist more pleasant is undisputed.

Both oral and topically applied fluoride are incorporated into tooth enamel. Fluoride protects the enamel, so it is less likely to dissolve under assault from the acid-producing bacteria that thrive in your mouth. Even adults can benefit from fluoride's tooth-toughening talents.

Fluoride is also taken up by bone tissue, making the tissue stronger, too. But studies using fluoride to strengthen bones weakened by osteoporosis have had mixed results. The latest studies, however, have found that a combination of slow-release fluoride and calcium did reduce the tendency for postmenopausal women to sustain fractures by 50 percent. For the full story on using nutrients to prevent and treat osteoporosis, see page 429.

Using Fluoride Safely

People who drink fluoridated water get about one milligram per liter of water. People who don't drink fluoridated water may get very little fluoride in their diets, unless they're big tea drinkers. One cup of tea offers one to three milligrams of fluoride.

Up to ten milligrams of fluoride a day from foods and water is considered safe for adults. You should not take more than four milligrams a day from supplements of rapid-release sodium fluoride, says Khashayar Sakhaee, M.D., professor of internal medicine at the Center for Mineral Metabolism and Clinical Research of the University of Texas Southwestern Medical Center at Dallas. That amount may be enough to help teeth, but it doesn't help restore weak bones, Dr. Sakhaee says.

Although fluoride supplements are available only by prescription, rapid-release forms are not safe to take in large amounts, Dr. Sakhaee says. Large amounts can cause bone pain and, in children, mottled, brown teeth.

The slow-release form of fluoride that has been used in studies to prevent osteoporosis is currently undergoing Food and Drug Administration review for safety and effectiveness. "If it passes, it will be available by prescription within a few years," Dr. Sakhaee says.

Iodine

Daily Value: *150 micrograms*

Good Food Sources: *Iodized salt, lobster, shrimp, cooked oysters, marine fish, seaweed, breads, milk*

Iodine is used by the thyroid gland to produce an important hormone called thyroxine. This hormone helps regulate energy production, body temperature, breathing, muscle tone and the manufacture and breakdown of tissues. Iodine deficiency usually results in an enlargement of the thyroid gland known as goiter, visible as swelling on the front of the throat.

Using Iodine Safely

Thanks to iodine-fortified salt, there's no need to worry about getting enough iodine. Most people get several times the Daily Value with no ill effects.

Manganese

Daily Value: *2 milligrams*

Good Food Sources: *Canned pineapple juice, wheat bran, wheat germ, whole grains, seeds, nuts, cocoa, shellfish, tea*

The word *manganese* is derived from the Greek word for magic. And this little-known trace mineral can apparently work its own magic in the body.

Manganese is an essential part of biochemical reactions that affect bone, cartilage, brain function and energy supply, explains Jeanne Freeland-Graves, R.D., Ph.D., professor of nutrition at the University of Texas at Austin. "This is one mineral that you will definitely be hearing more about in the future," she says.

Manganese helps your body build and maintain strong bones. It makes up a part of molecules known as mucopolysaccharides. These molecules are used to form collagen, the strong, fibrous connective material that builds tissues throughout the body, including bone and cartilage, the rubbery cushioning found where bones meet.

In bone, a mesh of collagen provides the framework on which calcium, magnesium and other bone-hardening minerals are deposited. Animals deficient in manganese have bone problems similar to those that develop in people with osteoporosis. Under a microscope, these animals' bones actually appear riddled with holes. Other animals that are manganese-deficient develop tendon problems.

In one study, women with osteoporosis had lower blood levels of manganese than women without osteoporosis. Another study found that supplements of calcium, manganese, zinc and copper helped stop bone loss, but the effect of manganese alone was not tested.

Manganese is also necessary for proper brain function. Low levels have been associated with seizure disorders such as epilepsy. Manganese also helps your body break down carbohydrates and fat for energy.

Manganese deficiency has never been detected in people eating normal diets. Whether that's because people are getting enough of the mineral through foods or because deficiency symptoms go unrecognized has yet to be determined, Dr. Freeland-Graves says. "Around the turn of the century, we were getting about eight milligrams a day from a diet based on whole grains, nuts and seeds," she says. Nowadays, people average two to three milligrams.

"A number of studies have shown that you need at least three milligrams and up to five milligrams of manganese a day to maintain a positive balance," Dr. Freeland-Graves says.

Using Manganese Safely

Research indicates that amounts of up to 10 milligrams of manganese a day are safe, Dr. Freeland-Graves says. There's no need to get more than 3.5 to 5 milligrams daily, she adds.

To get your manganese, stick to foods, which can provide you with enough of this and other trace minerals. "Canned pineapple juice is one of the best sources, with about three milligrams of manganese per cup," Dr. Freeland-Graves says.

Some multivitamin/mineral supplements contain manganese. If you decide to take a supplement that includes this mineral, look for one that offers no more than two milligrams of manganese chloride, a very absorbable form, Dr. Freeland-Graves says. Single supplements of manganese are not available, nor are they desirable, since taking too much of this trace mineral can be toxic.

Calcium supplements may interfere with your body's ability to absorb manganese. In one study, a dose of 800 milligrams of calcium inhibited the absorption of manganese. So if you're taking calcium supplements, you might consider eating manganese-rich foods at other times of the day, says Dr. Freeland-Graves. She also suggests taking calcium separately from a multivitamin/mineral supplement containing manganese.

Manganese toxicity has been seen in industrial exposure to the mineral and in people drinking contaminated well water. High amounts can cause symptoms similar to those of Parkinson's disease, including trembling, shuffling and slow movement.

Molybdenum

Daily Value: *75 micrograms*

Good Food Sources: *Beans, whole grains, cereals, milk and milk products, dark green, leafy vegetables*

Come on, you can spit it out: *mo-LIB-duh-num.* This trace mineral with the funny name is a component of three enzymes, which act in the body to get important chemical reactions going.

Molybdenum is part of sulfite oxidase, an enzyme that helps the body detoxify sulfites, compounds found in protein foods and used as chemical preservatives in some foods and drugs. People who can't break down sulfites have toxic buildups of this chemical in their bodies, explains Judith Turnlund, R.D., Ph.D., of the U.S. Department of Agriculture Western Human Nutrition Research Center in San Francisco. "Infants born with this disorder are very sick and usually don't live long," she says. These infants have a rare genetic disorder that inhibits molybdenum-containing enzymes in their bodies, and giving them extra molybdenum doesn't usually help, she says.

Some people are supersensitive to the sulfites used as additives, developing asthma and other life-threatening breathing problems. "Unfortunately, supplemental molybdenum would not be particularly helpful in reducing sulfite sensitivity in people with asthma," says Dr. Turnlund.

Molybdenum is also part of two other enzymes, xanthine oxidase and aldehyde oxidase. Both are involved in the body's production of genetic material and proteins. Xanthine oxidase also helps the body produce uric acid, an important waste product.

Physical signs of molybdenum deficiency are considered extremely rare, Dr. Turnlund says. Only one case, a man on long-term tube feeding, has ever been confirmed. Molybdenum deficiency is difficult to induce even in animals. "People eating fairly normal diets simply don't become deficient in this nutrient," Dr. Turnlund says. Most people get about 180 micrograms daily from foods.

Using Molybdenum Safely

Up to 500 micrograms of molybdenum a day has proven safe in long-term experiments, but there's no reason to take that much, Dr. Turnlund says. Amounts higher than 500 micrograms may interfere with your body's metabolism of copper, another essential trace mineral.

There's no need to get this trace mineral in supplement form, Dr. Turnlund says. Some multivitamin/mineral supplements do supply molybdenum. Stick to one that provides no more than 75 to 250 micrograms, Dr. Turnlund advises.

People with gout or high blood levels of uric acid should consult their doctors before taking supplements that contain molybdenum.

Vitamin A

Daily Value: *5,000 international units*

Good Food Sources: *Carrot juice, pumpkin, sweet potatoes, carrots, spinach, butternut squash, tuna, dandelion greens, cantaloupe, mangoes, turnip greens, beet greens*

Give 200,000 international units of vitamin A to a malnourished child in Indonesia, Nepal, India or Ghana, and it could save his life. Give 25,000 international units of beta-carotene, a vitamin A precursor, to an adult every day, and it could help prevent macular degeneration, which, after cataracts, is the leading cause of blindness in people age 50 and older. One study at Johns Hopkins School of Hygiene and Public Health in Baltimore showed that between 9,000 and 20,000 international units of vitamin A, given daily to men infected with HIV, may help slow the disease's progression to AIDS by about 40 percent.

What is this powerful substance? Actually, *vitamin A* is the generic name given to a group of naturally occurring molecules called retinoids. Study after study shows that your body uses these retinoids, which are powerful compounds drawn from plant and animal sources, to build or maintain an effective immune system.

Without an adequate amount of vitamin A, your body is vulnerable to a whole host of infectious creatures that can cause anything from measles to AIDS. Those who lack vitamin A on their defense teams also face increased risk of cancer and blindness.

Symptoms of a vitamin A deficiency include night blindness, difficulty recovering vision (after looking into the headlights of an oncoming car, for example), distorted color vision, dry eyes, loss of appetite, poor taste and smell and difficulty keeping your balance.

Fortunately, most people in the United States get enough vitamin A from their diets. Those most at risk are people who have cancer, tuberculosis, pneumonia, chronic nephritis, urinary tract infections or prostate disease, all of which may increase the body's demands for vitamin A. People who have digestive conditions that impair fat absorption—celiac disease and cystic fibrosis are two examples—are also at risk.

Vitamin A is a fat-soluble substance, which means that you should eat a food that contains a small amount of fat when you take it. You can get vitamin A directly from a supplement. Or you can get it indirectly by eating fruits and vegetables that are loaded with beta-carotene. Your body will turn beta-carotene into the vitamin A it needs.

Many doctors prefer the second route. There are two reasons: One, foods contain hundreds of other substances that may have healthful benefits; and two, although excessive amounts of vitamin A are usually toxic, large amounts of beta-carotene usually are not. There is one exception: Both vitamin A and beta-carotene can damage the liver in someone who drinks heavily.

Using Vitamin A Safely

For centuries, Arctic adventurers, Eskimos and even sled dogs have known that eating polar bear liver can make them sick.

The reason? It's loaded with enough vitamin A to poison a full-grown adult. A single meal consisting of a half-pound to one pound of polar bear liver contains a whopping 3 million to 13 million international units of vitamin A, which is 6 to 26 times the amount needed to cause acute vitamin A poisoning.

Only 500,000 international units of vitamin A, taken over a short period of time, can cause irritability, headaches, vomiting, bone pain, weakness and blurred vision. Regular use of even 50,000 international units a day can cause hair loss, weakness, headaches, enlarged liver and spleen, anemia, stiffness and joint pain. And at least one death has been reported from the regular use of 25,000 international units every day.

Women of childbearing age need to be particularly careful when supplementing vitamin A. Daily doses of 10,000 international units, an amount found in some multivitamin/mineral supplements, during the first three months of pregnancy have been linked to a high risk of birth defects. And 25,000 international units daily is known to cause spontaneous abortions when taken early in pregnancy. For these reasons, women who are pregnant should never take daily supplements of 10,000 international units or more, and other women of childbearing age should check with their doctors before taking that much vitamin A. They should also check their multivitamin/mineral supplements to make sure they contain less than 10,000 international units of vitamin A.

The bottom line? In different amounts and situations, vitamin A can be either a miraculous healing agent or a malicious, toxic compound. It's a good idea to consult your doctor before supplementing.

Vitamin B_6

Daily Value: *2 milligrams*

Good Food Sources: *Bananas, avocados, chicken, beef, brewer's yeast, eggs, brown rice, soybeans, oats, whole wheat, peanuts, walnuts*

For more than 30 years, learning about vitamin B_6 has consumed much of John Marion Ellis's life. This retired M.D. from Mount Pleasant, Texas, has conducted studies and written papers about it. He has assembled notebooks containing the latest clinical findings. And of course, both he and his wife faithfully take B_6 supplements.

"Vitamin B_6 is as important to your body as oxygen and water," says Dr. Ellis. "Except it takes six weeks for B_6 to get functioning in there like it should."

More and more research is accumulating to support this point of view, says Dr. Ellis. From carpal tunnel syndrome and memory loss to diabetes and premenstrual syndrome, the list of conditions for which vitamin B_6—also called pyridoxine—is gaining acceptance as a possible treatment is long.

Vitamin B_6 serves the important purpose of ensuring that biological processes, including fat and protein metabolism, take place in the body. "In the absence of B_6, metabolism is basically altered," says Michael Ebadi, Ph.D., professor of pharmacology and neurology at the University of Nebraska College of Medicine in Omaha.

Vitamin B_6 is also important in brain function. This nutrient is vital in helping to create neurotransmitters, the chemicals that allow brain cells to communicate with one another, says Dr. Ebadi. As a result, a lack of B_6 impairs your memory, causing trouble with your ability to register, retain and retrieve information.

When it comes to diabetes, a shortage of vitamin B_6 has been linked to something called glucose intolerance, which is an abnormally high rise in blood sugar after eating. It may also impair the secretion of insulin and glucagon, the hormone that tells your pancreas when to stop producing insulin.

Shortages of the B vitamins can also lead to nerve damage in the hands and feet. Some studies indicate that people with diabetes experience less of the numbness and tingling of diabetes-caused nerve damage if they get supplemental amounts of B vitamins such as B_6 and B_{12}.

As for carpal tunnel syndrome, "you couldn't say enough about carpal tunnel and vitamin B_6," says Dr. Ellis. "The evidence is that positive." He contends that swelling and inelasticity of the sheath surrounding a nerve in the wrist may be caused by a lack of B_6. "B_6 helps you get rid of the extra water gain that causes carpal tunnel," he says. Another theory, backed up by two European studies, suggests that B_6 somehow short-circuits an angry nerve's ability to transmit pain signals.

Dr. Ellis says his research shows that numbness, tingling, swelling and pain in the knees, shoulders and arms—what he calls menopausal arthritis—may also be caused by low vitamin B_6.

Other potential uses of vitamin B_6 on the horizon: ending asthma attacks by lowering the body's histamine levels and defending against atherosclerosis by reducing a chemical in the blood that damages arterial walls. "We're just beginning to scratch the surface of what this vitamin can do," says Dr. Ellis.

Using Vitamin B_6 Safely

Even the foods richest in vitamin B_6—such as bananas, avocados, brewer's yeast and beef—provide barely a single milligram of B_6. But that doesn't necessarily mean you'll need to reach for a supplement, since the Daily Value is only two milligrams.

And if you do opt for a supplement, you should use caution. Too much vitamin B_6 has been linked to serious nerve disorders as well as to oversensitivity to sunlight, which produces a skin rash and numbness.

In one study, people took 6,000 milligrams of vitamin B_6 daily over a two-month period; in another, people took 2,000 milligrams daily for two months or more. The results were the same: The people suffered from severe loss of neuromotor coordination and muscle weakness that stopped a few months after they quit taking B_6. As a result, experts suggest consulting your doctor before taking more than 100 milligrams of B_6 a day. They also recommend getting this vitamin as part of a B-complex tablet that supplies the Daily Values of all of the B vitamins.

People who are undergoing levodopa therapy for Parkinson's disease should avoid vitamin B_6 supplements altogether. It has been found to reduce the drug's effectiveness.

On the other hand, certain drugs can cause a vitamin B_6 deficiency: isoniazid, for tuberculosis; cycloserine, an antibiotic for tuberculosis; and penicillamine, for Wilson's disease, lead poisoning, kidney stones and arthritis. If you are taking any of these drugs, you might want to talk to your doctor before taking a B_6 supplement.

Vitamin B_{12}

Daily Value: *6 micrograms*

Good Food Sources: *Clams, ham, cooked oysters, king crab, herring, salmon, tuna*

Short of an accident, there are few faster ways to short-circuit your body than bypassing vitamin B_{12}. That's because B_{12}—also called cobalamin—is vital to the production of myelin, the fatty sheath that insulates nerve fibers, keeping electrical impulses moving through your body.

Because of the nutrient's important nerve-protecting function, a whole host of problems have been linked to low levels of vitamin B_{12}, including memory loss, confusion, delusion, fatigue, loss of balance, decreased reflexes, impaired touch or pain perception, numbness and tingling in the arms and legs, tinnitus and noise-induced hearing loss. Deficiencies of B_{12} have also been linked to multiple sclerosis–like symptoms and dementia. "In a severe deficiency, there is actually a degeneration of the myelin sheath. The stuff begins to literally erode," says John Pinto, Ph.D., director of the nutrition research laboratory at Memorial Sloan-Kettering Cancer Center and associate professor of biochemistry in medicine at Cornell University Medical College, both in New York City.

But that's only the beginning of vitamin B_{12}'s importance. Researchers have discovered that a deficiency raises blood levels of a substance known as homocysteine. In addition to being toxic to brain cells in high doses—raising serious questions about its possible role in Alzheimer's disease—homocysteine may be one of the primary causes of heart disease. "It has been shown to activate a clotting system that makes blood cells become a little more adhesive, a little more sticky, making them cling to arterial walls," says Dr. Pinto.

There's evidence that in some, the accumulation of homocysteine may be caused by a genetic defect, while in others, it's simply the result of a vitamin B_{12} deficiency. Such clotting and homocysteine buildup also seem to occur during folate and B_6 deficiencies.

Because vitamin B_{12} is also important for the production of red blood cells, a severe deficiency, called pernicious anemia, can lower energy levels.

"When you take B_{12}, if you do have so-called tired blood (a decreased number of red blood cells), almost immediately you will see a burst of activity in the bone marrow—more cells—and that will mean more oxygen-carrying capacity to tissues," says Dr. Pinto.

Because vitamin B_{12} is found in animal products, vegans—strict vegetarians who avoid dairy products and eggs as well as meats—are at risk for becoming B_{12}-deficient. In fact, one study documented cases of children of vegans whose growth was stunted because they did not get adequate B_{12}.

And even when they do eat meats and dairy products, nearly one-third of people over age 60 can't extract the vitamin B_{12} they need from what they eat. That's because their stomachs no longer secrete enough gastric acid, the stuff that breaks down food so that B_{12} can be stored in the liver and muscles until it's needed. Without gastric acid, even someone who gets adequate amounts of B_{12} in his diet may become deficient.

Using Vitamin B_{12} Safely

It's easy to get adequate amounts of vitamin B_{12} from food sources, because you need so little of it. So there's really no need to take a supplement unless your doctor tells you to do so.

Doctors often prescribe shots for those who have trouble absorbing vitamin B_{12}, however. A typical regimen for someone who has been low for a while might include a daily shot of 100 to 1,000 micrograms for one to two weeks, then a weekly shot that provides between 100 and 1,000 micrograms to normalize B_{12} stores. This is followed by monthly injections of 250 to 1,000 micrograms.

If you have absorption problems, doctors recommend using sublingual B_{12} tablets—normally placed under the tongue—or a B_{12} nasal gel. Both are available in health food stores. For those without absorption problems, oral tablets are available, but doctors recommend both sublingual tablets and nasal gel as alternatives.

Vitamin B_{12} supplements are considered extremely safe; even huge excess doses are harmlessly excreted in your urine. If you get injections, there may be some discomfort at the injection site, and in rare cases, sensitive people could have allergic reactions to B_{12}. If you have any of the following conditions, you should check with your doctor before using B_{12}: folate deficiency, iron deficiency, any kind of infection, Leber's disease, polycythemia vera or uremia.

Vitamin C

Daily Value: *60 milligrams*

Good Food Sources: *Pineapple, broccoli, peppers, cantaloupe, strawberries, oranges, kiwifruit, pink grapefruit*

Linus Pauling is gone—dead at the age of 93 from cancer. But at the Linus Pauling Institute of Science and Medicine in Palo Alto, California, and in research labs across the country, his scientific legacy lives on. Experts continue to investigate the healing potential of vitamin C, also called ascorbic acid.

"We're conducting research projects that explore the role of vitamin C in cardiovascular disease, cancer, HIV infection, cataracts, skin health and other physiological and pathological conditions," says Stephen Lawson, chief executive officer of the institute.

There's good reason to believe that further research will bear even more fruit. While skeptics continue to carp, already dozens of studies strongly suggest that vitamin C plays a role in preventing a variety of diseases. And there is a growing number of doctors who are using the nutrient to treat disease as well.

Vitamin C is thought to help protect the esophagus, oral cavity, stomach and pancreas—and possibly the cervix, rectum and breasts—from cancer. How does it do all of that?

Some forms of cancer are thought to be caused by what are called free radicals, naturally occurring renegade molecules that damage your body's healthy molecules (such as DNA, in the case of cancer) by stealing electrons to balance themselves. Vitamin C and other substances known as antioxidants neutralize free radicals by offering their own electrons, minimizing oxidative damage to DNA and other molecules, explains Balz Frei, Ph.D., associate professor of medicine and biochemistry at Boston University School of Medicine. Nitrites—potentially cancer-causing preservatives found in foods such as hot dogs and lunchmeats—and nitrates—found naturally in vegetables and drinking water—are also neutralized by vitamin C.

The long arm of vitamin C's antioxidant protection may also extend to heart health. In studies that looked at vitamin C and cholesterol levels, researchers found those who had high blood levels of vitamin C showed reduced risk of heart disease.

And in lab experiments, high concentrations of vitamin C have also been found to inhibit the growth of smooth muscle cells in artery walls. The abnormally high growth activity of these cells has been considered one of the initial steps in the development of cardiovascular disease, says Vadim Ivanov, Ph.D., head of the cardiovascular research program at the Linus Pauling Institute.

Vitamin C's role as an antioxidant may even help delay or prevent cataract formation. The nutrient may be beneficial because ultraviolet light and oxidative stress in the lens of your eye are thought to be leading causes of cataract formation. Vitamin C can help prevent the damage caused by oxidative stress.

Cold sufferers have raved for years about vitamin C's effect on what ails them. Research shows that high intake of this water-soluble vitamin actually supercharges some of your immune system's most important defense cells, helping them to move faster while tracking down potential pathogens such as bacteria and viruses. That means you may not be able to prevent a cold by taking vitamin C, but you can probably make it shorter and less severe. Not only that, but vitamin C has also been found to reduce the body's levels of histamine, a chemical released by the body that can dampen immune response, says Carol Johnston, Ph.D., associate professor of food and nutrition at Arizona State University in Tempe.

This antihistamine benefit may also be good news for folks suffering from asthma or allergies. Researchers at Harvard Medical School found that people who got at least 200 milligrams of vitamin C a day had a 30 percent reduced risk of bronchitis or wheezing compared with people who got about 100 milligrams of vitamin C a day.

Researchers at the Linus Pauling Institute have found that vitamin C inhibits replication of HIV, at least in infected cells in the laboratory.

One day, people with diabetes may also benefit from vitamin C. An animal study seemed to show that vitamin C helps regulate insulin release. And a human study showed that vitamin C prevents the sugar inside cells from converting to a chemical called sorbitol. This sugar alcohol, which accumulates in the cells, has been implicated in diabetes-related eye, nerve and kidney damage.

As if all of that weren't enough, vitamin C has long been known to protect gums, joints, ligaments, artery walls and skin. It also improves wound healing by aiding the production of collagen, the building block of tissues. "About one-third of your body's protein is collagen, which means you're in pretty bad shape without vitamin C," says Dr. Johnston.

Although most people have heard of vitamin C's healing benefits, many may be depleted of this important nutrient. In a study conducted at Arizona State University, Dr. Johnston found that 60 percent of the participants got about 125 milligrams of vitamin C a day, more than twice the Daily Value. Between 18 and 20 percent, however, were depleted, and roughly 3 percent had blood vitamin C levels that indicated they should be suffering from scurvy, a potentially fatal deficiency disease once common among sailors. "We saw in our population that the ones who were deficient ate less than one serving of fruits and vegetables a day, when it is recommended that you eat five to nine servings," says Dr. Johnston.

Early signs of vitamin C depletion include weakness and lethargy, followed by delayed wound healing. If stores are completely exhausted—a rare occurrence today—scurvy appears. Its symptoms include dementia, bleeding gums, tooth loss, hemorrhages and pain in muscles, bones and joints.

Using Vitamin C Safely

Scan the shelves in your local health food store, and you may see more forms and brands of vitamin C than new cars at a dealership.

But don't worry about which one to buy. At least one study shows that it doesn't seem to matter. Whether the vitamin C is top of the line or bargain basement, the amount that your body uses is the same. "I compared ones that are expensive with those that are dirt cheap—two bucks a bottle—and there was no difference," says Dr. Johnston. "In other words, additives like rose hips, manipulation like buffering and cost didn't have any impact on bioavailability." There may be one small difference, however: Buffered vitamin C could cause slightly less diarrhea in high doses than other forms.

And high doses do seem to be safe. Megadoses of vitamin C—between 500 and 2,000 milligrams every four hours—have been used to acidify urine, which affects the way some medications are absorbed. In no fewer than five clinical studies, folks who took 5,000 milligrams a day for more than three years reported no side effects. Dr. Pauling took megadoses of vitamin C every day for decades with no reported ill effects.

Doses of 500 milligrams a day have been linked to kidney stones in people who are prone to them, however. And as mentioned, large doses of vitamin C can cause diarrhea. (If you experience this reaction, experts recommend taking the vitamin in divided doses with meals throughout the day.)

Stress increases the body's need for vitamin C. So does nicotine. Because of this, the Food and Nutrition Board of the National Research Council has recommended that smokers get 100 milligrams of vitamin C per day.

The vitamin may also interfere with the absorption of tricyclic antidepressants, and it interferes with the results of certain diagnostic blood and urine tests, so you might want to mention your vitamin C intake to your doctor if you take these drugs or are going in for tests. People who have deficiencies in a red blood cell enzyme called glucose-6-phosphate dehydrogenase should not take large doses of vitamin C because it can damage their red blood cells and cause anemia. This deficiency is most common among people of African, Mediterranean or Asian descent. Some experts recommend limiting the use of chewable vitamin C tablets because they can cause enamel loss from the surface of the teeth and other dental problems.

Vitamin D

Daily Value: *400 international units*

Good Food Sources: *Herring, sardines, salmon, fortified milk, eggs, fortified cereals*

The *D* in vitamin D could very well stand for *different*. How else to describe the only nutrient that's both made by your body (vitamin D is synthesized through your skin by the action of ultraviolet light that's present in sunlight) and required in your diet?

Without it, another *D* word comes to mind: *devastating*. Children who don't get adequate vitamin D develop rickets, a condition characterized by flaring ankles and wrists that have noticeable knobby bumps and by weak, soft leg bones that bow under the child's own weight. Similarly, adults risk developing osteomalacia, a condition similar to rickets but occurring in developed bones. Some experts believe that not getting enough vitamin D can make osteoporosis worse. Osteoporosis is a bone-weakening disease that leads to fractures and tooth loss.

Vitamin D is responsible for getting the important bone builders calcium and phosphorus to the places in the body that they need to go to help bone grow in children and remineralize in adults. It does this first by making certain these minerals are absorbed in the intestines, second by bringing calcium from bones into the blood and third by helping the kidneys reabsorb the two minerals, says Binita R. Shah, M.D., professor of clinical pediatrics and director of pediatric emergency medicine at the State University of New York Health Science Center at Brooklyn. "When you see a case of rickets, the body is desperately trying to make bone, but adequate calcium and phosphorus aren't available. It's a poor effort. The result is a mass of unmineralized bone accumulation," says Dr. Shah.

Fortified milk is one ready source of vitamin D, although it takes a quart to provide the Daily Value. But you don't have to rely on diet alone to give you the vitamin D you need. Ten minutes of summer sun on your hands and face provides enough, says H. F. DeLuca, Ph.D., chairman of the Department of Biochemistry at the University of Wisconsin–Madison.

"It depends on where you are in relation to the equator, but in northern climates during the winter, the sun is at such an angle that the right rays don't penetrate the skin to make vitamin D," says Dr. DeLuca. "During the summer, you can store up quite a bit of vitamin D in your fat cells. If your diet is good, it will probably last you through the winter." Sitting next to a sun-filled picture window or driving in a car doesn't count; the glass filters out the rays you need.

Fortunately, kids are born with enough vitamin D to last them nine months. Adults aren't as lucky, as shown in a study at Columbia University in New York City. After evaluating the calcium and vitamin D status of elderly people who were entering nursing homes, researchers determined that a majority had low vitamin D levels. Nearly 85 percent had symptoms of osteoporosis.

"There is mounting evidence that vitamin D deficiency in elderly people is a silent epidemic that results in bone loss and fractures," reports Michael F. Holick, M.D., Ph.D., chief of the Section of Endocrinology, Diabetes and Metabolism and director of the General Clinical Research Center at Boston University Medical Center.

Vitamin D also plays a role in immune function, although it's still unclear just how that takes place.

Using Vitamin D Safely

When eight people in Massachusetts developed symptoms such as nausea, weakness, constipation and irritability just from drinking fresh vitamin D–fortified milk, doctors scratched their heads—that is, until they discovered that the milk had accidentally been fortified with more than 580 times the proper amount of vitamin D.

Such massive overfortifications are rare. But they're a good example of what can happen when you get too much vitamin D. Because the nutrient is stored in fat cells, long-term high doses can cause calcium to be deposited in the soft tissues of the body and can result in irreversible damage to the kidneys and cardiovascular system. Doses of 1,800 international units a day can cause stunted growth in infants and young children. High intake of vitamin D can even lead to coma.

Because vitamin D can be so toxic, you should never take more than 600 international units of vitamin D daily unless your doctor prescribes a higher dosage for you.

Vitamin E

Daily Value: *30 international units*

Good Food Sources: *Vegetable and nut oils, including soybean, safflower and corn; sunflower seeds; whole grains; wheat germ; spinach*

Vitamin E may well prove to be one of the most powerful nutrients on the face of the earth.

Studies indicate that it fights heart disease, prevents cancer, alleviates respiratory problems and boosts your immune system's ability to fight off infectious disease. It may also prevent some of the damage that diabetes does to the body, particularly to the eyes.

How does a simple vitamin achieve such complex results? Vitamin E works in a variety of ways, but a key mechanism seen in the laboratory is its ability to neutralize free radicals, naturally occurring unstable molecules that can damage your body's healthy molecules by stealing electrons to balance themselves.

And what happens in the laboratory seems to translate into what happens in real life. Two joint studies, which looked at more than 127,000 people, for example, reported that those who took vitamin E supplements for at least two years had about 40 percent less risk of heart disease than those who didn't.

"There's a lot of evidence to support the possible benefits of vitamin E, but these are the first studies to actually measure benefits in terms of less disease and fewer heart attacks," says Meir Stampfer, M.D., Dr.P.H., an investigator at the Harvard School of Public Health who was involved with the study.

Yet despite this vitamin's ability to prevent disease, somewhere between 69 and 80 percent of older adults do not get even the Daily Value of 30 international units. And Dr. Stampfer maintains that we might need many times that amount to prevent disease.

Vitamin E deficiency, however, is very rare. Infants with low birth weight are susceptible, as are people with conditions such as cystic fibrosis, which prevents the proper absorption of fat. Signs of deficiency can include neurological and reproductive problems.

Unless you want to drink two quarts of corn oil or eat a pound of sunflower seeds every day, the only way to increase your vitamin E intake is with supplements.

There are eight different forms of the vitamin. But the supplement labeled "d-alpha-tocopherol" is the one that will give you the biggest bang for your buck. It makes more vitamin E available to your body than any other form.

D-alpha-tocopherol loses its potency when exposed to air, heat and light, so make sure it's stored in a cool, dark place. It should be taken with a meal that contains fat; otherwise your body cannot absorb it adequately. It should not be taken at the same time as an iron supplement, since iron seems to destroy vitamin E before it can get down to business.

Using Vitamin E Safely

Some studies that have found vitamin E can prevent disease have also shown that getting somewhere between 200 and 800 international units is necessary to release its power.

Fortunately, the vitamin seems to be relatively safe, even at higher doses. Studies indicate that daily supplements of 800 and 900 international units have been taken without any reported problems. People who are taking anticoagulants (sometimes called blood thinners or heart medicine) should not take vitamin E supplements, however, because they can be harmful. Some experts think it's also a good idea for people who have had strokes or bleeding problems to consult their doctors before taking supplements. Vitamin E can also interfere with the absorption and action of vitamin K, which is involved in blood coagulation.

On the other hand, those who are taking anticonvulsants, cholesterol-lowering drugs, tuberculosis drugs, ulcer medication or the antibiotic neomycin should probably talk to their doctors about increasing the amount of vitamin E they take. All of these medications can increase the body's need for the nutrient.

Vitamin K

Daily Value: *80 micrograms*

Good Food Sources: *Cauliflower, broccoli and green, leafy vegetables such as spinach and kale*

Unless you were born within the past couple of minutes, your chances of having a vitamin K deficiency are pretty slim.

Your body needs such tiny amounts of this nutrient to help blood clot when you're injured—this is vitamin K's primary job—that you most likely get more than enough without making any effort at all. You can even manufacture your own vitamin K. About half of the vitamin K your body needs is normally produced by your own intestinal bacteria.

Babies are the big exception. They lack the bacteria necessary to produce vitamin K, and they're usually not up to a diet of green, leafy vegetables for quite a while. And although breast milk has a small amount of the nutrient, it's one of the few instances in which breast milk is simply not enough. So babies are generally given a shot of vitamin K at birth.

The only other folks who need an extra boost of supplemental vitamin

K are those who have a digestive disease such as cystic fibrosis, says James Sadowski, Ph.D., chief of the vitamin K laboratory at the Jean Mayer USDA Human Nutrition Research Center on Aging at Tufts University in Boston.

But there are some folks who are afraid that they get too much vitamin K. Many people who are taking anticoagulants, or blood thinners, to prevent heart attack and stroke actually cut down on the amounts of green, leafy vegetables they eat because they're afraid that their lettuce will trigger the same events that their medications are trying to prevent.

"This is absolutely wrong," says John W. Suttie, Ph.D., professor and chair of nutritional sciences at the University of Wisconsin–Madison. "Physicians tell a lot of people whom they put on anticoagulants to limit their vitamin K intakes. I don't know why they do this, but it's fairly common. It is not good advice."

Dr. Sadowski agrees. "If someone is on oral anticoagulants because he has had a heart attack, a stroke or blood clots in his legs, he should keep his vitamin K consumption at a fairly constant level every day. But it probably doesn't matter how much he's getting as long as it's pretty close to the same thing every day."

The reason? Every individual's anticoagulant dose is custom-tailored to his particular needs, says Dr. Suttie. Those needs are identified through a series of blood tests when the anticoagulants are started. The amount of anticoagulant then prescribed is intended to strike a very delicate balance, giving your body enough vitamin K to clot and heal wounds but not enough to clot and cause a heart attack.

Using Vitamin K Safely

Since your body can absorb vitamin K only when it's accompanied by dietary fat, it's best to eat your leafy greens with a food that contains at least some fat. A dollop of oil-based salad dressing on a bed of greens or even a serving of lettuce on a lean burger will make sure your vitamin K is there when you need it.

Zinc

Daily Value: *15 milligrams*

Good Food Sources: *Cooked oysters, beef, lamb, eggs, whole grains, nuts, yogurt*

When you think zinc, think productivity. From helping to create new skin and sperm cells to boosting the immune system, this mineral works overtime to produce the cells you need to keep healthy.

"Healing, growth, pregnancy, lactation are all situations where there is an increased need for zinc because of the need for more cells," says Adria Sherman, Ph.D., professor and chair of the Department of Nutritional Sciences at Rutgers University in New Brunswick, New Jersey.

A classic example is immune defense. Before your body can battle a foreign invader, zinc and chemicals called zinc-dependent enzymes work together to help build new immune system cells and whip them into fighting trim. That's why zinc is helpful in fending off viral infections.

By the same token, too much zinc—just 25 milligrams a day in one study—has been found to decrease immunity.

Zinc's quick cell replication skills come in handy when you have cuts or wounds. It's vital for the production of collagen, the connective tissue that helps wounds heal, says Richard Wood, Ph.D., associate professor in the School of Nutrition at Tufts University in Medford, Massachusetts, and chief of the mineral bioavailability laboratory at the Jean Mayer USDA Human Nutrition Research Center on Aging at Tufts University in Boston. "And when you don't get enough zinc, normal healing doesn't occur," he says.

Although research findings are slim, some doctors recommend zinc to treat enlarged prostate, a disease that disrupts the flow of urine in men. Zinc hasn't been tested in any large scientific studies, and until it is, many doctors will remain skeptical. It's important to work with a doctor knowledgeable in nutrition if you want to try zinc for prostate problems.

Even several key enzymes that protect and preserve your vision can't be formed without zinc. "Zinc and vitamin A interact in the eyes to maintain the normal process of dark adaptation, where the eyes adjust to low levels of light," says Dr. Wood.

The benefits of zinc aside, it's likely that most Americans simply don't get enough of this mineral. In fact, one study found that 30 percent of healthy elderly people are zinc-deficient. They may not be the only ones: In their zeal to eat low-fat diets, more people than ever are shunning red meat, and red meat is a solid source of this vital nutrient.

Another potential problem: Increased calcium intake, recommended to prevent osteoporosis, removes some zinc from the body, says Dr. Wood. The heavy plant emphasis of some vegetarian diets can interfere with zinc absorption, as can alcoholism, oral penicillin therapy and diuretics (water pills). Low levels of vitamin B_6 have also been found to reduce zinc absorption.

Signs of possible deficiency include impaired immunity, weight loss, bloating, loss of appetite, rashes and other skin changes, bedsores, hair loss, diminished sense of taste or smell, absence of menstrual periods and depression.

Using Zinc Safely

While it's best to get zinc from foods, you can choose from several zinc supplements. But be careful not to take too much. More is not necessarily better. Excessive amounts can cause nausea, headaches, lethargy and irritability. In fact, taking more than 2,000 milligrams of zinc sulfate has been known to cause stomach irritation and vomiting.

Even taking between 30 and 150 milligrams of zinc daily for several weeks interferes with copper absorption and can cause copper deficiency. (For this reason, doctors often recommend that those using zinc supplements take additional copper, in a ratio of 1 milligram of copper to 10 milligrams of zinc.) More than 30 milligrams of zinc a day can increase your risk of developing anemia. Such high doses have also been found to lower levels of HDL, the "good" cholesterol, while raising levels of LDL, the "bad" cholesterol. (A doctor may, however, recommend amounts this high to treat Wilson's disease, a condition involving excess copper in the body.) And increased dietary zinc has been shown to markedly decrease mental functioning in people with Alzheimer's disease. Because of these risks, doctors recommend that zinc supplements in excess of 15 milligrams a day be taken only under medical supervision.

Because zinc can cause stomach upset, it may be taken with food. Dairy products, bran products and foods high in calcium and phosphorus, such as milk, may decrease zinc absorption. Protein-rich foods such as lamb, beef and eggs enhance absorption.

Drugs Can Sabotage Your Nutrition

You're doing everything you can to eat right. You pay careful attention to getting all of the right nutrients, and that means you're probably taking vitamin and mineral supplements. And you're sure that you have all your nutritional bases covered. But do you really?

If you regularly take medication, either prescription or over the counter, you should be aware of the fact that some drugs are potential nutrition robbers. Nutrition researchers now know that drug-nutrient interaction is a potentially serious problem. Some drugs can remove nutrients from your body, prevent absorption of nutrients or affect the body's ability to convert nutrients into usable forms. In fact, medical experts have determined that of the top 25 drugs prescribed most often, 19 have the potential for causing serious nutrient deficiencies.

Pregnant and nursing women, infants and the elderly may be even more at risk. They may be more deficient in essential nutrients to begin with.

The table that follows lists some common prescription drugs and their nutrient interactions. If you're taking any of these drugs, you may want to check with your doctor to see if you should increase your intake of the nutrients that the medication affects.

How can you prevent nutrient deficiencies caused by medication? Here are several suggestions from Arthur I. Jacknowitz, Pharm.D., professor and chairman of the Department of Clinical Pharmacy at West Virginia University in Morgantown.

- Make sure you understand the patient information provided to you with your prescription drug. If you have any questions, ask the advice of your doctor or pharmacist.
- When you buy an over-the-counter product, read the label carefully. If you're confused about ingredients, don't hesitate to ask about them.
- Follow your doctor's instructions about when to take a medication.
- The actions of some drugs may be enhanced or lessened by certain foods and beverages. Don't be afraid to ask your doctor or pharmacist how drugs may interact with your favorite foods, especially if you eat large amounts of them.
- Eat a nutritionally well-balanced diet with a wide variety of foods.

(continued)

Drugs Can Sabotage Your Nutrition—Continued

Drug Class	Treatment for . . .
Antacids	Indigestion
Antibacterial agents	Chronic bronchitis, tuberculosis, urinary tract infections
Antibiotics	Bacterial infections
Anti-cancer drugs	Tumors
Anticoagulants	Blood clots
Anticonvulsants	Epilepsy, seizures
Antihypertensive agents	High blood pressure
Anti-inflammatory agents	Inflammation, swelling
Antimalarials	Malaria
Diuretics	High blood pressure, water retention
H_2 receptor antagonists	Peptic ulcers
Hypocholesterolemic agents	High blood cholesterol
Laxatives	Constipation
Tranquilizers	Depression, sleeping problems

Generic Name	May Interfere with . . .
Aluminum hydroxide, sodium bicarbonate	Calcium, copper, folate
Boric acid	Riboflavin
Isoniazid	Niacin, vitamin B_6, vitamin D
Trimethoprim	Folate
Gentamicin	Magnesium, potassium
Tetracycline	Calcium
Cisplatin	Magnesium
Methotrexate	Calcium, folate
Warfarin	Vitamin K
Phenobarbital, phenytoin, primidone	Vitamin D, vitamin K
Hydralazine	Vitamin B_6
Aspirin	Folate, iron, vitamin C
Colchicine	Vitamin B_{12}
Prednisone	Calcium
Sulfasalazine	Folate
Pyrimethamine	Folate
Furosemide	Calcium, magnesium, potassium
Thiazides	Potassium
Triamterene	Folate
Cimetidine, ranitidine	Vitamin B_{12}
Colestipol	Folate, vitamin A, vitamin B_{12}, vitamin K
Mineral oil	Vitamin D, vitamin K
Phenolphthalein	Potassium
Senna	Calcium
Chlorpromazine	Riboflavin

Part Two

Therapeutic Prescriptions for Healing

Age Spots

Going, Going, Gone

Ours is a culture with little appreciation for spots. None of us likes getting a spot on our record, on our reputation or on our shirt. And we certainly don't like seeing spots when we're looking into a mirror!

But as we age, many of us do begin to see spots, especially on our hands and faces. And whether we call them liver spots, age spots or sun spots, the reaction is likely the same: We want a spot remover.

Technically known as lentigines, age spots are the result of excess pigment being deposited in the skin during years of sun exposure. So along with treatment, dermatologists also recommend avoiding exposure to the sun.

Note: Though the majority of age spots are harmless blemishes that require no more than a trip to the dermatologist, early stages of skin cancer can masquerade as innocent-looking age spots. If any spot enlarges, thickens, changes color, bleeds or itches, have it checked by a doctor. For extra protection, also include a skin examination in your annual checkup.

The good news is, if your spots really are just age spots, dermatologists today have an assortment of treatments at their disposal that can fade them, if not remove them completely. These include topical application of tretinoin, a vitamin A acid known as Retin-A.

Fade 'Em Away with Retin-A

Originally developed as an acne medication to unplug clogged pores, Retin-A has found resounding success as an anti-aging ointment. Though not a fountain of youth, Retin-A works to eliminate fine wrinkles, blemishes and age spots by stimulating cell turnover in a metabolic process that still is not entirely understood, says Retin-A creator Albert Kligman, M.D., Ph.D., professor of dermatology at the University of Pennsylvania School of Medicine and an attending physician at the Hospital of the University of Pennsylvania, both in Philadelphia.

To remove an age spot, dermatologists often recommend applying the strongest dosage of Retin-A that you can tolerate directly on the spot. The area will proceed to peel, and after a few months, the spot should diminish and possibly even disappear.

If you're like the people who were in a research group at the University of Michigan Medical Center in Ann Arbor, you may even see results after just one month. In a ten-month study of 58 people with age spots, researchers found that the majority of people treated with Retin-A experienced lightening of these spots after one month. After ten months, 83 percent of those treated with Retin-A experienced lightening of their age spots, and 32 percent had at least one spot disappear.

Retin-A can be even more effective when used in combination with other treatments, says John F. Romano, M.D., clinical assistant professor of dermatology at New York Hospital–Cornell Medical Center and St. Vincent's Hospital, both in New York City.

"I often have people apply glycolic acid in the morning and Retin-A at night. Or I may combine it with a bleaching cream," says Dr. Romano.

Retin-A cream comes in a variety of concentrations, the weakest being 0.025 percent and the strongest being 0.1 percent. It's available only by prescription, so you'll need to work with your dermatologist to find the dosage that's right for you.

And because Retin-A continually sloughs off the outermost, dead layer of

Food Factors

Unfortunately, there are no magical foods that, if eaten, will fade age spots. There are, however, a few that can increase your sensitivity to the mother of age spots, the sun. Here's what you might want to avoid before playing in the sunshine.

Hold the lime. Certain fruits and vegetables—particularly celery, parsnips, carrots and limes—contain psoralens, chemicals that can increase your sensitivity to the sun. Unless you're sensitive to psoralens, eating these foods before going out in the sun is not likely to be a problem, says Douglas Darr, Ph.D., director of technology development at the North Carolina Biotechnology Center in Research Triangle Park. You'd best wash your hands—which are already susceptible to sun exposure and age spots—after handling these foods, however. Anyone's skin can be more susceptible to burning after direct contact with psoralens.

skin, it can not only eliminate existing spots but also nip new spots in the bud. The downside of this process is that an area of skin previously sheltered from evaporation and the elements is exposed. That's why a common side effect of Retin-A is dry, sun-sensitive skin that can be irritated and scaly. Though this effect typically diminishes with time, if you're using Retin-A, you'll likely need a moisturizer. Sunscreen is also a must once you start using Retin-A.

Protect Your Skin with Vitamin C

If vitamin D is the sunshine vitamin, then vitamin C is the sunblock vitamin, say some researchers—many of whom also proclaim it the healthy skin vitamin.

"In general, vitamin C is important for keeping the skin younger looking," says Lorraine Meisner, Ph.D., professor of preventive medicine at the University of Wisconsin Medical School in Madison. She recommends a safe daily vitamin C intake of about 300 to 500 milligrams to maintain skin quality.

Medical researchers have also found vitamin C to be of some help when applied topically. It has been shown to significantly reduce the amount of so-called free radical damage that occurs from sun exposure. Free radicals are naturally occurring unstable molecules that steal electrons from your body's healthy molecules to balance themselves. Unchecked, they can cause significant tissue damage. Antioxidants—vitamin C is one—neutralize free radicals by offering their own electrons and so protect the healthy molecules from harm.

"Since vitamin C prevents skin damage from sun exposure, it's reasonable to suspect that it can also prevent the consequences of that damage, including wrinkling and age spots," says Douglas Darr, Ph.D., director of technology development at the North Carolina Biotechnology Center in Research Triangle Park. Dr. Darr advocates using topical vitamin C as an adjunct to sunscreen.

One such topical vitamin C product is Cellex-C, a 10 percent vitamin C lotion. It's available without a prescription from dermatologists, plastic surgeons and licensed aestheticians (full-service beauty salon operators) and by mail order from Cellex-C Distribution, 2631 Commerce Street, Suite C, Dallas, TX 75226 (1-800-423-5592). For optimum sun protection, the lotion should be applied once a day, along with a sunscreen, according to Dr. Meisner, one of the developers of Cellex-C.

Also, though snacking on citrus fruits may help keep your skin healthier, don't count on being able to eat enough oranges to protect you from the sun, says Sheldon Pinnell, M.D., chief of dermatology at Duke University Medical Center in Durham, North Carolina, and another of the developers of Cellex-C. "The cream allows you to get 20 to 40 times the levels that you would achieve by ingesting vitamin C," he says.

Prescriptions for Healing

The only vitamin that has been proven to erase age spots is vitamin A, applied topically as the prescription drug tretinoin (Retin-A). But there are several nutrients that can do the next best thing: prevent the sun damage that leads to age spots. Here's what some experts recommend as the best dosages.

Nutrient	Daily Amount/Application
Oral	
Selenium	50–200 micrograms (l-selenomethionine)
Vitamin C	300–500 milligrams
Vitamin E	400 international units (d-alpha-tocopherol)
Topical	
Vitamin A	0.025%–0.1% cream (Retin-A), depending on skin type
Vitamin C	10% lotion (Cellex-C)
Vitamin E	At least 5% cream or oil, applied after sun exposure

MEDICAL ALERT: *Selenium can be toxic in daily doses exceeding 100 micrograms, so if you'd like to try this therapy to protect your skin, you should discuss it with your doctor.*

If you are taking anticoagulant drugs, you should not take oral vitamin E supplements.

Damage Control with Vitamin E

Vitamin E, an antioxidant vitamin added to everything from nail polish remover to shampoo, is also helpful in preventing sun damage.

Researchers have shown that vitamin E oil can prevent inflammation and skin damage if applied within eight hours of sun exposure. Because vitamin E itself produces free radicals when exposed to ultraviolet light, however, researchers recommend that you apply it following, not before, sun exposure.

Vitamin E oil can be bought over the counter in drugstores, as can vitamin E–fortified creams. Research has shown that if the cream or oil contains at least 5 percent vitamin E, it can also be effective in reducing post-sun damage.

You can also reap some of vitamin E's sun-protective properties by taking supplements, adds Karen E. Burke, M.D., Ph.D., a dermatologic surgeon and dermatologist in private practice in New York City. "It's highly effective as an anti-inflammatory agent, and it reduces sun damage to the skin," she says. Dr. Burke recommends that people take 400 international units of vitamin E in the form of d-alpha-tocopherol daily.

Good dietary sources of vitamin E include polyunsaturated vegetable oil, wheat germ, spinach and sunflower seeds.

Try Some Selenium Sun Protection

You might want to boost your dietary intake of the antioxidant mineral selenium as well, says Dr. Burke.

"Selenium can prevent solar damage, pigmentation and dark spots, but because the selenium content of soil varies across the country, not everyone is getting enough to be beneficial," says Dr. Burke, citing the Southeast in particular as an area deficient in selenium.

To quench the free radicals caused by sun exposure and to prevent skin damage, Dr. Burke recommends daily supplements of 50 to 200 micrograms of selenium in the form of l-selenomethionine, depending on where you live and your family history of cancer. Selenium can be toxic in doses exceeding 100 micrograms, so if you'd like to try this therapy to protect your skin, you should discuss it with your doctor.

To get more selenium in your diet, try tuna; a three-ounce can serves up a full 99 micrograms. Or treat yourself to an ounce of baked tortilla chips for a whopping 284 micrograms.

Aging

A Radical Solution

At age 38, Elizabeth lies on Litchfield Beach in South Carolina, sunscreen carefully smoothed over her wrinkle-free skin, her naturally dark hair tucked under a scarf and a pair of dense wraparound sunglasses shielding her lovely blue eyes from the morning sun.

Beside her is a cooler containing several bottles of springwater and a fresh fruit salad of watermelon, cantaloupe and honeydew for lunch. Next to her on the sand is a pair of well-used sneakers for the two-mile walk she takes along the water's edge every day.

Elizabeth knows that she's gorgeous. There are no wrinkles or stretch marks marring her perfect body. And she's determined that there will never be. She'll do whatever it takes to defy aging until the day she dies.

What are the odds that she'll make it? Better than they were a decade ago. Back then scientists had already found the reasons that we deteriorate into wrinkles, bags, age spots, flab and life-threatening conditions. The reasons were, and still are, genetics, disease, environmental factors such as smoking and diet and the aging process itself. Today these scientists also know that every single one of these factors may be directly influenced and perhaps even altered by getting enough of the right kinds of vitamins and minerals.

A Chemical Blitzkrieg

Both the diseases that contribute to aging and the physical and mental "damage" that we associate with old age seem to be triggered by a lifelong blitzkrieg of damaging molecules that affect us on many levels.

These molecules, sometimes called free radicals by scientists, are sent zinging through our bodies by cigarette smoke and chronic infection as well as by the normal cell metabolism that converts the carbohydrates and fat we eat into the energy required to power our cells. Yes, just eating your daily breakfast normally produces untold numbers of these harmful molecules. There's no way to avoid them completely.

Unfortunately, free radicals have the nasty habit of stealing electrons from your body's healthy molecules to balance themselves, in the process damaging cells and their DNA, the genetic blueprint that tells a cell how to do its job. And without a perfect copy of that DNA blueprint, a cell doesn't know what it's supposed to do. Yet biochemists estimate that every cell in the body is hit 10,000 times every day by free radicals patrolling the body.

The result?

Depending on how badly they're hit and how quickly they're returned to service by cellular repair squads, the cells may mutate or die, explains researcher Denham Harman, M.D., Ph.D., professor emeritus of medicine at the University of Nebraska College of Medicine in Omaha. And when either of these events happens, it may initiate the underlying biochemical processes that cause many of the diseases that accelerate aging: heart disease, high blood pressure, Parkinson's disease, cancer, cataracts, diabetes and even Alzheimer's disease.

Some scientists also believe that free radicals affect the aging process even more directly, says Dr. Harman, the man who first raised the possibility. In fact, he adds, "there's a growing consensus that aging itself is due to free radical reactions."

The idea is that there may be an accumulation of damage from the constant cellular bombardment by free radicals. A cell gets hit once, the cellular repair squads come to the rescue and cut out the damage to the cell's DNA blueprint, and the cell bounces back into action. But when the cell gets hit over and over again, there may come a point at which the repair squads can't patch everything back together the way it was. So the cell continues to do its job, but not as well as it had been.

If it's a skin cell, for example, you might end up with wrinkled skin rather than smooth, polished skin. If it's an eye cell, maybe you just can't see as clearly as you used to.

In any event, scientists have found that 40 to 50 percent of all of the proteins in an older person may be damaged by free radicals. Proteins are involved in a myriad of functions in the body, from guiding chemical reactions to supplying energy to maintaining the body's structures.

And that, plus the fact that laboratory studies indicate that damaged proteins shorten the life span of laboratory animals, has led some scientists to suspect that free radicals may directly cause aging.

Natural Antioxidants

Although millions of free radicals bombard your cells on a daily basis, the fact that it takes as long as it does for them to cause damage or disease is a tribute to the natural free radical–fighting systems with which you were born. "These systems are fighting free radicals every moment of every day," says Pamela Starke-Reed, Ph.D., director of the Office of Nutrition at the National Institute on Aging in Bethesda, Maryland.

Each system is ingeniously designed to produce an antioxidant, a naturally occurring chemical that neutralizes the free radical (or the oxidant, as it

Food Factors

Although a rich supply of vitamins and minerals is clearly a priority in any anti-aging program, here are three other factors to consider.

Love garlic. Not only can garlic help your body stay young by fighting heart disease and cancer, it may also prolong the life span of normal skin cells and help them maintain their youthful shape, according to preliminary laboratory studies.

Eat protein. Older people may sometimes have birdlike appetites, but the amount of protein that they need to stay active is elephantine.

A joint study conducted by researchers from the Jean Mayer USDA Human Nutrition Research Center on Aging at Tufts University in Boston, the Massachusetts Institute of Technology in Cambridge and Pennsylvania State University in University Park found that the average person over age 55 needs between 0.8 and 1 gram of protein per kilogram of body weight every day. This amount is nearly one-third more than nutritionists usually recommend. So a person weighing 150 pounds, or 68 kilograms, would need between 54 and 68 grams of protein a day.

Two great sources of protein are chicken and fish. A three-ounce portion of chicken breast and a three-ounce portion of tuna contain 27 and 25 grams of protein, respectively. Add a cup of skim milk to that, and you'll be consuming another 10 grams of protein.

Forgo fat. Medical research has shown that dietary fat is a prime generator of free radicals, the naturally occurring unstable molecules that damage your body's healthy molecules by stealing their electrons and, in the process, contribute to aging. Here's yet another reason to stick to a low-fat diet.

is sometimes called) by offering its own electrons. In doing so, the antioxidant helps preserve your body's healthy molecules.

Each antioxidant is designed to work in a different way in a different part of the cell, says Dr. Starke-Reed. Its marching orders come from the genetic instructions on your chromosomes, and its power comes from a ready supply of specific nutrients in your diet. One natural antioxidant is dependent upon the availability of copper, zinc and manganese. Another is dependent on iron, and a third is dependent on selenium.

How much do you need? "You want to keep everything in balance," says Dr. Starke-Reed. But since scientists are just beginning to understand what it takes to keep that balance, "the best that we can do right now is to tell people that they should be taking in at least the Daily Values of all essential vitamins and minerals," she says.

Supplementing the Body's Natural Antioxidants

Although the body produces natural antioxidants to neutralize free radical damage, it doesn't produce enough to handle the free radical bombardment generated by the modern world. Your body's natural antioxidant systems were simply not designed to handle rooms full of cigarette smoke, a diet loaded with fat and constant exposure to new and more virulent viruses.

This may change once scientists learn how to genetically alter our genes so that we produce more natural antioxidants. But in the meantime, we do have another option: enhancing our natural antioxidants with man-made antioxidants—in a word, supplements.

Laboratory studies indicate that antioxidant supplements, predominantly vitamins C and E plus beta-carotene and selenium, seem to be able to neutralize free radicals that sneak past the natural antioxidants produced in your cells, says Dr. Harman.

"Nobody really knows what the optimum levels are," he adds. "But I recommend daily doses of 200 to 400 international units of vitamin E and 1,500 to 2,000 milligrams of vitamin C, along with 25,000 international units of beta-carotene every other day. I also suggest that people take one 50-microgram tablet of selenium in the morning and one at night." Some people may experience diarrhea when taking high daily doses of vitamin C.

Will this actually slow the aging process? "Nobody knows," replies Dr. Harman. It does in laboratory animals. But it will be decades before the people who load up on antioxidants live long enough to answer that question for humans, he says.

Yet while we're waiting to find out, one thing seems absolutely clear: Those folks who take supplemental antioxidants or who enrich their diets with antioxidant-rich fruits and vegetables certainly seem to be preventing development of the diseases that can accelerate the aging process.

More than 50 studies conducted during the past decade demonstrated that high intake of foods rich in beta-carotene reduces the risk of cancer. More than 40 studies indicated that vitamin C does the same. And a review of studies that measured the amounts of antioxidants people eat revealed that the one-fourth of the American population consuming the most fruits and vegetables, the primary dietary sources of beta-carotene, vitamin C and selenium, had half of the rate of cancers of the lung, mouth, esophagus, stomach, pancreas, cervix and bladder compared to those who didn't consume as much.

Prescriptions for Healing

The exact amounts of vitamins and minerals required to slow aging and to prevent many of the diseases that accelerate aging is a hot topic of debate among scientists. Until more research provides further information, here's what the experts conducting the research suggest.

Nutrient	**Daily Amount**
Beta-carotene	25,000 international units, taken every other day
Selenium	100 micrograms, taken as 2 divided doses
Vitamin C	1,500–2,000 milligrams
Vitamin E	200–400 international units

Plus a multivitamin/mineral supplement containing the Daily Values of all essential vitamins and minerals

MEDICAL ALERT: *The high daily dose of vitamin C recommended here may cause diarrhea in some people.*

If you are taking anticoagulant drugs, you should not take vitamin E supplements.

What's more, people who got less of the antioxidant vitamins C and E and carotenoids such as beta-carotene were more likely to develop cataracts and macular degeneration, a vision-destroying disease that affects mainly older people. People who got plentiful supplies of these antioxidants were 37 percent less likely to have heart attacks.

So not only do antioxidants seem to prevent the diseases that accelerate us into old age, they also seem to be helping us to maintain quality of life.

Getting people to eat more as they age is important, says Jeffrey Blumberg, Ph.D., associate director and chief of the antioxidants research laboratory at the Jean Mayer USDA Human Nutrition Research Center on Aging at Tufts University in Boston. But what you eat is also important, he adds.

"In essence, eating a super high quality diet is crucial if you want to do all that you can to stay young longer," says Dr. Blumberg. "It's especially important to key in on good food sources of vitamins C and E and beta-carotene." Good sources include orange and yellow vegetables, fruits and whole grains.

"In addition, I'd go so far as to advise people who want to take steps to slow down the aging process to take a daily multivitamin/mineral supplement," he says. "The idea behind this is that you can die 'young' as late as possible."

Alcoholism

Repairing Nutritional Damage

You probably know someone with a drinking problem. In fact, maybe that person is you.

Problems with alcohol are fairly common in the United States. "Two-thirds of all Americans drink," says Charles H. Halsted, M.D., chief of clinical nutrition and metabolism at the University of California, Davis. "Sixty percent are light to moderate drinkers, but up to 10 percent drink excessively."

The light to moderate drinkers are probably in pretty good health, according to Dr. Halsted. (There is a wide range of opinion as to what constitutes moderate drinking; experts define it as anywhere from four drinks a week to one or two drinks a day.) "Moderate drinking is probably safe and may even be beneficial, since it lowers the risk of cardiovascular disease," he says.

But excessive alcohol consumption is another story. Excessive drinking on a daily basis—more than three drinks for a woman and more than six for a man—increases your risk of cancer and can damage the liver, pancreas, intestines and brain, says Dr. Halsted. It can cause diarrhea, osteoporosis, night blindness and anemia and can knock as many as 15 years off your life span. It can also cause nutritional deficiency diseases such as scurvy and pellagra. Although rare in this country, when scurvy and pellagra do occur, it's usually in alcoholics.

The Liquid Saboteur

How does alcohol damage your health? It hinders your body's ability to absorb, process, use and store the nutrients found in food—plus it tends to edge out food in your diet.

"The problem is that alcoholic beverages are devoid of vitamins and minerals," says Charles S. Lieber, M.D., director of the Alcohol Research Center for the National Institutes of Health/National Institute on Alcohol Abuse and Alcoholism in Bethesda, Maryland, professor of medicine and pathology at Mount Sinai School of Medicine in New York City and director of the Alcohol Research and Treatment Center, the liver disease and nutrition section and the gastrointestinal-liver training program at the Bronx Veterans Affairs Medical Center in New York. "Alcoholic beverages are full of empty calories. Yet if you're a heavy drinker, those empty calories replace other nutrients in the diet. In addition, alcohol has a direct, toxic effect on the gastrointestinal tract."

The result is that many, if not most, of the vitamins, minerals and other nutrients extracted from food during digestion cannot be absorbed through the intestinal wall and into the bloodstream. Compounding the problem is the fact that alcohol is toxic to the liver, the organ that processes nutrients. Normally the liver either stores the nutrients it receives or, after processing, sends them cascading back into your bloodstream to be used throughout your body.

But once the liver is damaged, your body's ability to use vitamins is significantly reduced. The liver is no longer able to process, store or use many of the water-soluble vitamins such as thiamin, B_6 and folate (the naturally occurring form of folic acid). And since a damaged liver produces less bile, a substance the body uses to prepare fat-soluble vitamins for absorption by the intestines, your body is no longer able to use vitamins A, D and E, either.

You also have to keep in mind that your liver manufactures the transportation system that escorts minerals throughout your body. It provides proteins on which minerals hitch rides to get to where they're needed. But if the liver is damaged, the minerals can't get out of the liver. The result can be a mineral deficiency throughout your body—and a potentially toxic buildup of minerals in the liver.

Antioxidant Protection

Although alcohol devastates the body both directly as a toxin and indirectly through nutrient loss, scientists are beginning to suspect that it may also affect the body by destroying or otherwise interfering with the body's use of the antioxidants vitamin C, vitamin E and selenium. Antioxidants are substances that protect your body's healthy molecules against damage by unstable molecules called free radicals.

In a study in France of 102 recovering alcoholics, researchers found that blood levels of vitamin C, vitamin E and selenium remained lower in the former drinkers, even after they ditched the booze and began eating balanced diets, than in a similar group of men who drank only occasionally. Researchers also found high concentrations of free radicals, those unstable molecules that damage your body's healthy molecules by stealing electrons in order to balance themselves.

Scientists are not ready to draw any definite conclusions, but it looks as though at least some of the damage caused by alcohol occurs simply because there aren't enough antioxidants in the blood to put a half nelson on those roving free radicals. Recovering alcoholics should pay special attention to getting the Daily Values of these important nutrients. The Daily Value for vitamin E is 30 international units, and for vitamin C, 60 milligrams. For selenium, the Daily Value is 70 micrograms.

Problem drinkers also have difficulty getting enough protein and calories to maintain a healthy weight. Aside from that, the main nutritional deficiencies caused by heavy drinking are of vitamin A, thiamin, folate, vitamin B_6, zinc and magnesium, says Dr. Halsted.

Vitamin A: Finding the Right Balance

Vitamin A deficiency occurs because alcohol metabolism promotes excretion of vitamin A in bile. So it should come as no surprise that a study of 28 alcoholics, done at the University of Illinois in Urbana, found that 57 percent had low levels of vitamin A. Vitamin A plays an important part in helping you to reproduce, to grow new cells, to fight infection and, because of its important role in the retina, to see at night. Another study found that half of alcoholics who have severe liver disease also have night blindness. (Among those who don't have severe liver disease, 15 percent have night blindness.)

Although it seems like common sense that the answer to a vitamin A deficiency is to simply pop a couple of pills, giving supplemental vitamin A to people with alcohol problems is tricky, cautions Dr. Lieber.

"Vitamin A can be toxic to the liver if taken in large amounts. But so is alcohol. So if you supplement vitamin A in an alcoholic, you have to be careful not to add insult to injury and enhance the toxic effects of alcohol," he says. "It's important to correct the deficiency. But at the same time, it's important to avoid any excess. There's a very small therapeutic window."

For a while, researchers wondered if they could avoid the toxic effects of supplementation and still prevent a vitamin A deficiency by prescribing beta-carotene, a nontoxic precursor of vitamin A that occurs naturally in

Food Factors

When alcohol replaces food in the diet, as it frequently does in people who have drinking problems, it speeds up the body's metabolism and can cause muscle breakdown and a protein deficiency that sabotages the body's ability to repair normal wear and tear.

That's why people with chronic drinking problems tend to lose weight, says Charles H. Halsted, M.D., chief of clinical nutrition and metabolism at the University of California, Davis. Here's what you can do to help correct the problem.

First, abstain. Not drinking is a prerequisite to correcting or restoring nutritional health.

Eat hearty. To counteract weight loss and protein deficiency, Dr. Halsted suggests that people with drinking problems eat between 2,000 and 3,000 calories a day. Most of those calories—about 60 percent—should be in the form of carbohydrates such as breads, pastas and other grains as well as fruits and vegetables. Another 15 percent of those calories should come from protein, and the remaining 25 percent should come from fat (10 percent from animal sources).

dark green, leafy vegetables and in orange and yellow vegetables. But for a drinker, beta-carotene has the same problem as vitamin A itself, says Dr. Lieber. Although it's seemingly nontoxic to everyone else in the world, too much beta-carotene can damage an alcoholic's liver just as easily as vitamin A.

To squeeze through that narrow therapeutic window between too little and too much vitamin A, Dr. Lieber recommends that people who drink excessively correct any vitamin A deficiency, when present, with a multivitamin/mineral supplement that does not exceed 5,000 international units of vitamin A for men or 4,000 international units for women. They should avoid any supplement with a higher dose of vitamin A as well as any preparation that has excess beta-carotene (more than about 10,000 international units), he says.

It's a short hop from helping to hurting with vitamin A, says Dr. Lieber. But sticking to a multivitamin/mineral supplement with no more than 5,000 or 4,000 international units, as explained above, should give you the most benefit at the least risk.

Think Thiamin for the Brain

The unsteady gait, confusion and poor memory that many of us associate with someone who drinks excessively is just as likely to be caused by a lack of thiamin as by too much to drink.

"Thiamin is an important player in the way the brain works," explains Dr. Halsted. Scientists feel that the vitamin is involved in the production and release of neurotransmitters—molecules that zip messages between brain and body—as well as in the transmission of electrical impulses along nerves.

And although the brain requires a continuous supply of thiamin, the body does not store it in any appreciable amount. Researchers report that 30 to 80 percent of alcoholics are deficient in thiamin.

Laboratory studies indicate that a thiamin deficiency from alcohol abuse disrupts the ability of brain cells to do their job, resulting in impaired function and cell death. This may eventually lead to Wernicke-Korsakoff syndrome, a brain disorder characterized by an unsteady gait and memory loss.

Some doctors prescribe 50 milligrams of thiamin a day to temporarily supplement the diets of alcoholics, but it's not known whether this can actually reverse the brain damage caused by a thiamin deficiency, says Dr. Halsted.

Prescriptions for Healing

Alcohol abuse causes damage to the liver, pancreas, intestines and brain. The process of reversing that damage begins when you stop drinking and start eating a balanced diet that provides at least the Daily Values of certain vitamins and minerals. Here's what doctors say that you need. If you find that you can't get these amounts from your diet, taking a general multivitamin/mineral supplement may help.

Nutrient	Daily Amount
Folic acid	400 micrograms
Magnesium	400 milligrams
Selenium	70 micrograms
Thiamin	50 milligrams
Vitamin A	4,000 international units for women 5,000 international units for men
Vitamin B_6	2 milligrams
Vitamin C	60 milligrams
Vitamin E	30 international units
Zinc	15 milligrams

Or a multivitamin/mineral supplement containing the recommended amounts of these vitamins and minerals

MEDICAL ALERT: *If you have a drinking problem, you should seek professional care.*

If you have heart or kidney problems, you should consult your doctor before taking magnesium supplements.

If you are taking anticoagulant drugs, you should not take vitamin E supplements.

Building with Bs

Aside from a thiamin deficiency, excessive drinking can also cause a deficiency of vitamin B_6, a nutrient needed to transmit nerve impulses. Doctors report that even a mild deficiency of vitamin B_6 alters brain waves and that a severe deficiency can cause convulsive seizures.

"Pyridoxine, or vitamin B_6, seems to be destroyed by alcohol," says Dr. Halsted. Over 50 percent of those who drink excessively seem to have deficiencies. Eating a well-balanced diet that includes the Daily Value of vitamin B_6—two milligrams—can correct the problem, says Dr. Halsted, but only if no further alcohol is consumed. Good food sources of vitamin B_6 include potatoes, bananas, chick-peas, prune juice and chicken breast.

Folate, another B vitamin, is also in low supply when people drink excessively, says Dr. Halsted. Since folic acid is one vitamin that does not significantly alter the taste of any beverage in which it's dissolved, some people have even suggested that manufacturers add folic acid to alcoholic beverages as they are bottled or canned.

Until that is done, however, a well-balanced diet full of folate-rich green, leafy vegetables or perhaps a multivitamin/mineral supplement containing the Daily Value of 400 micrograms of folic acid will help correct the deficiency, says Dr. Halsted.

Reversing a Mineral Deficiency

Because alcohol can derail the transportation system that escorts minerals such as zinc and magnesium out of the liver and into your bloodstream, researchers agree that anyone with a drinking problem also runs the risk of zinc and magnesium deficiencies.

Both zinc and magnesium are excreted in relatively large amounts when people are drinking excessively, says Dr. Halsted. They can be replaced by eating a well-balanced diet, he adds. Shellfish, pot roast and eggs are all good sources of zinc, while nuts, whole grains, vegetables and tofu are pretty decent sources of magnesium.

If you have heart or kidney problems, it's important that you talk to your doctor before taking magnesium supplements.

Vitamins Won't Correct the Addiction

There are three things you should remember about alcohol and nutrition, says Dr. Halsted.

First, there is no nutrient that will reduce the craving for alcohol, as some early scientific reports may have led people to believe. "The sum total of evidence seems to point more toward an addictive gene that causes the craving and results in excessive alcohol consumption," says Dr. Halsted. "So there's no way that nutrition will affect it."

Second, since nutrient levels can vary so widely from person to person, anyone who has a problem with alcohol should have his nutritional status individually evaluated by a doctor. If your doctor doesn't seem to know much about nutrition, you can contact the American Board of Nutrition for a referral to a doctor in your area who does. Write to the American Board of Nutrition, WEBB 234, 1675 University Boulevard, Birmingham, AL 35294-3360.

The third thing you should remember is this: "For the alcoholic, the only cure is abstinence," says Dr. Halsted. "There's no point in popping a vitamin pill or eating a balanced diet while you're still drinking. You can eat a balanced diet and take vitamins, but if you still drink in excess for 10 to 15 years, you run the risk of getting liver disease."

After you've stopped drinking, there is some good nutritional news, however. "A lot of the damage is reversible once you're on a regular, balanced diet that meets the Recommended Dietary Allowances for vitamins and minerals," says Dr. Halsted.

Allergies

Nutrients That Ease the Sneeze

Allergies are versatile. They can show up just about anywhere in your body and create an incredible variety of symptoms. They can affect your nose, eyes, throat, lungs, stomach, skin and nervous system. They can make you itch, wheeze and sneeze, make your nose run and your eyes weep, give you a headache or a bellyache and even bring on fatigue and depression.

So with all of these possible symptoms, what is it that makes an allergy an allergy? To put it another way, what exactly is going on in your body when you have an allergy?

Allergy symptoms occur when your body's immune system overreacts to substances in your environment. Most people can live with a little cat dander, dust or pollen, for example. (Some folks can live with a lot!) But people with allergies have immune systems that can react to just about anything that comes along. "It fights these foreign substances just as it would bacteria or viruses," explains Jeremy Kaslow, M.D., a Garden Grove, California, allergy specialist and associate professor of medicine at the University of California, Irvine.

The main causes of run-of-the-mill allergy symptoms are histamine and leukotrienes, biochemicals that your immune system releases. Your immune system is an incredibly complex system of several different kinds of cells working in tandem. The overly sensitive cells involved in allergies are mainly mast cells and basophils. Mast cells are found in tissues such as your skin, lungs, throat, stomach and intestines, while basophils hang out in your blood vessels. As you can see, these cells cover nearly every part of the body.

Why Your Nose Runs

Histamine is usually stored in granules inside mast cells. When a mast cell is exposed to a substance that triggers an allergic reaction, however, the cell releases its histamine into surrounding tissues.

"Histamine plays an important role in certain types of allergic reactions," Dr. Kaslow explains. "It causes small blood vessels to widen and become more permeable to fluid, allowing fluid to pass from the bloodstream into surrounding tissues, causing nasal congestion, runny eyes and nose and sometimes hives."

Histamine makes the smooth muscles in the walls of the lungs, blood vessels, stomach, intestines and bladder contract. That contraction brings on a wide range of symptoms. In the lungs, for example, histamine may cause wheezing. Histamine release also indirectly stimulates the production of thick, sticky mucus.

You can blame Mom and Dad for the fact that you're allergic; the tendency is inherited. But some doctors believe a healthy diet and certain nutritional supplements can balance your immune system, keeping it strong but not overreactive.

"To crack the underlying problem, you really need a healthy nutritional foundation that's based on diet," says Dr. Kaslow. "If you continue to eat poorly and simply take a few supplements, you aren't going to see much of a benefit."

With that in mind, here are particulars on the nutrients that may be helpful in fighting allergies.

Vitamin C Stops Histamine

There's no doubt that vitamin C can help tame allergic reactions, at least under laboratory conditions. Several studies have shown that high levels of vitamin C help reduce histamine release from mast cells and also make histamine break down faster once it is released. Not only that, but studies have also shown that vitamin C deficiency can send blood levels of histamine through the roof.

Only two studies have been done in humans, however. One small study, by researchers at Methodist Hospital in Brooklyn, found that people who took 1,000 milligrams of vitamin C every day for three days had significant reductions in blood levels of histamine.

In another study, Italian researchers found that people who had hay fever were better able to maintain the volume of air they could exhale if they were taking 2,000 milligrams of vitamin C a day. (In many allergic reactions, the

Food Factors

Some of the most serious allergic reactions—including deadly shock—can involve food. People with serious allergies usually find out through tests which foods they need to avoid. Components of certain foods may also help trigger allergies. Here's what you need to know.

Pinpoint your problem foods. If you suspect food is the culprit, see a specialist who can help you determine which foods are aggravating your symptoms, experts suggest. Peanuts, nuts, eggs, milk, soy and fish and other seafood have all been implicated in allergic reactions. And gluten, a protein found in wheat, rye, barley and oats, can cause allergy-related intestinal problems in some people.

Watch out for cross-reactions. Some people with inhalant allergies develop allergies to foods that contain similar substances.

"Someone who reacts to birch pollen, for instance, may get itching or swelling of the lips, tongue, throat or roof of the mouth if he eats apples," reports John W. Yunginger, M.D., professor of pediatrics at Mayo Medical School in Rochester, Minnesota. People allergic to ragweed, on the other hand, may react to melons, he says.

The foods most likely to cause reactions confined to the mouth: uncooked fruits, nuts and vegetables.

air passages narrow and restrict the flow of air into the body.)

Other studies have shown that vitamin C may also help dampen some of the inflammation associated with chronic allergies.

"My experience is that vitamin C can have modest beneficial effects for inhalant allergies and asthma if it's taken on a regular basis," says Richard Podell, M.D., clinical professor of family medicine at the University of Medicine and Dentistry of New Jersey/Robert Wood Johnson Medical School in Piscataway and author of *When Your Doctor Doesn't Know Best: Errors That Even the Best Doctors Make and How to Protect Yourself.*

Vitamin C has not been proved to help much if it's taken once symptoms begin, Dr. Podell says. "But if you take it before you're exposed to whatever is causing your allergies and allow it to get into your bloodstream, it is helpful, although it doesn't work as dramatically as do standard anti-asthma drugs," he adds.

He recommends taking the slow-release form of vitamin C—ester-C or calcium ascorbate—in 500- to 1,000-milligram doses twice a day. (If you take regular vitamin C, you'll see the best results if you take several hundred milligrams three or four times a day, he notes.)

Although the Daily Value for vitamin C is only 60 milligrams, these higher doses are considered safe for most people. Some people experience diarrhea with doses as low as 1,200 milligrams, however. If you experience any discomfort, you might want to cut back.

Extra Help from Bioflavonoids

Some vitamin C supplements contain added ingredients called bioflavonoids. These chemical compounds, which are closely related to vitamin C, have intrigued allergy researchers for decades. The chemical structure of bioflavonoids is similar to that of a drug called cromolyn, used in inhalers to reduce asthma-related inflammation.

Bioflavonoids may help reduce the body's release of symptom-producing histamine, explains Elliott Middleton, Jr., M.D., professor of medicine and pediatrics at the State University of New York at Buffalo.

"Unfortunately, experience with one of the common bioflavonoids, quercetin, suggests that it isn't readily absorbed," Dr. Middleton explains. "So its effect on allergic reactions in people is still to be clarified."

Researchers are still investigating the role of bioflavonoids in allergy prevention. For now, experts say, don't spend money on supplements; instead chow down on bioflavonoid-rich foods such as citrus fruits, cherries, dark

Prescriptions for Healing

For the best allergy-alleviating action, some doctors suggest adding these nutrients to a healthy, balanced diet.

Nutrient	Daily Amount
Magnesium	400 milligrams
Vitamin C	1,000–2,000 milligrams (ester-C or calcium ascorbate), taken as 2 divided doses
Plus a multivitamin/mineral supplement	

MEDICAL ALERT: *If you have heart disease or kidney problems, check with your doctor before taking magnesium supplements.*

Some people may experience diarrhea when taking more than 1,200 milligrams of vitamin C a day.

grapes, broccoli, red and green peppers and herb teas (stinging nettle is specifically recommended for allergies). You'll be getting a host of other helpful nutrients as well.

Magnesium May Ease Breathing

Some doctors who treat people with allergies recommend that their patients get the Daily Value of magnesium, which is 400 milligrams. That's because this essential mineral is known to help relieve bronchospasm, or constricted airways in the lungs. Magnesium has been used intravenously to help relieve the symptoms of life-threatening, drug-resistant asthma attacks. "Doctors who recommend it for simple nasal allergies are inferring that it may also help these symptoms," Dr. Podell explains.

One study, by researchers at Brigham Young University in Provo, Utah, found that laboratory animals severely deficient in magnesium had much higher blood levels of histamine when exposed to substances that trigger allergies than animals getting sufficient magnesium.

"The flow of calcium into and out of a cell helps regulate some cell function," explains Kay Franz, Ph.D., one the study's authors. "So it's possible that a magnesium deficiency changes the permeability of mast cell membranes, allowing calcium to more easily enter cells. When that happens, histamine is released."

"Magnesium deficiency definitely accentuates the allergic situation," says Terry M. Phillips, D.Sc., Ph.D., director of the immunogenetics and immunochemistry laboratory at George Washington University Medical Center in Washington, D.C., and author of *Winning the War Within*.

"In animals, magnesium deficiency causes the release of substances that can act on immune cells such as mast cells and basophils and make them hyperactive—more likely to release histamine," he says. Magnesium deficiency also causes other immune responses in the body that can lead to redness, swelling and pain.

You don't need to load up on magnesium to tame your sneeze and wheeze. If you do, you'll soon find your maximum tolerable dose: You'll end up with diarrhea. (That's why milk of magnesia is such a good laxative!)

Doctors suggest getting the Daily Value of magnesium, which is 400 milligrams. Studies show that women get only about half of that amount, while men generally fall short by about 100 milligrams. The very best sources of magnesium are nuts, beans and whole grains. Green vegetables are another good source, as are bananas. Most processed foods contain very little of this essential mineral. (If you have heart disease or kidney problems, definitely check with your doctor before taking magnesium supplements.)

Nutrients to Protect Mucous Membranes

Dr. Kaslow also recommends other nutrients: vitamin A (or its precursor, beta-carotene), selenium and zinc. That's because these nutrients play important roles in the health of mucous membranes, your body's internal skin.

"If you have healthy mucous membranes, your chances of having significant allergy problems will be less," Dr. Kaslow says. The mucous membrane is a layer of cells that secrete the slimy substance we all know and should love, because it contains an array of infection-fighting biochemicals. Mucus also shields cells from direct contact with pollen and other allergens, substances that trigger allergies.

"This mucus layer protects cells from the damaging effects of air pollution," Dr. Kaslow says. "Studies show that people who are exposed to both air pollution and allergens are more likely to have severe allergic reactions than those exposed only to allergens."

The allergic reaction itself also causes the generation of unstable molecules called free radicals, which injure your body's healthy molecules by stealing electrons to balance themselves. In the process, free radicals injure mast cells and may make them even more twitchy and prone to histamine release, Dr. Kaslow adds. Vitamins C and E, beta-carotene, selenium and other antioxidants all help to neutralize free radicals by offering their own electrons and so protect healthy molecules from harm.

Dr. Kaslow suggests nixing junk foods and eating more unprocessed foods to get an adequate supply of all of these nutrients. Some doctors recommend taking a multivitamin/mineral supplement that covers all the bases. For some people with allergies, avoiding certain foods can be dramatically helpful for all of their symptoms.

Alzheimer's Disease

Fighting the Memory Thief

Few health problems are as feared as Alzheimer's disease. The fourth leading cause of death in adults (after heart disease, cancer and stroke), Alzheimer's affects approximately four million Americans. And this figure is expected to more than triple by the middle of the next century.

Alzheimer's is a disease that sneaks up slowly, ever so quietly stealing away an elderly person's memory and personality, eventually eroding his ability to take care of himself. Elderly people with Alzheimer's are then forced to rely on family or health care professionals for survival. Is there no hope?

Actually, yes, there is. A cure is probably decades away. But even in the high-tech world of brain research, some of the most promising treatments on the horizon actually include the use of a few simple vitamins.

Investigating an Elusive Enemy

A look at what's going on in the brain of someone with Alzheimer's disease makes the memory loss and other personality problems at least understandable. Once-healthy brain cells get tangled into knots and die off.

Far less clear is just what's killing those cells. For years, research focused on microscopic plaques, made of a substance called amyloid, that slowly build up in the area of the brain responsible for memory and mental functioning. Once the plaques start hardening, the havoc begins.

As it turns out, amyloid probably has quite a few partners in crime—and at least one could be hiding in your family tree. Some forms of a blood protein called ApoE that normally ferry cholesterol through the blood also appear to cause more amyloid to be deposited in the brain and may help it harden, says Leonard Berg, M.D., chairman of the medical and scientific advisory board for the Alzheimer's Association and director of the Alzheimer's Disease Research Center at Washington University in St. Louis. And the evidence implicating one form, ApoE-4, as a risk factor for this disease is convincing. Folks with two ApoE-4 genes are eight times as likely to develop Alzheimer's as those who inherit only ApoE-2 or ApoE-3. In one study of 46 adults with Alzheimer's, 21.4 percent had the requisite two ApoE-4 genes compared with 2.9 percent who had no ApoE-4 genes.

Other researchers think zinc can potentially increase the amount of toxic amyloid deposited in the brain. In laboratory experiments, investigators at Massachusetts General Hospital in Boston found that a slight increase in zinc caused amyloid "to curdle into gluelike clumps" within just two minutes. More information is needed on the role of dietary zinc in Alzheimer's, according to the study's lead researcher, Rudolph Tanzi, M.D., director of the genetics and aging unit at Massachusetts General Hospital and Harvard Medical School. But now there is enough evidence to warn against megadoses of elemental zinc. Because increased dietary zinc has been shown to markedly decrease mental functioning in people with Alzheimer's, Dr. Tanzi suggests that they get no more than the Daily Value of 15 milligrams.

During studies in the 1960s, animals injected with aluminum developed tangles similar to those found in people with Alzheimer's. Since then, studies using advanced measuring devices have found increased concentrations of aluminum in brain tissue obtained from people who had died from Alzheimer's, says Daniel Perl, M.D., director of the neuropathology division at Mount Sinai School of Medicine in New York City. "We still don't know where the aluminum is from or what it's doing there, but we're trying to determine whether it has an active role," he says.

Brain Rust Sets In

No matter what the cause of Alzheimer's may ultimately be, some researchers are convinced that the oxidative damage your brain suffers over a lifetime also plays a role in the development of this disease. When the body burns oxygen to produce energy, the process also spawns chemically unstable molecules that are known as free radicals. These molecules steal electrons from your body's healthy molecules to balance themselves, damaging all kinds of cells, including brain cells, in the process.

A number of things contribute to the production of free radicals: pollution, cigarette smoke, alcohol—in other words, living in the late twentieth century. "What makes me think oxidative damage is important is that one of the main risk factors for Alzheimer's is getting old," says Dr. Berg. "Oxidative damage accumulates during aging just from normal metabolism of brain cells."

In fact, 10 percent of people ages 65 and older have Alzheimer's, while 20 percent of those over age 75 have the disease. A whopping 40 percent of those over age 85 have it.

Food Factors

Research has so far revealed very little about the impact of nutrition on Alzheimer's. If you are concerned about aluminum, you may wish to check out your water and cookware.

Watch your water. The possible connection between Alzheimer's and aluminum is still controversial and hotly debated. While many foods contain aluminum from leavening agents such as baking powder, concern over aluminum has often focused on water. Over 50 percent of the municipal water supplies in the United States use a form of aluminum to help remove contaminants. Does that mean you have to worry about aluminum in your drinking water? Perhaps.

"If the water is purified properly, there shouldn't be any problem," says Daniel Perl, M.D., director of the neuropathology division at Mount Sinai School of Medicine in New York City. If done properly, he explains, the process removes both the natural aluminum and that used for purification. "But the question is, how much of it is done properly? I'm reluctant to guess," he says.

If you are concerned about aluminum in your drinking water, you can have your water tested. One place to call is the National Testing Laboratory at 1-800-426-8378 or 1-800-458-3330. The laboratory's Watercheck tests for 74 chemicals, including aluminum, and for physical factors such as acidity.

One theory suggests that the oxidation process might make amyloid even more damaging—and might kill some brain cells on its own.

Further complicating the search for an Alzheimer's cure: ApoE-4, zinc, aluminum, oxidation and even inflammation may each play some small role in causing the disease in all people who have it. "There probably won't be a single solution," says Dr. Berg. "The same symptoms and the same plaques and tangles come about from multiple different causes."

Vitamin E Might Provide Some Protection

While researchers explore different approaches for conquering Alzheimer's, at least one research team has turned to a vitamin breakthrough in stroke treatment for answers.

Consider your cookware. One study found that cooking an acidic food in an aluminum pan raised the amount of aluminum in the food. Dr. Perl isn't recommending that you toss your aluminum pots; the research does not yet warrant that. He does have at least one aluminum frying pan. "And as I told *Newsweek*, my hands don't tremble when I reach for it," he says. Aluminum cans are not a problem, he adds. They're coated with plastic to prevent the acid from the soda or juice from breaking down the aluminum.

Fix some finger foods. What a difference a meat loaf sandwich can make! When a dietitian at a Toledo, Ohio, nursing home noticed that the facility's Alzheimer's patients were losing an unhealthy amount of weight, she reduced the number of foods in their diets that required the use of utensils—meats that needed cutting, for example—and added things such as meat loaf sandwiches, which were easy to handle.

A review of the patients' records, conducted by a food and nutrition professor at Bowling Green State University in Ohio, found that the dietary changes helped these people maintain their weight. The new foods also decreased frustration, increased morale and, as a result, increased consumption of food—always the best source of important vitamins and minerals.

During a stroke, damaged brain cells release a neurotransmitter called glutamic acid. This chemical causes a chain reaction that destroys more brain cells, releasing even more dangerous glutamic acid.

Exposing brain cells to vitamin E in the laboratory seems to shield them from the effects of a stroke, says David Schubert, Ph.D., professor of neurobiology at the Salk Institute for Biological Studies in San Diego. "Vitamin E actually has a protective effect on brain cells, limiting the number killed by the glutamic acid," he explains.

In another study, Dr. Schubert's laboratory showed that bathing brain cells in vitamin E protects them from a toxic protein found in amyloid plaques.

How? Just as soaking a peeled apple in lemon juice prevents oxidation from turning it brown, antioxidants such as vitamin E protect brain cells by neutralizing free radicals.

There's a hitch, however, in using vitamin E to prevent and treat Alzheimer's. Vitamin E doesn't cross what's called the blood-brain barrier very well. A natural protective mechanism, this barrier literally shields the brain from most substances. "It's a problem. Vitamin E is not the ideal com-

Prescriptions for Healing

Doctors are studying a couple of nutrients as potential treatments for Alzheimer's disease. Here's what they recommend, based on very preliminary research.

Nutrient	Daily Amount
Thiamin	5,000 milligrams
Vitamin E	400 international units

MEDICAL ALERT: Anyone with Alzheimer's disease should be under a doctor's care.

This amount of thiamin is thousands of times beyond the Daily Value and caused nausea in some people when it was tested. Make sure you get your physician's approval before trying this therapy.

If you are taking anticoagulants, you should not take vitamin E supplements.

pound to use in any type of therapy in this respect," says Dr. Schubert.

In the quest for a cure, however, researchers are attempting to fuse vitamin E with something like a steroid so that it can cross your blood-brain barrier more effectively, says Dr. Schubert.

It's too early to tell whether vitamin E supplements alone can help ward off Alzheimer's disease. But Dr. Schubert says there's enough potential to warrant taking supplements. "Vitamin E is pretty hard to get in your diet, because it's primarily in vegetable oils," he says. "And if you don't eat enough, the vitamin E in your blood and brain actually decreases as you get older. That can be elevated somewhat by vitamin E supplements."

Although you should see your doctor first, about 400 international units of vitamin E a day should be enough for most people, he says. The Daily Value for vitamin E is 30 international units.

The Thiamin Connection

While vitamin E researchers try to protect the brain against the ravages of amyloid plaques, those studying thiamin have taken a different approach: improving the memory of people with Alzheimer's.

In one study, 11 people with Alzheimer's symptoms were directed to take either 1,000 milligrams of thiamin or placebos (look-alike dummy pills) three times a day for three months. (This is a lot of thiamin, as the Daily Value is just 1.5 milligrams!) Tests before and after the study showed that memory improved slightly for those taking thiamin.

That might not seem like a particularly impressive finding. But people in the later stages of Alzheimer's disease generally experience a significant drop in mental functioning every six months. "We found some not very noticeable but clinically measurable positive results," says John Blass, M.D., director of the dementia research service at the Burke Medical Research Institute in White Plains, New York.

In another study inspired by Dr. Blass's work, researchers at the Medical College of Georgia in Augusta treated 18 Alzheimer's patients for five months with megadoses of thiamin ranging from 3,000 to 8,000 milligrams a day, with the dose changing from month to month.

At the end of each month, the participants were given a brief bedside exam that included questions about the date, the name of the hospital and the city, county and state, says Kimford Meador, M.D., head of the Section of Behavioral Neurology at the college. When the results were analyzed, Dr. Meador says, the research team discovered that some participants improved slightly the month they took 5,000 milligrams of thiamin a day.

"Overall, even in those whose scores dropped, they didn't drop as fast as they 'should have,' " says Dr. Meador. In other words, he would have expected people in the later stages of the disease to perform poorly, but while taking the vitamin, they were doing better than expected.

"In particular, on the bedside exam you can expect a three-point drop almost every four to six months. We didn't see that in these people," he explains. "Our people either maintained where they were or dropped a point or two—not as far as they should have. At this stage of the research, this is pretty much the best you can hope for."

Why might something like thiamin help protect memory? It's possible that thiamin helps make an important neurotransmitter called acetylcholine, which helps the nerve impulses that carry thought leap across the gaps between brain cells, more available in the brain, explains Dr. Meador. And acetylcholine is lower in people with Alzheimer's. Interestingly, research shows that thiamin deficiency in older folks may run as high as 37 percent, he says.

Does this mean that people with Alzheimer's could benefit from taking large doses of thiamin? Much more research needs to be done before answering that question for sure, says Dr. Meador. "The effect of the treatment is not tremendous in and of itself, but it looks like it's an innocuous treatment and of mild benefit," he says. "I'd like to stress that it's not a final answer and that we studied small numbers. But until something better comes along, why not?" Taking 5,000 milligrams of thiamin a day caused only mild nausea in some people, says Dr. Meador. If you or a family member would like to try this therapy, make sure you discuss it with your doctor.

Anemia

Getting Back in the Pink

The old doctors' joke—that the first order of business is to find the pale patient against the white sheet—makes one good point about anemia: It tends to drain the color out of you, as surely as it pulls the plug on your energy supply.

Anemia is a blood disorder that results from a shortage of hemoglobin in the red blood cells, the disk-shaped cells that carry oxygen to all parts of the body. No matter what kind of anemia you have—and there are several varieties—the symptoms tend to be the same. Along with being pale and fatigued, you can feel weak and short of breath, your heart rate may climb, and you may find it hard to concentrate.

These symptoms occur because without sufficient hemoglobin in the red blood cells, all parts of the body, including the brain, are starved for oxygen. And the heart tries to compensate by pumping more blood more often, explains Paul Stander, M.D., a doctor of quality management and director of medical education at Good Samaritan Medical Center in Phoenix.

Doctors can usually diagnose anemia by examining red blood cells under a microscope to determine their shape, size and number and by tests that measure levels of different blood components.

"Even after we've determined the type of anemia, it's important to figure out what's causing it," Dr. Stander says. Everything from excessive bongo playing (the constant impact on the hands damages blood cells) to arctic temperatures and toxic drugs can cause the disease.

"Nutritional deficiencies are a fairly common cause of anemia, too," Dr. Stander says. In addition to iron deficiency, a shortage of folate (the naturally occurring form of folic acid) or vitamin B_{12} can be a culprit. Rarely, the problem turns out to be an inadequate supply of copper, riboflavin or vitamin A, B_6, C or E.

Here's what studies show.

Iron Out an Oxygen Shortage

We've all heard about iron-poor blood, and for good reason. Iron deficiency is by far the most common cause of anemia. Up to 58 percent of healthy young women may be short on iron, although not always to the point of anemia.

The problem is that many women don't consume enough iron each day to make up for the 2.5 milligrams or so they lose each month during menstruation. Pregnant women need even more iron. Teens and women nearing menopause also often come up short.

Studies show that women ages 18 to 24 get about 10.7 milligrams a day, which is nowhere near the Daily Value of 18 milligrams.

An iron shortage leads to a reduction in hemoglobin, the iron-based protein in red blood cells that lets these cells pick up oxygen in the lungs and release it in tissues where oxygen is low. "It's simple enough," Dr. Stander says. "These cells simply can't transport the oxygen you need." The cells even look pale under a microscope.

If you do have iron-deficiency anemia, your doctor will initially prescribe large amounts of iron—often 200 to 240 milligrams a day, usually in a form called ferrous sulfate. (Experts caution against taking this much iron without medical supervision.) Avoid using over-the-counter preparations such as enteric-coated iron tablets or capsules containing slow-release granules, experts say. Both can interfere with the body's ability to absorb the iron. And make sure your doctor continues your treatment for a sufficient amount of time. Although your anemia will be corrected in 3 to 4 months, it takes an additional 6 to 12 months of therapy for your body's iron stores to be replenished.

The large amount of iron used to correct anemia is not available through food, says Sally Seubert, R.D., assistant professor of nutrition at the University of Texas Southwestern Medical Center at Dallas. "We still encourage women to eat more iron-containing foods, however," she says. Even liver, a food often avoided since *cholesterol* became a bad word, is recommended occasionally to anemic women, she says. "It's an unbeatable source of easily digested iron," she notes.

Getting Enough Copper

While you're stocking up on iron, you'll also want to make sure you're getting two milligrams of copper, the Daily Value.

Your body needs copper as well as iron to make hemoglobin. Although it's uncommon, copper deficiency can cause a kind of anemia similar to iron deficiency, Seubert says. Most people get less than 1.6 milligrams a day, the amount considered necessary to maintain proper copper balance in the body. Good food sources include shellfish, nuts, fruits, cooked oysters and dried beans.

And if you're taking zinc supplements, you'll want to pay special attention to your copper intake. That's because zinc actually interferes with copper absorption. For each 10 milligrams of zinc you take, you should make sure that you're getting 1 milligram of copper. (It's also worth noting that people who take more than 30 milligrams of zinc a day are at increased risk of developing anemia. So don't take more than this amount without medical supervision.)

The B_{12} Anemia

There's no doubt that a little bit of vitamin B_{12} can go a long, long way. The Daily Value is only six micrograms, the lowest requirement for any of the vitamins. But a dietary deficit of this nutrient causes major problems.

The anemia associated with vitamin B_{12} deficiency is called pernicious anemia. Until 1934, this form of anemia was invariably fatal. People survived for months or even years while growing ever weaker, but they eventually succumbed. Then in 1934, two Boston doctors won the Nobel prize in medicine for demonstrating that a diet rich in lightly cooked liver, which

A Little Bug'll Do You

Did you know that vitamin B_{12} is produced by bacteria? These "bugs" live in the intestines of animals and in the soil that clings to fresh grains, fruits and vegetables. If you've ever eaten a carrot straight out of the garden or taken a drink from a fresh mountain stream, you've probably gotten a little B_{12} along with it.

Such contaminants may add enough vitamin B_{12} to keep a strict vegetarian on the safe side of adequate, says Suzanne Havala, R.D., of the Vegetarian Resource Group in Baltimore.

Strict vegetarians, known as vegans, eat no meats, fish, poultry, eggs or dairy products, all good sources of vitamin B_{12}.

Several foods that vegetarians may eat—such as tempeh and miso, which are both fermented soybean products—were once thought to be good sources of vitamin B_{12}. Now, however, it is known that these foods contain inactive forms of the vitamin, which may actually inhibit the absorption of the form of B_{12} that is needed by the body.

Vegans can protect themselves from shortages of vitamin B_{12} by using B_{12}-fortified soy milk and eating fortified breakfast cereals or simply by taking an over-the-counter B_{12} supplement, Havala says. (The Daily Value for B_{12} is six micrograms.)

Because the body uses vitamin B_{12} very slowly, and because most people have considerable stores in their livers, it usually takes at least three to five years of a strict vegan diet for a B_{12} deficiency to appear. One important exception: Breastfed babies of vegan mothers have been reported to show signs of deficiency-related blood and nervous system problems within months of birth. So check with your doctor if you are a vegetarian and are currently breastfeeding.

contains a lot of B_{12}, could ward off the deadly deficiency.

Vitamin B_{12} is needed throughout the body to make DNA, a cell's genetic material. So a shortage leads to impaired cell production. Without adequate amounts of B_{12}, red blood cells suffer what is called maturation arrest, Dr. Stander explains. "They grow big, but they never mature into properly working red blood cells," he says. "Often they never make it out of the bone marrow, where they're made."

Fatigue is only one of several possible symptoms of pernicious anemia. Others include a burning tongue, tingling and numbness in the hands and feet, loss of appetite, irritability, mild depression, memory loss and vague stomach pains.

Today doctors know that usually it is not a shortage of this nutrient in the diet but an inability of the body to absorb vitamin B_{12} that causes deficiency problems.

As people get older, they may have reduced production in their stomachs of an enzyme called intrinsic factor. Intrinsic factor escorts any vitamin B_{12} that you've eaten across your intestinal lining into your bloodstream. As levels of intrinsic factor drop, less B_{12} gets absorbed, and what's stored in the body gets used up.

"Those who've had stomach surgery or who have Crohn's disease or other stomach or intestinal problems may also lose the ability to absorb vitamin B_{12}," Dr. Stander says.

Most people with vitamin B_{12} deficiencies need injections of B_{12} to bring levels back to normal. "And most will need injections for the rest of their lives," says Dr. Stander. Only the small percentage of people whose B_{12} deficiencies are caused by dietary shortages, such as strict vegetarians, will benefit from oral supplements or from getting more B_{12} from food to help meet the Daily Value of six micrograms.

Folate Shortage Can Cause Problems

They're called tea-and-toasters. And that's a fairly accurate description of the diets of some people who end up with anemia caused by a shortage of folate. Folate is a B vitamin found in brewer's yeast and in spinach and other dark green, leafy vegetables—the foliage foods from which this nutrient gets its name.

The body needs folate to make DNA. As with vitamin B_{12}, when folate is in short supply, blood cells never reach maturity. Instead, they become large, egg-shaped cells that just can't do their jobs right, Dr. Stander says.

Unlike vitamin B_{12}, folate is not stored in large amounts in the liver. The liver's supply is used up within two to four months, so symptoms of folate-related anemia can occur much more quickly than symptoms of vitamin B_{12} deficiency.

Blood tests can determine which vitamin is in short supply. "It's impor-

Prescriptions for Healing

Anemia is one disorder that you don't want to self-diagnose. See a doctor if you're tired all of the time. If he determines that you have a nutrition-related form of anemia, he may recommend one of these regimens.

Nutrient	Daily Amount
Copper	2 milligrams
Folic acid	400 micrograms for older people 1,000 micrograms for the general population 2,000–3,000 micrograms for pregnant women
Iron	200–240 milligrams
Vitamin B_{12}	6 micrograms for strict vegetarians

MEDICAL ALERT: *Talk to your doctor before taking more than 400 micrograms of folic acid daily, as high doses of this vitamin can mask symptoms of pernicious anemia, a vitamin B_{12}–deficiency disease.*

Most experts recommend that you consult your doctor before taking more than the Daily Value of iron (18 milligrams). Your doctor can prescribe the amount of iron that's appropriate for you based on a blood test. A daily intake of 25 milligrams or more for an extended period of time may cause undesirable side effects.

In people with vitamin B_{12} deficiencies caused by malabsorption problems, doctors give the vitamin by injection to bypass the faulty digestive system.

tant to make this distinction, since supplementing with folic acid when it's actually vitamin B_{12} that's needed can mask symptoms and lead to B_{12}-related nerve damage," Dr. Stander says. So check with your doctor before taking folic acid as a supplement.

People found deficient are given 1,000 micrograms of supplemental folic acid a day to replenish their tissues' supplies. Pregnant women may need as much as 2,000 to 3,000 micrograms, Dr. Stander says. Those amounts are much more than you can get from even the best food sources.

Some research indicates that older people, especially those in not-so-great health, are better able to maintain normal blood levels of folate if they get 400 micrograms a day. That's an amount found in many multivitamin/mineral supplements.

Food Factors

Eating the right kinds of foods is important for healthy blood. Here's what the experts recommend to keep anemia at bay.

Love your liver. Most doctors advise people to stay away from liver because it's so high in cholesterol. The single exception is that they often recommend it to people with anemia. A three-ounce serving of beef liver offers seven milligrams of easily absorbed iron and three milligrams of copper, along with hefty amounts of vitamin B_{12} and folate (the naturally occurring form of folic acid). "If you like liver, you can eat it once or twice a month without compromising a cholesterol-lowering regimen," says Sally Seubert, R.D., assistant professor of nutrition at the University of Texas Southwestern Medical Center at Dallas.

Choose iron-rich plants. People who prefer to get their iron from nonanimal sources can count on whole-grain and enriched flours and breakfast cereals, dark green, leafy vegetables such as kale, turnip greens and spinach and legumes such as lima beans, chick-peas and kidney beans to supply at least some of their needs. But strict vegetarians may need supplemental iron, Seubert says.

Stick to ironware. Select cast-iron pots and pans rather than stainless steel or aluminum, especially for long-cooking dishes such as soups and stews. They can add a little iron to your diet and perhaps provide an edge against deficiency, says Seubert.

Good food sources of folate include spinach, kidney beans, wheat germ and asparagus. If you're relying on greens to boost your supply of this nutrient, stick to salads and lightly steamed vegetables. Folate is destroyed by lengthy cooking.

Angina

Easing the Squeeze

Angina is actually a symptom, not a disease. This squeezing or dull, pressurelike pain—a kind of charley horse in the chest—is telling you that your heart muscle isn't getting enough oxygen to meet its needs. The pain is most likely to occur with exercise, stress or cold weather or after a big meal.

Just like the pain of a heart attack, angina can radiate to the left shoulder and down the inside of the left arm, straight through to the back and into the throat, the jaw, and even the right arm. The pain typically lasts for only 1 to 20 minutes. If it lasts longer or gets worse, get to a hospital—fast! You could be having a heart attack.

People who get angina usually have coronary heart disease. The spaghetti-size arteries that deliver blood to the heart muscle have been narrowed or clogged by plaque, which forms from cholesterol and scar tissue. Plaque reduces blood flow to the heart muscle and makes arteries more likely to go into spasm, which reduces the blood flow even more. And if a fatty deposit ruptures or develops a crevice or fissure where blood can enter, it invites clot-forming platelets to congregate at the scene. The end result of this whole mess can be a full-blown blood clot that obstructs blood flow and causes a heart attack.

"Drugs such as nitroglycerin, beta-blockers and calcium channel blockers offer predictable help," says Robert DiBianco, M.D., associate clinical professor of medicine at Georgetown University School of Medicine in Washington, D.C. "These drugs dilate blood vessels and reduce the heart's oxygen needs. Nitroglycerin and beta-blockers may also help protect the heart from the damage associated with oxygen deprivation in the early hours of a heart attack." Sometimes cholesterol-lowering drugs are prescribed.

Standard treatment also includes a diet that cuts total fat to less than 30 percent of calories and saturated (animal) fat to under 10 percent of calories—the same fat-trimming diet used to cut your risk of further artery clogging, Dr. DiBianco says.

Some medical experts take these low-fat guidelines to extremes. They recommend that no more than 10 percent of calories come from fat—a diet that in some cases makes cholesterol deposits shrink and that often reduces muscle spasms and clotting. They also call for nutrients that may help prevent atherosclerosis, such as vitamin E. And they add other nutrients, such as magnesium, which is thought to help the heart function better under less than ideal circumstances.

Here's what research shows may help.

Vitamin E: All-Around Heart Help

Vitamin E appears to play a role when it comes to beating heart disease. A study by Harvard University researchers found that men who took at least 100 international units of vitamin E daily for at least two years reduced their chances of developing heart disease by about 40 percent. (For the full story on vitamin E and other nutrients to prevent and treat heart disease, see page 285.)

Since angina is a symptom of heart disease, there's good reason to believe that vitamin E can help relieve angina pain. And in fact, British researchers found that people who had the lowest levels of vitamin E in their blood were 2½ times more likely to have angina than those who had the highest levels.

Vitamin E may work directly in helping to prevent the buildup of fatty plaque that restricts blood flow to the heart muscle, says Balz Frei, Ph.D., associate professor of medicine and biochemistry at Boston University School of Medicine. "It helps prevent the oxidation of LDL cholesterol (the 'bad' kind) in the artery wall, which is one of the first steps in the development of heart disease," he says.

Vitamin E also helps prevent blood-blocking clots in arteries by its action on platelets, disk-shaped components of blood that regulate coagulation, explains Dr. Frei. "Adequate amounts of vitamin E inhibit the tendency for platelets to stick to each other and to the inside walls of blood vessels," he explains.

The best amount of vitamin E to relieve angina? Doctors who recommend this nutrient suggest 100 to 400 international units a day. These large amounts require supplementation, since most people don't get much more than 15 international units a day from vegetable oils, nuts and seeds, the usual food sources for this vitamin.

Food Factors

To ax angina, choose foods that help keep your arteries free-flowing. Here are the details.

Trim fat to the bone. If you can get below 20 percent of calories from fat and see a big drop in your cholesterol levels, you may even begin to reverse clogged arteries, says Robert DiBianco, M.D., associate clinical professor of medicine at Georgetown University School of Medicine in Washington, D.C. The best way to go super low fat? Eat mostly vegetarian, with a meal or two of fish each week. Stick to low-fat or nonfat dairy products, and use olive oil or canola oil sparingly to season salads and other vegetables.

Eat some mucilage. No, not library paste. It's the gummy soluble fiber found in flaxseed, oat bran and many fruits. (The bulk laxative Metamucil has psyllium, one of these soluble fibers.) Mucilage soaks up cholesterol-laden bile acids, secreted into the intestines by the liver. Your cholesterol levels drop, so you're less likely to develop blockages in your coronary arteries, Dr. DiBianco explains.

Get stinky. Scientific studies have shown that the chemical components of onions and garlic help counteract increased platelet stickiness after a high-fat meal. Platelets are disk-shaped components of blood that can stick together and to artery walls, causing clots.

Go gingerly. This fiery spice also reduces platelet stickiness. Indian researchers found that two to three teaspoons of powdered ginger significantly inhibited platelet stickiness after a fatty meal.

Munch on mackerel. Omega-3 fatty acids, found in oily fish such as mackerel, tuna, salmon and sardines, help blood vessels relax, research suggests. These fatty acids help reduce levels of two potentially harmful types of blood fats: LDL cholesterol and triglycerides. They also reduce the tendency for blood to clot. "But this is not a food source to pile on, since fish oil is fat and contains nine calories in each gram," says Dr. DiBianco.

Prescriptions for Healing

For easing the pain of angina, some doctors recommend both a low-fat diet and these nutrients.

Nutrient	Daily Amount
Magnesium	400 milligrams
Selenium	50–200 micrograms
Vitamin E	100–400 international units

MEDICAL ALERT: *If you have angina, you should be under a doctor's care.*

People who have heart or kidney problems should not take magnesium supplements without medical supervision.

Selenium in doses exceeding 100 micrograms daily should be taken only under medical supervision.

If you are taking anticoagulants, you should not take vitamin E supplements.

Add On Some Selenium

There's also some evidence that selenium, a mineral that teams up with vitamin E, can offer protection from angina.

One study, by researchers in Poland, found that people with a particularly dangerous kind of angina called unstable angina were more likely than normal to have low levels of both vitamin E and selenium.

Another study found that people with heart disease who took 200 international units of vitamin E and 1,000 micrograms of selenium a day (a very high dose that requires medical supervision) had significant reductions in angina pain compared with patients taking placebos (blank pills).

Doctors who recommend selenium supplements to their heart patients generally stick to 50 to 200 micrograms a day. Supplements in excess of 100 micrograms should be taken only under medical supervision, however. (The Recommended Dietary Allowance is 70 micrograms for men and 55 micrograms for women.) To up your intake from foods, munch on whole-grain cereals, seafood, garlic and eggs.

Magnesium May Smooth Things Out

Magnesium is well-known for its ability to relax the smooth (involuntarily controlled) muscles. These include the muscles that wrap around blood vessels, bronchial tubes and the gastrointestinal tract. That's why magnesium seems to be helpful for disorders that may include muscle constriction, such as high blood pressure, Raynaud's disease, migraines and at least some kinds of angina.

In several studies, magnesium given intravenously was effective in stopping variant angina, spasms in the coronary arteries not related to a permanent blockage.

"Oral magnesium also seems to be helpful, at least for some kinds of angina," says Burton M. Altura, Ph.D., a leading magnesium researcher and professor of physiology and medicine at the State University of New York Health Science Center at Brooklyn.

Unfortunately, magnesium deficiency seems to be all too common in people with heart disease. Studies show that up to 65 percent of all people in intensive care units and 20 to 35 percent of people with heart failure come up short on magnesium.

Magnesium deficiency can be induced by drugs meant to help heart problems, Dr. Altura says. Some types of diuretics (water pills) cause the body to excrete both magnesium and potassium, as does digitalis, a commonly prescribed heart drug. Signs of magnesium deficiency include nausea, muscle weakness, irritability and electrical changes in the heart muscle.

If you have angina, talk to your doctor to see if your diet is adequate in magnesium. Your doctor might suggest making changes in your diet to increase the magnesium content. If you're still low on magnesium, he may recommend magnesium supplementation, Dr. Altura says. How much magnesium you need to take depends on the results of a so-called magnesium loading test, Dr. Altura explains. For this test, you take a large dose of magnesium, and the doctor checks the amount of magnesium in your urine to see how much your body retains. "Not everyone needs to take the same amount," Dr. Altura says.

Although magnesium is considered to be a fairly safe mineral, even in high doses, don't take supplemental magnesium without medical supervision if you have kidney or heart problems. You could have a dangerous buildup of magnesium in your blood, or your heart could slow down too much.

The Daily Value for magnesium is 400 milligrams. Based on his research, Dr. Altura has calculated that 70 percent of men get only 185 to 260 milligrams daily, while 70 percent of women get 172 to 235 milligrams daily.

Diets rich in vegetables and whole grains are much higher in magnesium than diets that include lots of meats, dairy products and refined foods.

Asthma

Opening Up for Easier Breathing

Want to know exactly what asthma feels like?

"Pinch your nose shut and breathe through a straw," suggests Nancy Sander, president of the Allergy and Asthma Association/Mothers of Asthmatics. Then try climbing a flight of stairs or chasing after something fast—say, a frisky toddler. You'll soon be gasping for air the way someone with asthma does during an attack. "It's a frightening experience," Sander says.

The usual setup for an attack combines an allergic (or supersensitive) immune system, an inherited trait, with exposure to environmental allergic triggers such as animal dander, mold spores and pollen or to environmental irritant triggers such as air pollution, cold air and cigarette smoke. Other activators can include respiratory infections, colds, laughter, crying, anger, exercise and stress.

There are two major components of asthma. One is noisy—the wheezing, coughing, choking, can't-catch-your-breath feeling. That's the part most people call an asthma attack, or bronchospasm and congestion.

The second part of asthma is quiet. It is called inflammation—the part of asthma that is always present but not always noticed. Just as a sunburn may not be evident until long after you've come in from the sun, airway inflammation is not noticeable until the damage has become so extensive that an asthma attack begins.

During an asthma attack, the muscles surrounding the lungs' bronchial tubes contract, narrowing airways and making it hard to breathe.

People with chronic asthma also have inflammation in their lungs. The membranes lining the inner walls of the air passages become swollen and leaky. And the glands within these walls produce excess mucus. "That makes it harder for the lungs to do their job of gas exchange, picking up oxygen from the air and dumping carbon dioxide out the body," explains Ronald

Simon, M.D., head of the Division of Allergy and Immunology at Scripps Clinic and Research Foundation in La Jolla, California.

Asthma is usually treated with drugs that open airways and reduce inflammation as well as by avoiding substances that trigger attacks. For some people, that means finding a new home for a family pet, exchanging the wall-to-wall carpeting for linoleum or steering clear of cigarette smoke, car and truck exhaust and chemical fumes.

Dietary counseling for asthma, especially in young children, may include testing for possible problem foods. But it doesn't often include recommendations for vitamin or mineral supplements, experts say.

Nevertheless, some research suggests that certain nutrients may play roles in asthma by reducing airway sensitivity and dampening inflammation.

Here's what research shows. (*Note:* If you're feeling well enough to reduce your dosage of asthma medication, do so only under medical supervision, experts warn. Stopping asthma drugs abruptly could lead to problems.)

Magnesium Makes a Difference

"Magnesium has properties that may help people with asthma," says John Britton, M.D., a senior lecturer in the respiratory medical unit at City Hospital in Nottingham, England.

This essential mineral helps reduce inflammation by stabilizing immune cells—mast cells and T lymphocytes—so that they are less likely to break down and dump their irritating contents in the lungs, Dr. Britton explains. It also helps the body eliminate certain lung-irritating chemicals. And magnesium helps produce anti-inflammatory biochemicals, called prostacyclins, in the body.

"All of these functions could help relieve congestion, constriction and hypersensitivity in people with asthma and other lung problems," Dr. Britton says.

A study by Dr. Britton and his colleagues found that people who got about 480 milligrams of magnesium a day from foods could expel more air from their lungs than people getting only about 200 milligrams of magnesium a day. (The volume of air that can be expelled is considered an important indicator of healthy lungs.) People getting the larger amount of magnesium were also twice as likely to be able to tolerate the maximum dose of an airway-constricting spray, Dr. Britton says.

"Further studies are needed to confirm that magnesium can help control asthma," Dr. Britton says. But he and other researchers agree that it's a good idea to get the Daily Value of magnesium, which is 400 milligrams. Studies show that most people fall short.

"I recommend a diet of whole, unprocessed foods such as nuts, beans and whole grains," Dr. Britton says. He also suggests "a pint a day of stout, another good source of magnesium." Actually, he adds, any beer will do.

Food Factors

Reactions to protein or additives in certain foods are the strongest links between asthma and food. Additional factors such as salt and caffeine may also play roles. Here's what you need to know.

Aim for an ideal body weight. "People with asthma who are overweight have trouble breathing. The extra weight makes it more difficult for them to breathe, especially when they exert themselves, because of the abdomen pressing against the diaphragm," explains dietitian Lana Miller of the National Jewish Center for Immunology and Respiratory Medicine in Denver. "The number one issue is being at a good weight. It's a concern for 95 percent of all people with asthma."

People taking oral steroids need to be particularly vigilant against weight gain, she says, since these drugs can stimulate appetite and cause fluid retention.

Beware the guacamole. Thanks to laws that require sulfites to be listed on labels, it's fairly easy these days for people with asthma to avoid this potentially deadly food preservative. Dried or canned fruits and vegetables, instant food mixes and wine are the store-bought foods most likely to contain large amounts of sulfites, says Martha White, M.D., director of research and pediatrics at the Institute for Asthma and Allergy at the Washington Hospital Center in Washington, D.C.

It's still possible, however, to get unsuspected sulfites. Potatoes, shellfish, shrimp, salads and guacamole (avocado dip) are often treated with sulfites. And imported beers and wines may not list sulfites on their labels, Dr. White says. "People are most likely to be unexpectedly exposed to sulfites when eating out," she says. This is because they have no control over food processing or preparation.

Call ahead to find out which, if any, foods on a restaurant's menu contain sulfites, she suggests.

If you are considering trying magnesium supplements, be sure to check with your doctor first if you have heart or kidney problems.

Interestingly, magnesium is sometimes given intravenously to treat serious asthma attacks. Large doses of magnesium relax the muscles around blood vessels and airways. Intravenous magnesium is helpful for a person having a life-threatening asthma attack called status asthmaticus, which does

Stay away from salt. People taking oral steroid drugs for their asthma may need to monitor their sodium intakes because of problems with fluid retention, says Miller.

Your best strategy for cutting back on salt is to avoid processed foods. "Foods with more than 400 milligrams of sodium per serving are considered high-sodium items," says Miller. Canned soups, packaged macaroni and cheese, cottage cheese and lunchmeats are all high in sodium.

Switch to fish. The oil in fatty fish such as mackerel, salmon and swordfish has anti-inflammatory effects that may help some people with asthma. In a study by British researchers, people with asthma who took 18 capsules of fish oil a day had fewer breathing problems a few hours after being exposed to a symptom-inducing inhalant. Some doctors suggest that each week, you simply replace a meal or two of beef or poultry with fish.

Know your trigger foods. Some people, especially children, have asthma attacks soon after eating foods such as peanuts or other nuts, eggs, fish, shellfish, milk, soy, wheat or bananas, says Dr. White.

People who believe they have such food allergies—or who eliminate certain foods from their children's diets in the hope of improving symptoms—should make sure their diets remain balanced, she emphasizes. "If you are eliminating dairy products, for instance, it's important to take calcium supplements," she says.

Drink your milk. Unfortunately, some parents still adhere to the old myth that milk and dairy products create mucus in the lungs, says Miller. There is simply no valid reason to deprive children with asthma of these foods, which are so important for building healthy bones, she admonishes.

not respond to the usual drugs. Apparently the trick is to get the magnesium into the body fast, say doctors from Wilford Hall Medical Center in San Antonio, Texas.

Vitamin C May Ease Wheezing

People with asthma sometimes take supplements of vitamin C because they believe in its legendary virus-fighting powers. There's some proof that vitamin C does indeed reduce the duration and severity of colds, an important benefit for people with asthma, whose symptoms often worsen with respiratory infections.

But vitamin C may do more than ease sneezing and sniffles.

A study by researchers at Harvard Medical School found that smokers who got at least 200 milligrams of vitamin C (three oranges' worth) a day had a 30 percent reduced risk of bronchitis or wheezing compared with people who got about 100 milligrams of the vitamin a day.

Another study by the same researchers found that vitamin C helps maintain healthy lungs. People getting about 200 milligrams of vitamin C a day did best on tests that measured their lungs' capacity to expand and draw in oxygen.

"This study suggests that a high dietary intake of vitamin C–rich foods is associated with improved levels of lung capacity," says study co-author Scott Weiss, Ph.D., associate professor of medicine and associate physician in the Channing Laboratory at Brigham and Women's Hospital in Boston. "Getting enough vitamin C may prove to play an important role in reducing your risk of chronic lung disease, including asthma."

In several other studies, taking vitamin C well before symptoms appeared reduced people's tendency to have asthma attacks while exercising.

Vitamin C may protect the lungs in a number of ways, says Vahid Mohsenin, M.D., a researcher in the John B. Pierce Laboratory at Yale University.

First, it helps shield lungs from the damaging effects of chemicals in smoke or smog-laden air. It neutralizes these chemicals so that they can't hurt cells. That's important, because exposure to air pollution often makes asthma worse, Dr. Mohsenin says. Vitamin C can also neutralize the harmful chemicals produced by the body as a result of the inflammation that occurs with asthma, helping to prevent a vicious cycle of increasingly severe attacks.

Vitamin C also seems to act as a natural antihistamine, which means that it helps reduce the lungs' sensitivity to histamine, a biochemical released

Prescriptions for Healing

Most doctors use drugs, not vitamins and minerals, to treat asthma. Those who do provide nutritional therapy usually combine it with drugs and with avoiding exposure to substances that can trigger an asthma attack. These are the nutrients that some doctors recommend.

Nutrient	Daily Amount
Beta-carotene	25,000 international units
Magnesium	400 milligrams
Niacin	100 milligrams
Selenium	100 micrograms
Vitamin B_6	50 milligrams
Vitamin C	500–1,000 milligrams
Vitamin E	800 international units

MEDICAL ALERT: *If you have asthma, you should be under a doctor's care.*

If you're feeling well enough to reduce your dosage of asthma medication, do so only under medical supervision, experts warn. Stopping asthma drugs abruptly could lead to problems.

If you have heart or kidney problems, you should check with your doctor before taking supplemental magnesium.

It's a good idea to talk to your doctor before taking the amount of vitamin E recommended here. If you are taking anticoagulant drugs, you should not take vitamin E supplements.

by cells during allergic reactions. "Vitamin C also reduces lung sensitivity to methacholine, a biochemical that causes airways to constrict," Dr. Mohsenin says. And vitamin C interferes with the body's production of prostaglandins and leukotrienes, two potentially harmful biochemicals that can promote inflammation and constriction of the airways, he says.

Doctors recommending vitamin C to their patients with asthma who exercise prescribe 500 to 1,000 milligrams a day. That amount is considered well within the safe range, but higher doses can cause diarrhea in some people.

Antioxidants Shield Lungs

Researchers who say vitamin C is helpful for asthma point out that other nutrients with similar antioxidant properties could be beneficial. These nutrients include vitamin E, selenium and beta-carotene, a yellow pigment found in carrots, cantaloupe and other fruits and vegetables. "Laboratory work indicates that all three help reduce inflammation-producing biochemicals," says Dr. Simon.

So far, however, only one study has actually looked at any of these nutrients as supplements for people with asthma. In that study, by researchers in Sweden, people with asthma who took 100 micrograms of selenium daily for 14 weeks had stronger lungs and were less sensitive to airway-constricting inhalants than when they were taking placebos (dummy pills).

Selenium is needed in the body to produce glutathione peroxidase, an enzyme that helps protect cells by breaking down biochemicals associated with inflammation.

"It's too soon to say for sure whether supplementing a regular diet with selenium will help people with asthma," Dr. Simon says. People who want to try it can safely take 100 micrograms, the amount found beneficial in the Swedish study, he says. (The Daily Value is 70 micrograms.)

Studies have shown that people generally get about 100 micrograms a day from the average healthy diet. Don't overdo it with selenium, say nutrition experts. A daily intake of 200 micrograms from foods and supplements is considered the upper limit of the safe range.

People who want to take other antioxidant nutrients can safely supplement with up to 800 international units of vitamin E and 25,000 international units of beta-carotene a day, Dr. Simon says. It's a good idea to talk to your doctor before taking more than 600 international units of vitamin E daily.

Bs to the Rescue

Some B vitamins—notably vitamin B_6 and niacin—have also been reported to help people who have asthma. One study of children with asthma found that doses of 100 or 200 milligrams of B_6 a day dramatically reduced the frequency, duration and severity of asthma attacks. A later study, however, conducted by researchers at the National Jewish Center for Immunology and Respiratory Medicine in Denver, found that adults with severe asthma did no better while taking 300 milligrams of B_6 than a similar group who were taking placebos.

Still, some doctors recommend 50 milligrams of supplemental vitamin B_6 a day for their patients with asthma. And one study by researchers in South Africa found that people taking theophylline, a common asthma drug, along with 15 milligrams of B_6 a day were less likely to suffer from the side effects of the drug—irritability, anxiety and faintness. Doses of more than 100 milligrams of B_6 a day can cause nerve irritation, so don't take more than that amount without medical supervision.

Several studies have observed that niacin supplements reduce the incidence of wheezing, perhaps because this nutrient prevents the release of histamine. Harvard University researchers, for instance, found that people who got the most niacin in their diets were significantly less likely to have bronchitis or wheezing than people who got the least. In addition, lower blood levels of niacin were linked to increased wheezing.

Doctors who recommend niacin to their patients with asthma suggest about 100 milligrams a day.

Some studies suggest that in addition to the nutrients mentioned above, calcium, zinc, copper and vitamin D may all play supporting roles in easing the symptoms of asthma. Whew! "There's no doubt in my mind that people with asthma can do better in the long run if they eat a healthy diet," says Sander.

Bedsores

Nourishing Skin under Pressure

You would think that a couple of thousand years would be enough time to find a way to beat an ailment as common as bedsores. Evidence of these painful lesions has been found in ancient Egyptian mummies, but today we're still struggling to prevent bedsores from forming on people who are confined to bed.

Clearly, the quality of mattresses has improved since the rule of King Tut. So why are bedsores still such a problem? Because bedsores, also known as

Food Factors

Though they're called bedsores, your nutrition—along with change of position—is more important than your mattress when it comes to avoiding these painful lesions. Here is what most experts recommend to keep your skin healthy and free of bedsores.

Get protection from protein. "Protein is very, very important for healing skin," says Mitchell V. Kaminski, Jr., M.D., staff surgeon at Thorek Hospital and Medical Center and clinical professor of surgery at the University of Health Sciences/Chicago Medical School. "You really need to increase your protein intake when you're dealing with pressure ulcers."

Researchers at the University of Maryland at College Park gave supplements containing either 14 or 24 percent protein to 28 people with pressure ulcers. The researchers found that those who received the higher-concentration supplements experienced significant decreases in the surface areas of their pressure ulcers, while those receiving only 14 percent experienced almost no changes.

To prevent or treat bedsores, Dr. Kaminski recommends that people get about 0.68 gram of protein per pound of body weight. That's about double the amount of protein you would typically need. To get enough protein to prevent bedsores, a 140-pound woman who is at risk, for example, would need 95 grams of protein, or about the amount found in four three-ounce cans of tuna.

"If it's too difficult to get that much protein from foods, liquid protein drinks work just as well," says Dr. Kaminski. These are available in your local pharmacy.

pressure ulcers, have less to do with beds and lots to do with nutrition, say the experts. And that, sadly, is something that can still be pretty poor even in this day and age, especially among the elderly.

"The bottom line is that a malnourished person is predisposed to developing a pressure ulcer," explains Mitchell V. Kaminski, Jr., M.D., staff surgeon at Thorek Hospital and Medical Center in Chicago and clinical professor of surgery at the University of Health Sciences/Chicago Medical School. Dr. Kaminski has researched and written extensively on the nutrition–pressure ulcer connection. "In fact, the more malnourished a person is, the more severe the ulcer. I believe that malnutrition may be the most significant component in the development of the type of pressure ulcer commonly seen in Americans today," he says.

Anatomy of a Bedsore

Essentially, a bedsore occurs as the result of skin being suffocated beneath the body's weight. When someone lies or sits in one position for a long time, as is the case with people who are bedridden with illness or who use wheelchairs, the skin over bony prominences such as the hips and tailbone is squeezed against hard surfaces. This squeezing cuts off the blood supply that delivers oxygen and nutrients to the tissues. Eventually the smaller blood vessels clot, and a sore red patch appears, which, left unchecked, can crack open and develop into a craterlike, painful wound. In worst-case scenarios, the tissues can erode deeply, exposing muscle or bone.

One of the best ways to avoid bedsores is by continually changing positions. Doctors recommend moving every 15 minutes, if possible, or at least every two hours if you're in a bed or every hour if you're in a chair. It doesn't take much time for a bedsore to develop, especially when skin is thin and frail, when wound healing is slower and when movement is limited, as is the case with many elderly people.

That's why good nutrition is essential. The healthier and thicker your skin is, the better it can withstand the weight of your body and the less likely you are to get a bedsore.

Note: Though nutritional supplementation may expedite healing, it's very important that any bedsore that develops be treated under a doctor's supervision. And anyone who has diabetes must be especially alert for this condition. Bedsores can get worse very, very quickly.

Multivitamin Protection

Some doctors recommend multivitamin/mineral supplements for most people who are at risk for developing pressure ulcers, because it ensures that they get the appropriate nutrient intakes every day.

A multivitamin/mineral supplement is especially important for older people who are confined to bed or to wheelchairs. They are frequently deficient in a wide array of vitamins, notes Dr. Kaminski.

Prescriptions for Healing

Research shows that strong skin and physical activity are your best defenses in the fight against bedsores. Here's what many experts recommend to toughen up and heal your skin.

Nutrient	Daily Amount
Vitamin C	1,000 milligrams
Zinc	15 milligrams
Plus a multivitamin/mineral supplement	

MEDICAL ALERT: *It's important that any bedsore be treated under a doctor's supervision.*

Vitamin C Plays a Major Role

One of the most common single vitamin deficiencies among the elderly is vitamin C. Too little of this vitamin opens the door to thinning skin, capillary fragility and, consequently, bedsores.

Some studies even indicate that vitamin C deficiency may be the key nutritional factor in bedsore development. Researchers studying 21 elderly people with hip fractures at St. James's University Hospital in England reported that of the 10 who eventually developed bedsores, all had vitamin C deficiencies. In fact, their vitamin C levels were just half of those of the people in the study who did not develop sores, even though other vitamin levels were similar.

"Vitamin C deficiency can double your healing time," says Dr. Kaminski. "I routinely put my patients who are being treated for or who are at risk for pressure ulcers on 1,000 milligrams of vitamin C a day. Vitamin C won't help if there is no deficiency, but the extra vitamin won't hurt, either."

Zinc Speeds Healing

Like vitamin C, zinc has been linked in studies to preventing bedsores and helping them to heal.

"If there is a zinc deficiency, healing time is retarded by 50 percent," says Dr. Kaminski. "Like vitamin C, supplemental zinc won't do any good if there is no deficiency. But zinc deficiency is so common that I routinely supplement it as well."

The Daily Value for zinc is 15 milligrams, an amount that you can get from either foods or supplements. To add some superior food sources of zinc to your diet, try eating more seafood and shellfish, wheat germ and whole-grain breads and cereals.

Beriberi

Getting Enough Thiamin

The legend goes something like this: A nineteenth-century Dutch shipboard physician, studying the effects of a strange disease in the Far East, calls for his next patient. But instead of seeing someone walking through the door, he hears a faint cry of "Beriberi!"

Roughly translated from Sinhalese, a language of the tiny country of Sri Lanka, the response means "I can't, I can't!" The would-be patient literally couldn't muster enough muscle to get up to see the doctor. And his response became the name of the mystery disease.

Years later, this disease, which involves a gradual decline in neuromuscular coordination, was linked to a deficiency of thiamin. Although rice and whole grains—dietary staples in that part of the world—naturally contain thiamin, the process of refining them for consumption removes the nutrient. The result: Those folks who live on the devitalized rice and grains become thiamin-deficient. The deficiency soon leads to symptoms such as leg swelling and numbness, fluid buildup in the heart, severe muscle wasting, irritability and nausea.

Adding thiamin to rice and flours has all but eliminated most forms of beriberi in the United States. "Even things such as white bread and doughnuts—foods you wouldn't consider very healthy at all—are of some benefit anyway, because they contain thiamin," says Robert Keith, R.D., Ph.D., professor in the Department of Nutrition and Food Science at Auburn University in Alabama.

Prescriptions for Healing

These days, cases of beriberi are rare in the Western world. When doctors do encounter patients with this thiamin-deficiency disease, they administer the vitamin intravenously or intramuscularly.

Intravenous thiamin is given only in cases of severe deficiency. In less severe cases, doctors prescribe oral thiamin, along with other B-complex vitamins.

Nutrient	Daily Amount
Thiamin	50–100 milligrams, given intravenously or intramuscularly for 7–14 days

MEDICAL ALERT: *If you have symptoms of beriberi, you should see a doctor for proper diagnosis and treatment.*

Dealing with Alcohol Abuse

But what fortification eliminates, alcohol precipitates. The most common cause of beriberi in the Western world is alcohol abuse. "Your body's thiamin stores are simply used up during the metabolism of ethanol," explains Dr. Keith.

As a result, some alcoholics go on to suffer from a beriberi-like disease known as Wernicke-Korsakoff syndrome, which includes symptoms such as severe memory loss, unsteady gait and loss of appetite, says Gary E. Gibson, Ph.D., professor of neuroscience at the Burke Medical Research Institute in White Plains, New York. "If you dramatically reduce thiamin intake, you reduce the ability of the brain to use glucose. And if you reduce that, you have impaired mental ability," he explains. Severe thiamin deficiency not only kills the brain cells responsible for memory but also may lead to an increase in a protein that has been linked to Alzheimer's disease, says Dr. Gibson.

When doctors encounter severe thiamin deficiency these days, they administer the vitamin intravenously or intramuscularly, usually in doses of 50 to 100 milligrams daily for 7 to 14 days. For the full details on using nutrients to treat alcoholism, see page 69.

Birth Defects

Eating Right for Two

Conception is the quick and easy part. From then on, the fertilized egg has to go through an intricate nine-month-long process of cell growth, division, migration and specialization, all geared toward producing a living, breathing bundle of joy.

That single fertilized egg cell must grow and divide to produce several billion cells. At the same time, all of the individual cells being formed receive directions to move toward specific regions of the embryo, perhaps where an arm or an eye will be. They also receive signals to differentiate, so some become, say, nerve cells, while others become bone cells. The process is complicated enough that it's a wonder couples turn out as many perfect babies as they do.

When things do go wrong, it's due to any number of different factors. Doctors now know that certain drugs, x-rays, exposure to environmental toxins, infections such as German measles and inherited genetic abnormalities can all cause a wide range of birth defects if the embryo is exposed at certain critical stages of development. So, too, can nutritional shortages.

"What percentage of birth defects in humans is associated with nutritional deficiencies isn't known," says William McGanity, M.D., professor of obstetrics and gynecology at the University of Texas Medical Branch at Galveston. "In about half of all cases of birth defects, however, the cause is not known, and in many of those cases, poor nutrition is believed to be one of the factors, either acting directly or interacting with other factors."

Nutrients such as protein, calcium, magnesium, iron and folate (the naturally occurring form of folic acid) are literally the building blocks for a new being.

"Studies of animals have confirmed that a severe shortage of any one of several different vitamins can lead to birth defects," Dr. McGanity says. These vitamins include thiamin, riboflavin, niacin, pantothenic acid, folate and vitamins A, B_6, B_{12}, C, D, E and K. Shortages of these nutrients are known to cause a wide range of birth defects in animals, including cleft palate, hydrocephalus (water on the brain), Siamese twins and kidney, limb, eye and brain malformations.

So far, however, deficiency of only one vitamin, folate, has been firmly linked to human birth defects, Dr. McGanity says. Whether any other vitamin will prove to play as crucial a role as this one remains to be seen. "Right now there doesn't seem to be any other nutrient that has as small a margin of safety as folic acid," Dr. McGanity says.

Here's what research shows.

Folic Acid: Right from the Start

As early as 1965, researchers suggested a relationship between folate deficiency and major central nervous system problems. That connection was suspected after reports of very serious birth defects in babies born to women taking anticonvulsant drugs that interfered with folate metabolism.

Those serious birth defects, called neural tube defects, are enough to turn the blessed event into a nightmare.

In a developing baby, the neural tube is a fold of tissue running the length of the embryo. This tube is what develops into the central nervous system, or the brain and spinal cord. When the neural tube fails to close at the top, the baby is born with only a very small brain or with no brain, Dr. McGanity says. The baby usually dies within a few hours or days.

When the neural tube fails to close at the base of the spine, the baby is born with a condition called spina bifida, a defective fusion of the vertebrae in the lower back. In severe cases, spina bifida causes crippling paralysis of the lower extremities.

It wasn't until the 1980s that the cause and effect really started to get nailed down. In two separate studies, researchers in Britain found that women who had given birth to one baby with a neural tube defect (which put them at high risk for having another) were much less likely to have a second baby with the same problem if they took folic acid supplements prior to becoming pregnant and during pregnancy.

In fact, in the high-risk group of the second study, the incidence of neural tube defects was cut by more than 80 percent.

Other later studies, in 1992 and 1993, showed that folic acid supplementation prior to conception could prevent first-time neural tube defects.

"Folic acid is important for fetal development because it's needed for the fetus to make DNA, the genetic material found in every cell," Dr. McGanity says. When it's lacking, cell production lags. "Requirements for this vitamin are much higher in the fetus than in the mother because of the rapid rate of cell growth and division," he explains.

Food Factors

Eating for your baby means paying particular attention to eating right.

Hop on the wagon. The devastating effects of alcohol on a developing fetus are now well-known.

The best course of action is to plan your pregnancy and stop drinking all alcohol for at least a few weeks before you conceive, says William McGanity, M.D., professor of obstetrics and gynecology at the University of Texas Medical Branch at Galveston. And you should definitely lay off once you know you're pregnant. If you're having trouble stopping, get help.

Fill up at the produce section. Early childhood brain cancer is rare, admittedly. But some preliminary research suggests that it may be linked to what a mom eats during the time she's pregnant, report researchers at the University of Pennsylvania in Philadelphia.

They found that women who ate the most vegetables, fruits and fruit juices—two to three servings of each per day—and, accordingly, got higher amounts of vitamin C, beta-carotene and folate (the naturally occurring form of folic acid) were less likely to have children who developed early childhood brain cancers than women who ate few of these foods.

"It's possible that in some cases, poor maternal nutrition may set the stage for the development of cancer in offspring," says the study's main author, Greta Bunin, Ph.D., professor of pediatrics at the University of Pennsylvania. In fact, one of these cancers, primitive neuroectodermal tumors, develops from cells that line the neural tube. This is the same area of cells found to be so dependent on adequate folate for proper spinal cord and brain development.

Forget the franks. A study by researchers at three different cancer centers and hospitals in the United States found that the children of women who ate hot dogs at least once a week during pregnancy were more than twice as likely to develop brain tumors as children whose mothers eschewed franks.

Although little is known about the cause of these childhood cancers, it is known that certain food preservatives and nitrites are converted to nitrosamines in the body, Dr. Bunin explains. "In animals, nitrosamines (*N*-nitroso compounds) have been linked to nervous system cancers," she says.

Prescriptions for Healing

If you're pregnant or planning to become pregnant within the next year, you should see an obstetrician/gynecologist to plan your course.

Why so far in advance? Because if you're overweight or underweight, you may need to lose or gain a few pounds. And if you have diabetes or some other chronic disease, you'll want to make sure it's well under control.

You'll also want to start taking folic acid supplements three months before you stop using contraceptives.

Here's what doctors recommend to help prevent birth defects.

Nutrient	Daily Amount
Folic acid	400 micrograms 4,000 micrograms for women who've had a baby with spina bifida

Pregnant women should also take these nutrients for general health.

Nutrient	Daily Amount
Calcium	1,200 milligrams
Iron	30 milligrams

Plus a multivitamin/mineral supplement containing the Recommended Dietary Allowances for pregnant women

MEDICAL ALERT: *While doctors routinely recommend iron supplementation for women who are pregnant, you should talk to your doctor before taking more than the Daily Value, which is 18 milligrams. A daily intake of 25 milligrams or more for an extended period of time may cause undesirable side effects.*

Neural tube formation happens early in pregnancy, during the third and fourth weeks. Usually, that's about the time a woman first becomes aware that she's pregnant. "That's why it's important to start taking folic acid before you get pregnant," Dr. McGanity says. Studies show that folic acid offers the most protection when it's started at least three months prior to becoming pregnant and continued for at least three months into the pregnancy.

The results of these studies were strong enough for U.S. public health officials to make two recommendations.

First, they recommend that women who've had a baby with spina bifida take 4,000 micrograms of folic acid daily before and during pregnancy. (That is a very large dose and can be obtained only with a prescription.)

Second, they recommend that all women of childbearing age make sure to get the Daily Value of 400 micrograms of folic acid a day, even if it means taking a supplement to do so.

There's good evidence that many women aren't getting anywhere near 400 micrograms of folate a day from foods, say researchers at the University of California, Davis.

They found that even sensible eaters—those following the U.S. Department of Agriculture's Food Guide Pyramid, getting two to three servings of fruits and three to four servings of vegetables a day—consume only 190 micrograms of folate a day. (Public health officials are still debating the merits of fortifying foods with folic acid to increase intake, but the British aren't. They have already added it to cereals and other items.)

"I advise women to plan their pregnancies, to take folic acid supplements prior to conceiving and to continue for three months into their pregnancies in order to significantly reduce the chances of the fetus having a neural tube defect," Dr. McGanity says. You'll want to start taking folic acid supplements at least three months before you stop using contraceptives.

Taking a Little Insurance

Doctors say that pregnant women need extras of just about every other nutrient as well, including vitamin A, thiamin, riboflavin, vitamin B_{12}, calcium, phosphorus, magnesium and iron. But dietary surveys indicate that mothers-to-be tend to come up short, consistently getting well below the Daily Values of seven nutrients: vitamins B_6, D and E, folate, iron, zinc and magnesium.

That's why Dr. McGanity recommends a multivitamin/mineral supplement that includes no more than the Recommended Dietary Allowances for pregnant women. (There are no Daily Values for pregnant women.) "Use of a supplement as additional insurance is worthwhile and is not potentially damaging," he says.

Not all obstetricians recommend a multivitamin/mineral supplement, however. "Doctors working in the public sector of medicine are more likely to realize the potential benefits of supplements, since they see women who are at higher than normal risk for nutritional deficiencies," Dr. McGanity says. Most likely to be at risk: teenagers, vegetarians and women who are lactose-intolerant, who are having twins (or more!) or who smoke or use drugs or alcohol.

If your doctor doesn't recommend a multivitamin/mineral supplement, ask him about taking one, especially if you don't eat as well as you should, Dr. McGanity advises. Some doctors also recommend additional amounts of iron and calcium to prevent the anemia and bone loss that can accompany pregnancy. (The Recommended Dietary Allowances for pregnant women are 30 milligrams of iron and 1,200 milligrams of calcium daily.)

On the other hand, you don't want to overdo it with supplements. If you're taking large amounts of any vitamin or mineral, get your doctor's okay to continue before you become pregnant. Iron, for example, can cause undesirable side effects when taken in daily doses of 25 milligrams or more for an extended period of time.

In large amounts, fat-soluble vitamins A and D can cause birth defects. "During your pregnancy, you should get no more than twice the Recommended Dietary Allowances of these nutrients from foods and/or supplements," Dr. McGanity says. "If you're drinking plenty of milk and eating margarine and butter, you'll easily get the amounts you need of these nutrients without supplementation." In addition, women of childbearing age should talk to their doctors before taking vitamin A in daily doses of 10,000 international units or more.

Bladder Infections

Flushing Out Trouble

For some women, the symptoms are all too familiar: burning and stinging during urination and the persistent urge to go, go, go, even when they have just gone. Their urine may be cloudy, smelly and sometimes tinged with blood. The usual problem: a urinary tract infection, caused by bacteria that have worked their way up the urethra into the bladder and settled in for the duration.

Urinary tract infections are second only to colds when it comes to infections in women, whose anatomy sets the stage for trouble. (In men, urinary tract infections are much less common but potentially more serious, because they're often tied to prostate problems.)

Women who get bladder infections, particularly women who don't seem to be able to shake them, may have a problem with the cells lining the bladder, says Robert Moldwin, M.D., assistant professor of urology at Albert Einstein College of Medicine in New York City and an attending physician at Long Island Jewish Medical Center in New Hyde Park, New York. Somehow these cells have undergone a change that makes it easier for bacteria to stick to the bladder wall as well as to the vaginal wall. Once the bacteria are on the vaginal wall, it's easy for them to migrate to the bladder.

"Normally, any bacteria that get into the bladder are flushed right back out, but in this case, they're not," Dr. Moldwin says.

Doctors recommend a number of moves to minimize the risk of infection for women who develop recurrent infections. Urinate before and soon after sex, for example. And think twice about using a diaphragm. Women who rely on this birth control method are two to three times more prone to recurrent infections than nonusers, since the diaphragm causes irritation of the vaginal surface, which allows bacteria to adhere, according to Dr. Moldwin.

Spermicidal jellies can also contribute to bladder infections, upsetting the normal balance of "friendly" bacteria in the vagina and the surrounding area. Also, jellies may irritate the vagina, set up inflammation and let bacteria adhere to the vagina, from where they migrate to the bladder, adds Dr. Moldwin.

Most doctors treat urinary tract infections with antibiotics, which usually work just fine. "And we often tell patients with recurrent problems to take one antibiotic pill each time they have sex," Dr. Moldwin adds.

In addition to these measures, some doctors suggest the following nutritional therapy.

Acidify with Vitamin C

Some doctors believe that pushing the urine's pH (acid-alkaline) balance a bit toward the acid side helps treat a bladder infection by slowing the growth of bacteria in the bladder. "Some doctors recommend vitamin C supplements for this," Dr. Moldwin says. It is unclear how this has an effect, and there are no studies to prove it, but it seems to help some women, he adds.

"Vitamin C also is likely to be prescribed when a woman is taking a

Food Factors

Drinking more water is about the only dietary move doctors agree on when it comes to urinary tract infections. Some recommend more acid foods, since acidic urine can inhibit bacterial growth. Others think this is impractical, because the acid balance of urine can change from hour to hour. "Women may need to experiment with foods to see what sort of diet is least bladder-irritating for them," says Robert Moldwin, M.D., assistant professor of urology at Albert Einstein College of Medicine in New York City and an attending physician at Long Island Jewish Medical Center in New Hyde Park, New York. Alkaline foods can help in treating symptoms such as urgency and frequency but can't treat specific bacterial infections, he adds.

Here is what's recommended. (*Note:* These dietary measures won't cure an established infection, but they may help thwart a recurrence or make urinating more comfortable.)

Drink up. Perhaps the single most important dietary measure you can take to prevent urinary tract infections (and to speed your recovery from them) is to drink lots of water—about six to eight eight-ounce glasses a day. Keeping yourself well-hydrated helps flush bacteria out of your bladder.

Guzzle cranberry juice. Women have long touted cranberry juice for its ability to prevent bladder infections. Now there's scientific proof for this old wives' tale. But remember, if you have an infection, this won't help much in its treatment, adds Dr. Moldwin.

In a study by Harvard Medical School researchers, 153 older women (average age 78) were divided into two groups. One group was given ten ounces a day of either ordinary cranberry juice sweetened with aspartame; the other got a drink prepared to look and taste exactly like cranberry juice. Urine samples were collected every month for six months. Those who drank the real juice tested positive for infection only 42 percent as often as those who drank the fake juice.

urinary antiseptic drug such as methenamine mandelate (Uroqid-Acid) or methenamine hippurate (Hiprex), which work best when urine is acidified," Dr. Moldwin says. These drugs are most likely to be prescribed as long-term

"In the past, the theory was that cranberry juice makes the urine more acidic and discourages the growth of bacteria," explains Jerry Avorn, M.D., associate professor of medicine at Harvard Medical School and the study's main researcher.

"In this study, however, urine did not become more acidic, which lends credence to another theory that something in cranberry juice prevents bacteria from sticking to interior tissues of the bladder, making them easy to flush out and unable to multiply," Dr. Avorn explains.

Blueberry juice has a similar effect, Israeli researchers have found. But other types of juices that were tested—grapefruit, orange, guava, mango and pineapple—do not have the anti-adhesive component.

Stay neutral. Some doctors believe that acid foods slow down resolution of a bladder infection because the acid may irritate an already inflamed bladder. So they recommend neutralizing your urine with a low-acid diet, including antacids or a teaspoon of baking soda mixed in a glass of water two times a day.

Ferret out food foes. If you think something in your diet exacerbates flare-ups, suggests Kristene Whitmore, M.D., chief of the Department of Urology at Graduate Hospital in Philadelphia and co-author of *Overcoming Bladder Disorders*, try eliminating these possible culprits: caffeine-containing foods (coffee, tea, chocolate, cola and some drugs), guava juice, citrus fruits, apples, cantaloupe, grapes, peaches, pineapple, plums, strawberries, tomatoes, spicy foods, alcoholic beverages, carbonated beverages and vinegars. It might also help to eliminate foods that contain the amino acids tyrosine, tyramine, tryptophan and aspartate. They include aspartame, avocados, bananas, beer, cheeses, chicken livers, chocolate, corned beef, lima beans, mayonnaise, nuts, onions, prunes, raisins, rye bread, saccharin, sour cream, soy sauce and yogurt.

therapy to prevent recurrent or antibiotic-resistant infections.

Doctors who recommend vitamin C to prevent or treat bladder infections usually suggest a daily dose of 1,000 milligrams. You would have to eat

Prescriptions for Healing

Vitamins aren't the first thing most doctors reach for when it comes to treating or preventing urinary tract infections. But some do recommend vitamin C, especially if you're taking a drug that works better when the urine is acidic. You can split the dose and take half two times a day, according to Kristene Whitmore, M.D., chief of the Department of Urology at Graduate Hospital in Philadelphia and co-author of *Overcoming Bladder Disorders*.

Nutrient	Daily Amount
Vitamin C	1,000 milligrams

about 14 oranges a day to get that much. In fact, oranges and orange juice aren't your best sources of vitamin C in this case, and not only because you would OD on OJ.

"Because of the way your body metabolizes it, orange juice does not acidify your urine as efficiently as supplements," says Kristene Whitmore, M.D., chief of the Department of Urology at Graduate Hospital in Philadelphia and co-author of *Overcoming Bladder Disorders*.

You can check the acidity of your urine with chemically treated nitrazine strips, a sort of litmus paper that's available in many pharmacies. Follow the directions on the package.

Bruises

Fading Out the Black and Blue

Trip over a crumpled rug, and you've got one. Bump into the bedpost, and you've got one. Forget you left that bottom drawer open, run right into it as you hurry to answer the phone and—ouch!—you've got a really bad one.

Food Factors

When it comes to bruising, vitamins C and K seem to be getting the lion's share of attention. Some researchers, however, believe that bioflavonoids—chemical compounds related to vitamin C and found in fruits and vegetables—may deserve a second look.

Say okay to citrus. Eating plenty of oranges and other citrus fruits can boost your level of rutin, a bioflavonoid that was singled out by researchers in the 1950s as one that could help strengthen fragile capillaries and minimize the bruising that often accompanies this condition.

"It's important to remember, however, that though this compound may prevent some bruises from occurring, it isn't good for the treatment of a bruise after it has occurred," says Varro E. Tyler, Ph.D., professor of pharmacognosy at Purdue University School of Pharmacy in West Lafayette, Indiana.

Rutin is also found in plentiful supply in buckwheat. So here's a good excuse to enjoy a hearty breakfast of buckwheat pancakes.

We've all had our share of bruises. It takes just one good, swift blow, and the blood vessels beneath your skin rupture, spilling blood into the surrounding tissues and creating the colorful palette of blacks, blues, purples, yellows and greens we know as a bruise. For the bruise to heal, the body must reabsorb all of that spilled blood, which, depending on the extent of the damage, could take days or even weeks.

Though bruising is no more than a minor, albeit uncomfortable, inconvenience for most of us, for others, particularly the elderly, it can be a Technicolor nightmare. As skin ages, it becomes thinner and more fragile, a condition that is exacerbated by years of sun exposure. As a result, the underlying blood vessels are more vulnerable to damage. For this reason, older people frequently develop what is known as purpura senilis—bruises on their hands, arms and sometimes legs that occur from the slightest contact and that take months to heal.

"Virtually everybody in their seventies and eighties develops this problem to some extent," says Melvin L. Elson, M.D., medical director of the Dermatology Center in Nashville, co-author of *The Good Look Book* and editor of *Evaluation and Treatment of the Aging Face.*

If you're prone to bruising, basic first-aid treatment can help you heal. Apply an ice pack, wrapped in a towel, on and off for the first 24 hours, followed by warm compresses the next day. If you really want to give bruises the old heave-ho and make yourself less "bruisable" in the future, however, the mineral zinc and a dollop of cream fortified with vitamin C or vitamin K are the way to go, say many experts. For extra protection, they advise boosting your dietary intake of these nutrients as well.

Vitamin K to Chase the Blues Away

Vitamin K, named for the German word *koagulation*, has long been used to promote blood clotting and prevent bleeding, particularly in cases of aspirin poisoning or blood-thinner overdose. It's also a favorite among plastic surgeons, who use large doses on their patients to prevent post-surgery bruising.

Now these benefits are accessible to the general public as well. Research shows that applying vitamin K topically can fade away bruises, even those occurring from purpura senilis.

In a study of 12 people with significant bruising, Dr. Elson, a longtime vitamin K investigator, applied vitamin K cream to one arm of each patient and an identical cream without vitamin K to the other. After one month, the arms treated with vitamin K had significantly fewer bruises than those treated with plain ointment.

"We also had people use vitamin K cream on one side of a bruise but not on the other and found that the side treated with vitamin K healed in 5 to 7 days, while the untreated side took 11 to 13 days to heal," says Dr. Elson.

Moreover, vitamin K strengthens blood vessel walls, so it also makes you less prone to bruising, explains Dr. Elson, who has developed a 1 percent vitamin K cream called Vitamin K Clarifying Cream. "I've had elderly patients tell me that for the first time since they're older, they can go outside with short sleeves on," he says. Vitamin K Clarifying Cream is available only through a physician, so if you'd like to try some "bruise guard," check with your doctor.

The logical question, of course, is: If vitamin K works when you rub it on, can you also ward off bruises by eating more vitamin K–rich foods such as green, leafy vegetables, fruits, seeds and dairy products? "There's no absolute proof, but studies seem to indicate that you can," says Dr. Elson.

Even though getting plenty of vitamin K—the Daily Value is 80 micrograms—may be helpful, when you have a bruise or an area prone to bruising,

Prescriptions for Healing

Some experts agree that certain vitamins and minerals can not only heal bruises but also prevent them. Though these nutrients work best at clearing up bruises when applied as topical creams, oral supplements may be helpful in warding off bruising as well. Here's what some doctors recommend.

Nutrient	Daily Amount/Application
Oral	
Vitamin C	500–1,000 milligrams
Vitamin K	80 micrograms
Zinc	15 milligrams
Topical	
Vitamin C	10% lotion (Cellex-C)
Vitamin K	1% cream (Vitamin K Clarifying Cream)

MEDICAL ALERT: *Frequent inexplicable bruising, although rare, may be a sign of a clotting disorder or an immune problem or a side effect of some medication. If you find yourself bruising easily and frequently, you should see your doctor.*

you want large doses of vitamin K right where you need them, and the best way to get them there is topically, says Dr. Elson.

Vitamin C Can Help

Vitamin C, the scurvy-fighting nutrient that's abundant in citrus fruits and broccoli, may also help strengthen the collagen (skin tissue) around your blood vessels and help battle bruises.

"Although studies still need to be done, there is some evidence that supplemental vitamin C at the level of 500 to 1,000 milligrams per day is quite useful against the bruising of old age," says Sheldon Pinnell, M.D., chief of dermatology at Duke University Medical Center in Durham, North Carolina.

"The medical literature indicates that beginning at age 55 or 65, people can become vitamin C–depleted," says Dr. Pinnell. "It's not clear whether this depletion is caused by a lack of intake or a problem with absorption, but it appears that supplemental vitamin C can take care of it."

For even better results, try a topical form of vitamin C, says Dr. Pinnell, who, along with his colleagues, has developed a 10 percent vitamin C lotion called Cellex-C. During tests where they applied the lotion to one side of the faces of people with some discolored spots but not to the other, the preparation produced a "dramatic diminution" of bruising injury, says Dr. Pinnell. "By using the lotion, you get 20 to 40 times the level of vitamin C that you could achieve by ingesting the vitamin."

The lotion may be especially useful for the elderly, says Dr. Pinnell, as they are at particular risk for vitamin C deficiency and for the skin problems such as bruising that occur as a result. Cellex-C is available without a prescription from dermatologists, plastic surgeons and licensed aestheticians (full-service beauty salon operators) and by mail order from Cellex-C Distribution, 2631 Commerce Street, Suite C, Dallas, TX 75226 (1-800-423-5592).

Zinc Lends a Helping Hand

Although its role in bruise healing is not as well-researched or well-defined as those of vitamins C and K, the mineral zinc is known to lend a hand in wound healing and may help with bruises as well.

"Zinc is important in wound healing and skin repair, but it's probably more important for older people," says Lorraine Meisner, Ph.D., professor of preventive medicine at the University of Wisconsin Medical School in Madison.

You can get your Daily Value of zinc (15 milligrams) by filling your plate with shellfish and other seafood as well as with whole grains and lean meats. In fact, just one steamed oyster contains a whopping 12.7 milligrams of zinc.

Note: Frequent inexplicable bruising, although rare, may be a sign of a clotting disorder or an immune problem or a side effect of some medication. If you find yourself bruising easily and frequently, see your doctor.

Burns

◆◆◆

Repairing the Damage

A roaring fireplace. A cup of hot tea. Glowing candlelight. Ah, the perfect ingredients for quiet conversation, romantic musings . . . and a good burn.

In fact, we burn ourselves so frequently that we even categorize the injury by degree: first, second or third. It's first-degree if it is red and painful, with no blisters, and goes away after seven to ten days (a minor sunburn, for example); second-degree if it oozes or blisters and has a raw, moist surface that is painful to touch; and third-degree if it leaves the skin charred and white or cream-colored.

Because third-degree burns damage nerve endings, they may be less painful than other burns. But don't be fooled. Third-degree burns can be life-threatening and require immediate medical attention, as do large first- and second-degree burns. First- and second-degree burns that are smaller than a quarter on a child or a silver dollar on an adult, however, can usually be treated at home.

For the best burn treatment outside a hospital, the old standbys still apply: Submerge the burned area in cool water, apply burn ointment and wrap it in a clean bandage. And for even better results, you might consider adding a new twist to this old remedy: nutritional supplements. Research indicates that certain vitamins and minerals can not only speed the healing of a burn but also minimize the scarring once the burn is gone.

The Anatomy of a Burn

To understand the nutrient connection, it helps to first understand what happens when you get a burn.

After a significant burn (one that is roughly 20 percent or more of the body's surface), the body's energy demands increase 1½ to 2 times, tissues deteriorate quickly, fat deposits decrease, and proteins start to break down, all of which leaves the body nutritionally bankrupt.

Burning yourself on a moderately hot pan handle will certainly (and

Prescriptions for Healing

Doctors agree that good nutrition is important for healing burns of all sizes. Here are the nutrients they recommend as key fire fighters when you're nursing a minor burn at home.

Nutrient	Daily Amount/Application
Oral	
Beta-carotene	5,000–25,000 international units
Vitamin C	250–1,000 milligrams
Vitamin E	30 international units
Zinc	15 milligrams
Topical	
Vitamin E	Oil from a capsule or a water-soluble cream (Gordon's Vite E Creme, Aloe Grande Creme or Lazer Creme), applied once a burn has healed to prevent scarring

MEDICAL ALERT: *You should seek immediate medical attention for any serious burn.*

If you are taking anticoagulant drugs, you should not take oral vitamin E supplements.

thankfully) not elicit such a tremendous response. But even on the small scale of a minor burn, experts say, it's important to get enough of the proper nutrients—especially vitamins A, C and E and the mineral zinc—to promote healing.

"There isn't scientific evidence to back up the need for a special diet for people with nonsignificant burns," says Randolph Wong, M.D., a plastic and reconstructive surgeon and director of the burn unit at Straub Clinic and Hospital in Honolulu. "But based on common sense, I don't discount the benefits of increasing your intakes of these nutrients to be sure that you're getting the Daily Values."

Burns Eat Vitamin E

When it comes to nutrition, burn studies around the globe are yielding similar results. Certain vitamins known as antioxidants are vital contributors to burn healing because they fight free radicals. Free radicals are unstable molecules that steal electrons from your body's healthy molecules to balance themselves, and in the process, they do all kinds of damage to your body's cells. Though everyone forms some free radicals through normal activities such as breathing and sun exposure, their production is accelerated by injury, especially burns. Antioxidants such as beta-carotene and vitamins C and E neutralize free radicals by offering their own electrons and so protect healthy molecules from harm.

Although your body is armed with a hefty supply of antioxidants, free radical activity is so rampant after a serious burn that your supply is quickly depleted, giving free radicals free rein.

In fact, researchers at the University of Texas Medical Branch at Galveston and Shriners Burns Institute, also in Galveston, found that the vitamin E levels of 13 people admitted with serious burns were only about one-fourth of the levels of people who had not suffered burns. Plus the people with burns had more than twice the free radical activity of those without burns. To make matters worse, the vitamin E levels among the people with burns continued

Food Factors

Because burns speed up your metabolism, your nutritional needs go into overdrive. You need more vitamins and minerals as well as more protein. Here's what doctors use for major burns and what may help for those that are less serious.

Pack in the protein. The best nutritional plan for people with significant burns is a high-calorie, high-protein diet in the hospital. With minor burns, your body doesn't use nearly as much energy for healing as it does with serious burns, so you probably don't need extra calories. But "common sense indicates that you probably want to step up your protein intake," says Randolph Wong, M.D., a plastic and reconstructive surgeon and director of the burn unit at Straub Clinic and Hospital in Honolulu. Prime protein sources include tuna, turkey, lean beef and chicken.

to drop throughout their two-week hospital stays, leaving them more vulnerable to cell damage and scarring.

Sunflower oil, wheat germ oil and safflower oil are among the best foods for boosting your dietary vitamin E. And if you're nursing a minor burn, you might want to take a multivitamin/mineral supplement to be sure you receive the Daily Value of 30 international units, which experts say is all you need to maintain healthy levels of this antioxidant while treating a minor burn.

For extra protection against scarring, you can also slather vitamin E on your healed burn, says Dr. Wong. "We use vitamin E as an antioxidant to control the amount of scarring on the skin," he says. "People can rub on the oil from a vitamin E capsule to help heal a small burn, or they can use a water-soluble vitamin E cream such as Gordon's Vite E Creme, Aloe Grande Creme (both from Gordon Laboratories) or Lazer Creme (from Pedinol)."

Vitamin C Mends Damage

Another free radical scavenger that can help increase healing after a burn is vitamin C. In fact, one of vitamin C's major duties is to build collagen (skin tissue) in the body, says Michele Gottschlich, R.D., Ph.D., director of nutrition services at Shriners Burns Institute in Cincinnati. And collagen building is just what you need following a burn!

As evidence of vitamin C's skin-healing power, researchers in the burn center of Cook County Hospital of the University of Illinois at Chicago found that laboratory animals supplemented with high doses of vitamin C following major burns lost significantly less fluid from open, leaking burns than those not supplemented with vitamin C. Quick healing is especially important because people frequently lose many vital nutrients before a burn heals over.

The Daily Value for vitamin C is 60 milligrams. But most experts agree that this amount is woefully inadequate for optimum health, particularly when the body has an added stress such as a burn. Instead, most experts recommend between 250 and 1,000 milligrams as a safe daily intake. Supplementation can help you boost your vitamin C levels, as can eating plenty of broccoli, spinach and citrus fruits.

Bet on Beta-Carotene

Another nutrient that swings into action following a burn is beta-carotene, an antioxidant that converts to vitamin A in the body.

In fact, after studying 12 men and women admitted for major burns

(burns over 20 percent of their bodies), researchers at the University of Michigan Hospitals in Ann Arbor concluded that people undergoing burn treatment should get supplements of beta-carotene, along with vitamins C and E. When the men and women weren't getting supplements, the researchers found, their beta-carotene levels fell below normal, which lowered their defenses against free radical damage.

Orange and yellow fruits and vegetables, such as carrots and cantaloupe, are packed with beta-carotene. Experts recommend a daily intake of between 5,000 and 25,000 international units. One large carrot contains about 20,000 international units of beta-carotene; one-third cup of mashed sweet potatoes contains about 5,000 international units.

Zinc for Healing

Zinc, a mineral found in foods such as oysters, wheat germ and Alaskan king crab, has been receiving attention lately for its role as a wound healer. And studies are finding that as with the antioxidant nutrients, levels of zinc decrease after a major burn.

"Zinc is an important mineral in healing burns, large or small," says Dr. Gottschlich, who relies on supplementation for people suffering from serious burns. "For small burns, getting your nutrients by eating the right foods is probably good enough."

The Daily Value for zinc is 15 milligrams, an amount you can easily surpass by treating yourself to a half-dozen steamed oysters. Other zinc-rich foods include beef, lamb, peanuts, wheat germ and bran flakes.

Cancer

Prevention Starts on Your Plate

Let's face it: It's really hard to see a light side of cancer. Even jokes about this deadly disease can't help but remind us of our mortality.

But one of the brightest sides of cancer these days is that so much of it seems to be preventable. Many experts believe that at least 50 percent of cancer cases could be averted with changes in diet. But because changing their diets is not an easy thing for people to do, some experts believe that

(continued on page 136)

Food Factors

Just about everything that goes in your mouth can play a role, positive or negative, when it comes to cancer. Vitamins and minerals are only part of the story. Experts offer these additional dietary suggestions to reduce your risk.

Eschew the fat. A high-fat diet ups your odds for most kinds of cancer.

Experts say that an optimum cancer-preventive diet should contain no more than 20 to 25 percent of calories from fat. That's about half of the amount of fat that most Americans eat.

To reach that goal, stick mostly with fruits and vegetables, whole grains and beans, fish and shellfish, lean meats and low-fat or nonfat dairy products.

Change the one-third rule. Experts used to suggest that you get no more than one-third of your daily fat allotment from each of these sources: saturated fats, polyunsaturated fats and monounsaturated fats.

Saturated fats, which are hard at room temperature, include animal fats—lard and butter, for example—and hydrogenated vegetable oils, the white stuff that comes in a can. (Lots of processed foods are made with hydrogenated vegetable oils; make sure you read the labels carefully.)

Polyunsaturated fats include most vegetable oils, such as corn, safflower, sunflower and soy. Monounsaturated fats include olive oil, canola oil and the fat found in avocados.

But there is growing evidence that monounsaturated oils can help prevent certain kinds of cancer. That is why some researchers are beginning to suggest that the one-third rule be changed. They recommend that you get no more than one-fourth of your daily fat allotment from saturated fats, another one-fourth from polyunsaturates and the remaining half from the healthy monounsaturates. You can increase your use of monounsaturates by switching to olive oil or canola oil or by mixing them equally with polyunsaturated oils when you cook.

Use the freshest oils you can find, at least one expert recommends. Never use rancid oil; if it smells "off," toss it. Oils become rancid as they oxidize and produce damaging free radicals. Buy your oil in small quantities and keep it refrigerated.

Go on green. While beta-carotene has gotten most of the attention, evidence suggests that other components in vegetables may prove as powerful at licking cancer. One of them, lutein, is found in broccoli, green peas, celery, kale and spinach.

Watercress may also fight cancer. In one study, a compound in watercress called PEITC appeared to prevent lung cancer in experimental animals exposed to cigarette smoke.

Don't forget the tomatoes. While they don't contain much beta-carotene, tomatoes are packed with lycopene, a close relative with suspected health benefits. A study from Italy found that people who ate seven or more servings a week of raw tomatoes were 60 percent less likely to develop cancer of the stomach, colon or rectum compared with people who ate two or fewer servings a week. Besides tomatoes, ruby red grapefruit and sweet red peppers are good sources of lycopene.

Be a tea tippler. It turns out that tea contains substances called polyphenols that, in laboratory animals at least, have been proven to have cancer-preventing properties. "These substances act as antioxidants and neutralize cell-damaging free radicals just as vitamins do," explains Zhi Y. Wang, Ph.D., associate research professor in the Department of Dermatology at Columbia University College of Physicians and Surgeons in New York City.

Both green and black tea are rich in polyphenols. Based on his research, Dr. Wang suggests that you use regular tea, which naturally contains caffeine, rather than artificially decaffeinated tea, because regular tea has better cancer-protecting effects.

Gobble up garlic. This pungent bulb wards off more than evil spirits. A study from researchers at Pennsylvania State University in University Park found that garlic inhibits breast cancer cell formation. And Iowa researchers found that eating garlic at least once a week cut women's risk of colon cancer by one-third compared with women who never ate garlic.

Compounds in garlic, onions and chives—all members of the allium vegetable family—are involved in the production of enzymes that neutralize cancer-causing chemicals.

(continued)

Food Factors—Continued

Fill up on fish. There's some evidence that omega-3 fatty acids from fish such as mackerel and salmon help deter cancer. In one study, laboratory animals fed a diet high in fish oil were less likely to have breast cancer spread to their lungs. And researchers at Baylor College of Medicine in Houston found that people who consumed large amounts of fish oil daily were less likely than normal to develop the kind of cell damage associated with skin cancer during exposure to ultraviolet light.

Save the red meat for rare occasions. Women in one study had a greater risk of precancerous colon polyps as the proportion of red meat in their diets rose. Women with the highest dietary ratios of red meat to chicken and fish had a risk of polyps that was almost twice that of the women with the lowest ratios.

Women who normally eat beef, pork or lamb every day could more than halve their risk of colon cancer by eating red meat just once a month and substituting fish or chicken on other days, report Harvard University researchers.

Have a soyburger. Animal and human cell studies have shown that soybeans contain several chemicals that have proven anti-cancer activity. One such chemical, genistein, may protect against prostate cancer by inhibiting the male hormones that promote the growth of prostate cancer, say researchers at the University of Alabama in Birmingham. Soy may also help prevent breast cancer, research suggests.

In addition to tofu, try soy milk or cheese, miso and tempeh.

Fiber up. In the bowel, fiber bulks up the stool, increases acidity and reduces the concentration of potential cancer-causing bad guys. When fiber intake goes up, colon cancer rates go down. A high-fiber diet also seems to fight hormone-related cancers such as prostate and breast cancers.

Most Americans eat about 12 grams of fiber a day. Experts suggest increasing your fiber intake to 20 to 35 grams a day. You'll be well on your way to that amount if you eat a bowl of high-fiber cereal, a serving of beans, three slices of whole-grain bread, four servings of fresh vegetables and two pieces of fruit a day.

Remember rosemary. The extract from this fragrant herb is such a strong preservative that it's used in the food industry to keep foods fresh. Studies have found that animals eating even small amounts of rosemary each day are protected from cancer.

"Even using just a fraction of a teaspoon of the dried leaves every day could have potential health benefits," says Chi-Tang Ho, Ph.D., professor in the Department of Food Science at Rutgers University in New Brunswick, New Jersey. Try rosemary on chicken, potatoes and Italian foods.

Can the Spam. Cooked sausages, cured pork, deviled ham, meat spreads, dried beef, beef jerky, hot dogs, lunchmeats, smoked fish: All contain nitrites. These are preservatives that break down in the body into cancer-causing nitrosamines. So save these foods for no more than an occasional treat, experts recommend.

And when you do indulge, down vitamins C and E with your meal. Vitamin C neutralizes nitrosamines, while vitamin E inhibits their formation.

Don't get too sweet. Diets rich in sugar can increase your risk of cancer, studies show. Experts point out that a high-sugar diet is likely to also be high in fat and low in fiber and other nutrients.

Go easy on the alcohol. Drinking by itself can increase the risk of cancer two to three times. But mix even moderate levels of alcohol with smoking, and your risk of mouth and throat cancers skyrockets 15-fold, according to one study. Alcohol may directly irritate tissues, and it may induce marginal nutritional deficiencies that drop the body's defenses against cancer.

According to the American Institute for Cancer Research in Washington, D.C., if you choose to drink, you should drink in moderation. Moderate drinking for a man is two 12-ounce beers, two 4-ounce glasses of table wine or two shots of straight spirits a day. For a woman, moderate drinking means no more than one of these drinks per day.

Be a cabbage head. Compounds found in cabbage, broccoli, brussels sprouts and cauliflower help the body lower levels of a type of estrogen that is thought to stimulate breast cancer. Other beneficial compounds in these vegetables may rev up production of cancer-blocking enzymes.

supplements may be needed to make up for existing nutritional deficiencies.

"There's no one magic bullet to prevent cancer, but there are dietary changes you can make that, when combined, will certainly reduce your risk of cancer," says Patrick Quillin, R.D., Ph.D., certified nutrition specialist, nutritional director for the Cancer Treatment Centers of America, headquartered in Arlington Heights, Illinois, and author of *Beating Cancer with Nutrition.*

The sooner you make those dietary changes, the better your chances of never having to battle this deadly foe, Dr. Quillin says. "Cancer usually develops slowly, over many years, and goes through a number of stages," he adds.

Nutrition is most likely to have an impact on the early precancerous stages known as initiation and progression. These stages include potentially stoppable, even reversible, changes in a cell's genetic material, which are often the result of damage caused by chemical reactions in the body. Once the genetic changes are complete, however, and the now cancerous cell begins to multiply, nutrition is no longer a sole therapy option.

Researchers are still figuring out the exact details of a cancer-preventing diet, and they probably will be for a long time to come. Sometimes contradictory findings remind us that much remains to be learned about nutrition and cancer. Nevertheless, certain nutrients stand out as valiant warriors in the war against cancer. Here's what research shows.

Vitamin C Shields Cells

Sure they're tasty, but there's another reason that you might want to down a glass of freshly squeezed orange juice, slice a red pepper over your green salad and nibble a handful of fragrant strawberries. You'll be getting lots of vitamin C, potentially potent protection against cancer.

"Approximately 90 population studies have examined the role of vitamin C–rich foods in cancer prevention, and the vast majority have found statistically significant protective effects," reports researcher Gladys Block, Ph.D., of the University of California, Berkeley. "Evidence is strong for cancers of the esophagus, oral cavity, stomach and pancreas. There is also substantial evidence of a protective effect against cancers of the cervix, rectum and breast."

One review that looked at the results of several population studies found that women with the lowest risk of breast cancer were getting about 300 milligrams of vitamin C a day, the equivalent of about 4½ oranges or about three cups of orange juice. Their risk was reduced by about 30 percent.

In a study from Latin America, an area with one of the highest rates of cervical cancer in the world, women who got more than 314 milligrams of vitamin C a day had 31 percent less risk of developing cervical cancer than women whose intakes were under 153 milligrams a day.

And in a study from New Orleans, people getting at least 140 milligrams of vitamin C in their diets (about two oranges' worth) every day were only half as likely to develop lung cancer as those getting less than 90 milligrams a day.

"Vitamin C is a potent antioxidant," explains Balz Frei, Ph.D., associate professor of medicine and biochemistry at Boston University School of Medicine.

What's an antioxidant?

"Vitamin C," explains Dr. Frei, "along with certain other nutrients, has the ability to neutralize free radicals, harmful molecules in the body that can be produced during chemical reactions that involve oxygen."

Free radicals steal electrons from your body's healthy molecules to balance themselves, and in the process, they can harm a cell's membrane and genetic material. Antioxidant nutrients such as vitamin C offer free radicals their own electrons and so save cells from oxidative damage. "Free radical damage can occur as the result of normal body processes as we age and can also be the result of exposure to cancer-promoting chemicals," Dr. Frei explains.

Vitamin C helps prevent mouth, throat, stomach and intestinal cancers by neutralizing cancer-promoting nitrosamines. Nitrosamines are produced during the digestion of nitrites and nitrates. Nitrites are preservatives found in especially high concentrations in meats such as hot dogs and ham, while nitrates are naturally present in vegetables.

Vitamin C helps maintain a healthy immune system, an additional cancer-fighting talent. Plus it may help build up vitamin E, another anti-cancer nutrient, to proper fighting form.

Most experts believe that the average daily intake of vitamin C, 109 milligrams for men and 77 milligrams for women, isn't enough to provide optimum cancer protection. Although vitamin C supplements can easily boost your intake, eating vitamin C–rich foods such as citrus fruits and other tropical fruits, broccoli and brussels sprouts provides additional cancer protection with nutrients such as folate (the naturally occurring form of folic acid), beta-carotene, bioflavonoids and fiber. In fact, evidence of anti-cancer activity is considerably stronger for vitamin C–rich fruits and vegetables than for vitamin C itself.

The amounts of vitamin C supplementation that doctors recommend to optimize the potential for cancer protection vary widely, from 50 to 5,000 milligrams or more a day. Most, however, stay within 250 to 1,000 milligrams a day, taken in two or three divided doses.

Prescriptions for Healing

If you have cancer, you should be under a doctor's care. The high doses of vitamins and minerals recommended here should be taken only under knowledgeable medical supervision and are not substitutes for standard cancer treatment.

Some doctors recommend these nutrients, in a range of amounts, as part of a program to prevent or treat cancer.

Prevention

Nutrient	Daily Amount
Beta-carotene	10,000–25,000 international units
Folic acid	400–800 micrograms
Selenium	50–200 micrograms (l-selenomethionine)
Vitamin C	250–1,000 milligrams, taken as 2 or 3 divided doses
Vitamin E	400–600 international units
Plus a multivitamin/mineral supplement	

Treatment

This program is used by the Cancer Treatment Centers of America, a national health care organization headquartered in Arlington Heights, Illinois, and dedicated exclusively to the treatment of cancer. The centers combine nutritional, psychological and pastoral programs with traditional and innovative therapies in developing comprehensive, individualized treatment regimens for their patients.

Vitamin E for Extra Protection

Wheat germ, almonds and sunflower seeds: Sure, they're crunchy and delicious, great on yogurt or hot cereal, but they also provide healthy amounts of yet another nutrient that may help protect against cancer—vitamin E.

Nutrient	Daily Amount
Beta-carotene	100,000 international units
Folic acid	400 micrograms
Selenium	800 micrograms (l-selenomethionine)
Vitamin B_{12}	1,000 micrograms
Vitamin C	2,000–12,000 milligrams
Vitamin E	400 international units (mixed natural tocopherols), plus additional amounts of dry vitamin E (tocopherol succinate)
Plus a multivitamin/mineral supplement	

MEDICAL ALERT: *Talk to your doctor before taking more than 400 micrograms of folic acid daily, as high doses of this vitamin can mask symptoms of pernicious anemia, a vitamin B_{12}–deficiency disease.*

Selenium supplements in excess of 100 micrograms should be taken only under medical supervision.

Start with a low dose of vitamin C and work up to the higher amount. Large doses can cause diarrhea in some people.

If you are taking anticoagulant drugs, you should not take vitamin E supplements.

Studies using experimental animals have consistently shown that vitamin E can help protect cells from damage that can lead to cancer. "Population studies have had mixed findings, however, probably because most people don't get enough vitamin E from foods to get much cancer protection," Dr. Quillin says. More recently, population studies that have also looked at long-term intake from vitamin E supplements have found protective effects.

In the Iowa Women's Health Study, for instance, researchers found that women who developed colon cancer consumed the smallest amounts of vitamin E, averaging less than 36 international units a day. Women who got almost twice that much of the vitamin—about 66 international units from supplements—had only one-third of the risk of developing this cancer compared with those with low intakes.

Another study, by researchers at the National Cancer Institute in Rockville, Maryland, found that people who said they regularly used vitamin E supplements had half of the normal risk of oral cancer of people who did not take vitamin E supplements.

Studies that have looked at blood levels of vitamin E have also found evidence of protective effects. British researchers, for example, found that women who had the highest blood levels of vitamin E had only one-fifth of the risk of breast cancer compared with women who had the lowest blood levels of vitamin E.

"Like vitamin C, vitamin E has the ability to protect biological molecules from the kind of chemically induced damage that can lead to cancer," Dr. Frei says. "Because it is fat-soluble itself, vitamin E is particularly good at protecting fatty cell membranes from oxidative damage."

"Strong cell membranes may be particularly important in the colon, because the bacteria there produce a lot of free radicals, the unstable molecules believed to harm DNA and promote tumor growth," adds Roberd Bostick, M.D., assistant professor of epidemiology at Bowman Gray School of Medicine of Wake Forest University in Winston-Salem, North Carolina, and co-investigator of the Iowa Women's Health Study.

Vitamin E may also stimulate and enhance the immune system so that it attacks budding cancer cells and inhibits the production of nitrosamines, Dr. Bostick says.

Based on its possible protective effects against some types of cancer, a growing number of researchers believe that vitamin E may prove to be a key player in any cancer prevention plan. Many recommend 400 to 600 international units a day. Such large amounts are impossible to get through dietary sources alone. Even a diet that contains good sources, such as wheat germ and safflower oil, provides only about 30 to 40 international units of vitamin E a day. "Only supplements can provide these large amounts," Dr. Quillin notes.

Calcium Takes On Colon Cancer

Generally, any vitamin or mineral that's good for fighting one kind of cancer is good for all kinds. Occasionally, however, one nutrient earns star status for its ability to prevent just one form of cancer. Such is the case with calcium. This mineral seems to be emerging as something of a hero in the fight against colon cancer. That's because population studies suggest that people who get lots of calcium-rich foods in their diets are less likely than normal to develop colon cancer.

Calcium may thwart colon cancer by binding with cancer-promoting fats and bile acids, the digestive fluid secreted by the liver, says Bernard Levin, M.D., professor of medicine and vice-president for cancer prevention at the University of Texas M. D. Anderson Cancer Center in Houston. This neutralizes their toxic effects and causes them to be excreted without harming intestinal cells, he says.

"These effects seem to be strongest in people at highest risk for colon cancer, those eating high-fat diets," Dr. Levin says. People who eat low-fat diets, whose risk may already be low, don't benefit as much from additional calcium.

Several studies of people at high risk for colon cancer, such as those with a prior history of polyps, benign growths that can lead to cancer, also suggest that calcium may help reduce the possibility of abnormal growth in the cells lining the colon.

Don't count on miracles, however, Dr. Levin warns. "The effects are fairly modest and occur only at amounts well above normal intake," he says. Most studies used 1,250 milligrams a day, while the average daily intake of calcium is less than 800 milligrams. The Daily Value for calcium is 1,000 milligrams.

Dr. Levin advises eating a diet low in fat, high in fiber and loaded with fruits and vegetables. Then if you like, he says, you can add enough calcium-rich foods (and supplements, if necessary) to push you over the 1,000-milligram mark. He also suggests that you avoid any tobacco and excessive alcohol.

Incidentally, fortified dairy foods such as milk may provide additional protection. Fat-soluble vitamin D, best known for helping to escort calcium into the bloodstream, may also play a role in protecting cells from cancer-inducing genetic damage, says Dr. Levin.

Selenium: Vitamin E's Partner in Protection

Lots of evidence points to the fact that when selenium intake goes down, cancer rates go up. It seems that getting enough of this essential mineral cuts your risk of most kinds of cancer—lung, skin, breast, prostate and other types.

Researchers at the University of Limburg in the Netherlands measured the selenium content of people's toenails. (Strange as it may seem, toenail levels of selenium are considered a good indicator of long-term selenium intake.) They found that the people whose toenails had the highest levels of selenium had half of the rate of lung cancer compared with those whose toenails were low in selenium.

Selenium's protective effect was most apparent in people who weren't eating much in the way of beta-carotene and vitamin C.

In another study, people with the lowest blood levels of selenium were more than four times as likely to develop skin cancer as people with the highest levels.

"Selenium acts as an antioxidant, which means that it helps protect cells from harmful free radical reactions that occur when skin is exposed to sunlight or when lungs are exposed to cigarette smoke and pollutants," reports Karen E. Burke, M.D., Ph.D., a dermatologic surgeon and dermatologist in private practice in New York City. Selenium acts together with vitamin E, with selenium protecting within the cells and vitamin E protecting the outer cell membranes, she adds.

The Daily Value for selenium is 70 micrograms. The average daily intake from food is slightly more than 100 micrograms.

For cancer prevention, nutrition-oriented doctors, including Dr. Burke, recommend 50 to 200 micrograms of selenium a day (depending on what part of the country you live in and your personal and family history of cancer), taken in the form of l-selenomethionine. This is the organic form of selenium, which means it is more easily absorbed, with less possibility of adverse side effects.

To treat cancer, doctors at the Cancer Treatment Centers of America use up to 800 micrograms of selenium daily. In very large amounts, selenium can be toxic. Experts recommend that selenium supplements in excess of 100 micrograms be taken only under medical supervision.

Good food sources of selenium include whole-grain cereals, seafood, Brazil nuts, garlic and eggs. "Foods that are processed lose their selenium," Dr. Burke says. Brown rice, for example, has 15 times the selenium content of white rice, and whole-wheat bread contains twice as much selenium as white bread.

The Beta-Carotene Connection

The real heroes in the war against cancer are fruits and vegetables, hands down. "Studies consistently show that people who eat plenty of fruits and vegetables are less likely to develop cancer than those who avoid fruits and vegetables," Dr. Block reports.

And when fruits and vegetables are broken into their individual nutrients, several components seem to stand out as particularly protective against cancer. One of them, beta-carotene, is the yellow pigment found in a variety of fruits and vegetables.

One study, for instance, found that during the year prior to being diagnosed with cancer, men who got less than 1.7 milligrams (about 2,800 international units) of beta-carotene a day—the amount in about one inch of carrot—were twice as likely to develop the disease as men who got more than 2.7 milligrams (about 4,400 international units) per day.

In another study, breast cancer risk almost doubled in postmenopausal women who ate the fewest carotene-rich foods compared with women who ate more of those foods. The risk appeared to drop off sharply once women reached a beta-carotene intake of more than 5,824 international units per day. That's the amount in a little less than one-third of a carrot or three six-ounce glasses of vegetable juice cocktail.

And in yet another study, researchers at the University of Arizona in Tucson found that more than 70 percent of people with a precancerous condition called oral leukoplakia who took 30 milligrams (about 50,000 international units) of beta-carotene a day for six months reduced the size of their oral lesions. The lesions of 18 of the 25 people in the study decreased in size by 50 percent or more, and there were four complete remissions.

"Laboratory studies support beta-carotene's anti-cancer role," says Norman Krinsky, Ph.D., professor of biochemistry in the Department of Biochemistry at Tufts University School of Medicine in Boston. "Animals who are given large doses of beta-carotene prior to being exposed to a cancer-causing chemical are less likely to develop cancerous tumors."

In other cases, beta-carotene has slowed the progression of precancerous lesions and has even helped reverse precancerous cell changes, possibly by promoting the cell's repair of genetic material.

Beta-carotene is just one of the disease-fighting compounds known as carotenoids. Plentiful in fruits and vegetables, carotenoids are potent antioxidants. They help thwart the harmful ways of those pesky free radicals just as vitamins C and E do.

(continued on page 146)

What If You Already Have Cancer?

Most research regarding nutrition and cancer is geared toward preventing the disease. Some doctors, however, believe that optimum nutrition can help people with cancer live longer and better.

Doctors who consider nutritional therapy an important addition to cancer treatment tend to go far beyond the usual three squares a day recommended by hospital dietitians. Many recommend a low-fat, low-sugar, low-salt, mostly vegetarian diet for their cancer patients who are doing well.

"Those who are losing muscle weight, however, may not do well on such a diet and may need additional protein and fat," says Patrick Quillin, R.D., Ph.D., certified nutrition specialist, nutrition director for the Cancer Treatment Centers of America, headquartered in Arlington Heights, Illinois, and author of *Beating Cancer with Nutrition*. In hospitals, people with cancer who are losing weight get either protein-rich "whey shakes" or a unique form of total parenteral nutrition, feeding via a tube inserted into a vein.

Most nutrition-oriented doctors also recommend vitamin and mineral supplements. Doctors at the Cancer Treatment Centers of America, for instance, recommend that all of their patients take Immuno Max, a multivitamin/mineral supplement developed at the centers that contains several times the Daily Values of numerous nutrients. The supplement is available by calling 1-800-490-8555 or by writing to Shelby Health Systems, 3455 Salt Creek Lane, Arlington Heights, IL 60005. They also prescribe a daily regimen of 2,000 to 12,000 milligrams of powdered buffered vitamin C; 400 international units of vitamin E as mixed natural tocopherols and additional amounts of dry vitamin E (tocopherol succinate); 100,000 international units of beta-carotene; 800 micrograms of a low-toxicity form of selenium, l-selenomethionine; and 2 grams of eicosapentaenoic acid and 400 milligrams of gamma-linolenic acid, both fatty acids that in laboratory studies have been found to slow tumor growth.

Some doctors at the centers also prescribe non-nutrient supplements such as 200 milligrams of coenzyme Q_{10}, 2 to 12 grams of arginine, 1 to 5 grams of glutamine and a large assortment of herbs. If you wish to add supplements to your cancer therapy, consult your doctor or health care provider and let him know about the kinds and amounts that you are taking.

There's a small but growing body of scientific literature on the benefits of nutritional supplementation in reversing established cancers. One intriguing study, however, did find longer life spans in people who received nutritional therapy similar to that offered by the Cancer Treatment Centers of America.

That study, by Abram Hoffer, M.D., Ph.D., and Linus Pauling, Ph.D., looked at people with cancer who were receiving state-of-the-art treatment such as chemotherapy or radiation.

Those who continued eating as they had before they found out they had cancer had an average life span of 5.7 months. Of those receiving nutritional therapy (high-dose vitamins and minerals as well as information on food selection), 20 percent were considered poor responders. Still, their survival time was almost twice that of the patients not receiving nutritional support. The 80 percent considered good responders had an average life span of six years.

"This group included people with tough-to-treat cancers—lung, pancreas and liver," Dr. Quillin points out. Women with cancer of the breast, ovaries, cervix or uterus did best. Their average life span was ten years, a 21-fold improvement over those who did not get nutrition therapy.

In another study, conducted by researchers at West Virginia University School of Medicine in Morgantown, men with bladder cancer who took large doses of vitamin A (40,000 international units), vitamin B_6 (100 milligrams), vitamin C (2,000 milligrams), vitamin E (400 international units) and zinc (90 milligrams), in addition to a multivitamin/mineral supplement that provided the Recommended Dietary Allowances and their regular treatment, had a 40 percent reduction in tumor recurrence compared with men getting only the Recommended Dietary Allowances of these nutrients. This study also showed that after five years, the men taking large amounts of nutrients went for a significantly longer time without tumor recurrence.

"The take-home lesson in all of this," Dr. Quillin says, "is that nutrition is not a magic bullet against all cancers. Nutrition should not be used as a sole therapy. But nutrition can dramatically improve the quantity and quality of life and chances for complete remission for people with cancer."

In the body, some of the beta-carotene we eat is converted to vitamin A, an important regulator of cell growth and differentiation, Dr. Krinsky adds. "That means vitamin A helps cells mature into their final forms, which helps prevent cells from developing into cancer," he explains.

Unfortunately, a study from Finland found that longtime heavy smokers who took beta-carotene supplements of 20 milligrams (about 33,000 international units) a day were more, not less, likely to die from lung cancer. Although some doctors believe that finding is purely chance, others think it warrants careful consideration.

"This was such a well-designed study, with so much statistical power, that we can't ignore it," says Jerry McLarty, Ph.D., chairman of the Department of Epidemiology and Biomathematics at the University of Texas Health Center at Tyler and lead researcher in an ongoing study of beta-carotene and lung cancer. "Certainly, more research needs to be done to get to bottom of this."

Some researchers say that the study was too little, too late, that the men given the supplements may have already had early lung cancer, still undetectable on x-rays. "Certainly, the finding of this study supports the argument that vitamin supplements alone cannot undo the damage wrought by years of bad habits or act as a substitute for eating well," Dr. McLarty says.

An increasing number of nutritionally oriented doctors are recommending supplements of beta-carotene to help prevent cancer, usually 10,000 to 25,000 international units daily. One 7½-inch carrot contains about 20,000 international units of beta-carotene.

"We recommend these supplements not because they have been proven to prevent cancer but because we believe some beta-carotene is better than none," says David Edelberg, M.D., facilitator of the American Holistic Center/Chicago, one of the country's largest alternative medicine practices. "Unfortunately, the reality is that many people don't eat enough vegetables each day to get even this relatively small amount of beta-carotene."

Even doctors who recommend beta-carotene supplements, however, urge you to load up on orange, yellow and dark green, leafy vegetables such as carrots, spinach, kale, sweet potatoes, winter squash and cantaloupe. Having even a single serving of any of these foods every day puts you ahead of the national average when it comes to beta-carotene.

"These foods also contain other, less-studied compounds that may prove to be at least as protective as beta-carotene against breast cancer and other forms of cancer," Dr. Krinsky explains.

For people who've had lung cancer, some doctors may recommend up to 500,000 international units of beta-carotene, says Dr. Quillin. These amounts

Nutrition and Cancer Medications

When it comes to nutrition, cancer can do a double whammy on your body. The disease itself can cause nutritional deficiencies; so can the medications used to treat it.

Both cancer and its treatments can cause loss of appetite, nausea, intestinal absorption problems and increased metabolism (calorie burning), all of which can lead to malnourishment and weight loss. "If you have cancer, it's important that your doctor recognize these problems and correct them if possible," says Patrick Quillin, R.D., Ph.D., certified nutrition specialist, nutrition director for the Cancer Treatment Centers of America, headquartered in Arlington Heights, Illinois, and author of *Beating Cancer with Nutrition*. Malnutrition is a major cause of cancer deaths.

Studies show that certain nutrients can help protect the body's healthy cells from the damaging effects of chemotherapy without interfering with, and sometimes even enhancing, these drugs' antitumor activity. In one animal study, vitamin E given prior to treatment with bleomycin, a common cancer drug, helped prevent the lung tissue scarring this treatment can cause.

In animal and human studies, niacin, vitamin C and selenium also showed promise in reducing chemotherapy's toxicity and tissue damage. So did the supplements cysteine and coenzyme Q_{10}. These two are nonessential nutrient factors, and they protect the body against free radicals, naturally occurring unstable molecules that damage your body's healthy molecules by stealing electrons to balance themselves. If you are slated for chemotherapy, you may wish to discuss taking these nutrients with your health care professional. Don't start nutritional therapy on your own without informing your doctor.

are considered nontoxic, but you should discuss taking this much with your doctor or health care provider, he adds.

Folic Acid's Cancer-Stopping Power

Kale, spinach, romaine lettuce: These leafy greens are packed with a number of cancer-crushing nutrients. One in particular, folate, appears to help protect cells from cancer-inducing genetic damage from certain chemicals.

"Folate deficiency can induce damage to the genetic material in a cell, which can in itself lead to cancer and which also makes the cell more vulnerable to cancer-causing chemicals," explains Tiepu Liu, M.D., Dr.P.H., research assistant professor at the University of Alabama School of Medicine in Birmingham. Folate deficiency also makes it harder for a cell to repair its genetic material, which also sets the stage for cancer, Dr. Liu says.

In one study, researchers at the University of Alabama found that smokers treated with ten milligrams (10,000 micrograms) of folic acid and 500 micrograms of vitamin B_{12} each day had significantly fewer precancerous cells than an untreated group. (Vitamin B_{12} was added because smokers tend to be deficient in B_{12} and because folic acid needs B_{12} to be active.)

And in a more recent study, Japanese doctors also found that folic acid and vitamin B_{12} provide impressive protection. Smokers who took 10 to 20 milligrams (10,000 to 20,000 micrograms) of folic acid and 750 micrograms of B_{12} daily had significant reductions in the number of potentially precancerous cells found in abnormal spots in the passageways of their lungs. The spots were checked with a lung-scanning scope several times over the course of one year. Seventy percent of initially abnormal spots were reclassified as normal by the end of the year, and not one lesion had gotten worse. In contrast, a control group that took no supplements fared this way: 77 percent of their spots remained the same, 5 percent got worse, and 18 percent got better.

And Harvard Medical School researchers found that men getting 847 micrograms and women getting 711 micrograms of folic acid daily had one-third less risk of precancerous colon polyps compared with men getting 241 micrograms and women getting 166 micrograms a day.

Researchers at the University of Alabama also found that among women who were exposed to a potentially cancer-causing virus, those whose blood levels of folate were low were five times as likely to develop disturbing cervical cell changes (cervical dysplasia) as women with higher folate levels.

"We speculate that adequate amounts of folate may help protect a cell's genetic material from invading viruses," Dr. Liu says. Unfortunately, studies so far show that in women who already have cervical dysplasia, supplemental folic acid is unable to reverse the condition, Dr. Liu adds. For more information on vitamin therapy for cervical dysplasia, see page 173.

The amount of folic acid given in the University of Alabama study of smokers, 10,000 micrograms, is far above the Daily Value for folic acid, which is 400 micrograms. Some doctors believe people should be getting at least 400 to 800 micrograms of folic acid a day to prevent cancer. To get that amount, you'd have to fill up on the very best food sources: dark green, leafy vegetables, oranges, beans, rice and brewer's yeast.

Doctors who treat cancer with nutrition recommend about 400 micrograms of folic acid, along with 1,000 micrograms of vitamin B_{12}, every day, Dr. Quillin says. Vitamin B_{12} is available from food sources such as seafood and green, leafy vegetables. Supplements may also be helpful.

Finding a doctor who uses folic acid to treat rather than prevent cancer can be difficult. Because methotrexate, an early anti-cancer drug, worked by interfering with folate metabolism, there has been concern among cancer specialists that folic acid could fuel cancer growth. Not so, says Dr. Quillin. In animal studies, folic acid did not increase cancer growth. And according to him, a folate deficiency increases the likelihood that a cancer will spread to other parts of the body. Doctors at the Cancer Treatment Centers of America include 400 micrograms of folic acid in their treatment regimens.

Be aware that high doses of folic acid can mask symptoms of pernicious anemia, caused by vitamin B_{12} deficiency. It's best to work with a doctor if you plan to take much more than the Daily Value of folic acid.

Canker Sores

Soothing a Sore Mouth

Never is the statement "Out of sight, out of mind" less true than in the case of a canker sore. From the outside, you can't see that little white ulcer with the red border on the inside of your mouth. Others can't tell anything is amiss. But you sure know it's there every time you open your mouth to talk or—ouch!—eat.

Aphthous stomatitis, the technical name for a canker sore, is a bit of a medical mystery. No one really knows why some people frequently get these stinging lesions on their tongue and gums and inside their cheeks. Heredity does seem to play a role, as do stress, certain foods and abrasions, such as those caused by dentures.

Left alone, canker sores will generally clear up in 10 to 14 days, but there's no need to suffer in silence that long. Doctors can recommend a prescription medicated gel containing hydrocortisone, which is soothing and may speed healing, or even an over-the-counter ointment such as Blistex to numb the pain. And if you're prone to canker sores, there are some nutri-

Food Factors

You already know about certain foods from experience. That salty, sharp-edged potato chip, for example, is sure to hurt when it bumps up against a canker sore. And you wouldn't think of giving it that opportunity. But do you know that some foods can actually trigger a new sore? Here's what oral health experts recommend eating (or not eating).

Avoid citrus. Acidic foods such as tomatoes and citrus fruits can both aggravate an existing sore and stimulate an outbreak, according to research gathered by the American Academy of Otolaryngology–Head and Neck Surgery. If you're prone to canker sores, go easy on things such as grapefruit and lemonade.

Eat more yogurt. Eating yogurt each day keeps canker sores away, says Julian Whitaker, M.D., founder and president of the Whitaker Wellness Center in Newport Beach, California. If you're prone to canker sores, he recommends eating at least four tablespoons of yogurt daily to prevent outbreaks. To heal an outbreak, he recommends eating at least one eight-ounce container a day. To work, Dr. Whitaker says, the yogurt must contain active *Lactobacillus acidophilus* cultures. (If the yogurt contains these cultures, it will say so on the label.)

tional strategies that may prevent these nasty critters from becoming repeat offenders. Here's what many experts recommend.

Vitamin C for Relief

Though studies have not yet been done to prove their effectiveness, vitamin C supplements get their share of kudos. Oral health experts tout this vitamin as an effective means of preventing canker sores.

"Actually, it works against cold sores and canker sores," says Craig Zunka, D.D.S., past president of the Holistic Dental Association and a dentist in Front Royal, Virginia. "But since you can't feel a canker sore coming on, you have to take vitamin C every day instead of just at the onset of an outbreak, the way you can with cold sores."

For optimum prevention, many experts recommend taking 500 milligrams a day, every day, especially for people who are under a lot of stress or who smoke. To treat a new sore, take 1,000 milligrams of vitamin C right away, then follow up with 500 milligrams three times a day until the sore has cleared up, says Dr. Zunka. (Some people may experience diarrhea when taking more than 1,200 milligrams of vitamin C a day.) "Just be sure you take vitamin C with bioflavonoids," notes Dr. Zunka, "because plain vitamin C will not work as well." Bioflavonoids are chemical compounds closely linked to vitamin C.

Although oranges and grapefruit are excellent sources of both vitamin C and bioflavonoids, too much citrus can backfire and trigger canker sore outbreaks in people prone to these pesky lesions. So oral health experts say that supplementation is your best bet if you are prone to them.

Prescriptions for Healing

Only time is guaranteed to make canker sores go away. But if you want to speed healing and avoid new outbreaks, some experts say these nutrients might help.

Nutrient	Daily Amount/Application
Oral	
Vitamin C with bioflavonoids	500 milligrams to prevent sores
	1,000 milligrams, taken at the first sign of a sore; then 1,500 milligrams, taken as 3 divided doses, until the sore heals
Plus a multivitamin/mineral supplement containing the Daily Values of folic acid, iron and vitamin B_{12}	
Topical	
Vitamin E	Oil from 1 capsule, applied directly to the sore

MEDICAL ALERT: Vitamin C in excess of 1,200 milligrams a day may cause diarrhea in some people.

Take a Multi for Your Mouth

If you find that your canker sores have become more like intrusive weekend guests than occasional party crashers, you may need more than just a boost of vitamin C. According to research, you may have any of a number of different nutrient deficiencies.

Although research is inconclusive, several studies have linked deficiencies of folate, iron and vitamin B_{12} to recurrent canker sores, and some doctors believe that upping your intake of these nutrients might be beneficial for prevention.

Your best bet, say oral health experts, is to cover all your bases by taking a multivitamin/mineral supplement that includes the Daily Values of these nutrients.

Squeeze on Vitamin E

If, despite your best efforts, a canker sore puts in a bothersome appearance, a little vitamin E may be just what the doctor ordered. Only this time, suggests Dr. Zunka, instead of tossing back a vitamin E supplement or filling up on vitamin E–rich foods, crack open a vitamin E capsule and slather the oil directly on the sore for immediate pain relief.

Cardiomyopathy

Heart-Protecting Nutrients

Cardiomyopathy is a special form of heart disease. It's a breakdown of the muscle tissue in the heart. This muscle tissue, known as the myocardium, becomes inflamed, then scarred and fibrous. As a result, the walls of the heart may become thick and hard or thin and weak. The heart sometimes enlarges and beats faster, trying to play catch-up because it isn't pumping blood efficiently.

People with cardiomyopathy may become breathless when they're active and sometimes even when they're doing nothing at all. They may tire easily, develop ankle swelling and have chest pains.

Compared with coronary heart disease, which is the most common form of heart disease, cardiomyopathy is rare. But it's one of the main reasons peo-

Food Factors

Other than eating a well-balanced diet that's high in whole grains, fruits and vegetables, there's just one more thing you need to be concerned about if you have cardiomyopathy. Here's what experts recommend.

Don't get pickled. Alcohol abuse can cause cardiomyopathy by depleting the body of nutrients and having a direct toxic effect on the heart, says Robert DiBianco, M.D., associate clinical professor of medicine at Georgetown University School of Medicine in Washington, D.C. Limit yourself to no more than two drinks a day. And don't "save up" your drinks for the weekend. Binge drinking is particularly hard on hearts, not to mention friends and family.

ple become candidates for heart transplants. That's because traditionally, there hasn't been a whole lot available for cardiomyopathy. Most doctors use drugs to provide some relief by reducing demands on the heart.

"These drugs are indispensable and have been shown to be remarkably effective in some people," explains Robert DiBianco, M.D., associate clinical professor of medicine at Georgetown University School of Medicine in Washington, D.C.

Unlike coronary heart disease, cardiomyopathy isn't always caused by fat-clogged arteries, although it can be, Dr. DiBianco says. It may be caused by a virus or another type of infection, such as Lyme disease or AIDS; an inherited metabolic disorder; exposure to toxic chemicals such as cobalt, lead or carbon monoxide; sensitivity to commonly used drugs; toxins such as alcohol or cocaine; or heart damage caused by a disease such as diabetes.

Poor nutrition also seems to play a role in the development of some forms of cardiomyopathy or in worsening its symptoms.

Several of the "classic" deficiency diseases—pellagra (niacin deficiency), beriberi (thiamin deficiency) and kwashiorkor (protein deficiency)—can cause cardiomyopathy. So can imbalances of calcium and magnesium, which play important roles in proper heart function.

And shortages of other nutrients, particularly selenium and vitamin E, make the heart more vulnerable to damage.

Here's what research shows can help this potentially life-threatening problem.

Coenzyme Q_{10}: Good for Your Heart?

Many cardiologists would consider it unproven, harmless at best—that is, if they've even heard of coenzyme Q_{10}.

"Today in medicine, most doctors don't know anything about it yet," says Karl Folkers, D.Sc., Ph.D., professor and director of the Institute for Biomedical Research at the University of Texas at Austin. (The American Heart Association says it has "no official statement" about coenzyme Q_{10}.)

But a growing number of nutrition-oriented doctors say that supplements of this little-known nutrient (it isn't exactly a vitamin) are absolutely essential for people with heart failure. They say it has allowed their patients to live longer, more active lives, has saved some people who would otherwise have died waiting for donor hearts and has even allowed some to take their names off the transplant list.

"In some people, the improvement is clear, often dramatic," says coenzyme Q_{10} researcher Peter Langsjoen, M.D., a cardiologist in private practice in Tyler, Texas, with a special interest in nutrition.

Some studies, mostly from Japan, have looked at coenzyme Q_{10}'s role in cardiovascular disease, says Dr. Folkers. They include two double-blind, placebo-controlled studies, which are considered the most reliable. The studies showed that coenzyme Q_{10} has clinical benefits for 70 percent of the patients having congestive heart failure, says Dr. Folkers. Coenzyme Q_{10} is normally concentrated in the heart muscle, and levels drop when the heart begins to fail.

"Bear in mind, however, that some studies done in the United States found no benefits with coenzyme Q_{10} and were never published," says Robert DiBianco, M.D., associate clinical professor of medicine at Georgetown University School of Medicine in Washington, D.C. "Unless such studies are done and published, American doctors will remain rightly skeptical."

Coenzyme Q_{10} is an essential ingredient in the body's production

Selenium Shields Hearts

Until 1979, researchers didn't know for sure that the mineral selenium is essential for human nutrition. That year, evidence came from Chinese scientists who reported an association between low selenium intake and a condi-

of energy. Dr. Folkers says it has "bioenergetic activity," meaning that it participates in biochemical reactions that provide energy. In cardiomyopathy and other kinds of heart failure, supplements of coenzyme Q_{10} are thought to help the remaining muscle cells do their jobs more efficiently, Dr. Langsjoen says.

Coenzyme Q_{10} is manufactured by the body and stored in your organs: liver, kidneys and, you guessed it, heart. Dr. Folkers believes that people with low levels of coenzyme Q_{10} aren't getting enough of the vitamins necessary to convert the amino acid tyrosine to coenzyme Q_{10}. These vitamins include niacin, vitamin B_6, vitamin B_{12}, vitamin C and folate.

There are also coenzyme Q_{10} supplements, available in drugstores and health food stores. Dr. Langsjoen typically prescribes 120 to 360 milligrams of coenzyme Q_{10} a day, taken in doses of no more than 180 milligrams at a time. (This means that if you are taking more than 180 milligrams a day, you need to divide the dose). This fat-soluble nutrient needs to be taken with a bit of fat or oil (although some supplements are in an oil base, similar to vitamin E capsules). Dr. Langsjoen has his patients chew the tablets along with a spoonful of peanut butter. Dosage is determined by measuring blood levels of coenzyme Q_{10}. (Your doctor can order this test by sending your blood to a lab for analysis.)

"Generally, people who have heart failure begin to see an improvement in symptoms in about four weeks, although some people may take as long as three months," Dr. Folkers says. Maximum improvement occurs after six months, which is longer than ordinary drugs take to exhibit an effect, he says.

If you're interested in taking coenzyme Q_{10}, find a doctor who's familiar with its use or ask your own doctor to study up, Dr. Langsjoen suggests. Those using this nutrient in research or practice report no toxicity.

tion called Keshan disease, a form of cardiomyopathy that affects primarily children and women of childbearing age.

People in certain parts of China were getting little selenium in their diets because the soil in their region contains almost none. Since plants don't require selenium, they can grow in selenium-poor soil. But they offer no selenium to the people and animals who eat them, so there is simply no good food source, plant or animal, in the region. In fact, some animals suffered from the same heart condition, and it was Chinese veterinarians who first made the connection between human cardiomyopathy and selenium.

"Chinese doctors soon found that selenium supplements could prevent this potentially fatal problem," says Orville Levander, Ph.D., a research leader at the U.S. Department of Agriculture Beltsville Human Nutrition Research Center in Maryland.

Selenium deficiency alone doesn't seem to cause cardiomyopathy, however, Dr. Levander says. "Researchers now think this condition develops only in selenium-deficient people who have been exposed to certain viruses that zero in on the heart muscle."

Dr. Levander and his colleague, Melinda Beck, Ph.D., professor at the University of North Carolina at Chapel Hill, found that a particular kind of virus called Coxsackie remained its mild-mannered self in laboratory animals that were getting enough selenium. But in selenium-deficient lab animals, it caused extensive heart damage.

"Selenium seems to help protect the heart muscle from viral damage," Dr. Levander says. "We don't know exactly how, but it seems to be related to its antioxidant properties." Viral invasions cause the generation of free radicals, unstable molecules that steal electrons from healthy molecules in your body's cells to balance themselves, thus damaging the cells. Antioxidants disarm free radicals by offering up their own electrons, saving cells from harm.

Most researchers in the United States don't think Americans are deficient enough in this mineral to develop cardiomyopathy, Dr. Levander says. Chinese researchers found it takes only a small amount, about 20 micrograms a day, to prevent cardiomyopathy. Most Americans get well above that amount, averaging 108 micrograms a day.

But some research shows that so-called adequate amounts of selenium may not be high enough to provide optimum antioxidant or immunity-stimulating protection. That's why some doctors recommend selenium supplements of 50 to 200 micrograms a day.

If you're concerned about deficiency, ask your doctor to check your blood level of selenium, Dr. Levander says. If your blood level is low, you may need to take supplements. Supplements of more than 100 micrograms a day should be taken only under medical supervision, however, since selenium can be toxic in large amounts. Stop taking selenium if you develop a persistent garlic odor on your breath and skin, loss of hair, fragile or black fingernails, a metallic taste in your mouth, or dizziness or nausea with no ap-

Prescriptions for Healing

Even if you decide to try certain nutrients for your heart condition, don't toss away your heart drugs! Doctors who use nutritional therapy for cardiomyopathy say drugs are still necessary for some people. Here are the nutrients they recommend.

Nutrient	Daily Amount
Magnesium	400 milligrams
Selenium	50–200 micrograms
Vitamin E	400 international units

MEDICAL ALERT: *If you have cardiomyopathy, you should be under a doctor's care.*

If you have a kidney problem or heart disease, it's important to take magnesium supplements only under medical supervision.

Selenium supplements of more than 100 micrograms a day should be taken only under medical supervision. In large amounts, selenium is toxic.

If you are taking anticoagulant drugs, you should not take vitamin E supplements.

parent cause. These symptoms mean that you're getting too much.

Generally, fruits and vegetables don't contain much selenium. On the other hand, seafood and, to a lesser extent, meats are rich in easily absorbed selenium. Grains and seeds, garlic and mushrooms also offer some selenium, depending on where they are grown.

Vitamin E Adds Antioxidant Protection

If you're concerned about giving your heart all of the protection you can, you'll want to add vitamin E to your arsenal.

"In animal studies, cardiomyopathy problems are more likely to be worse in the animals with simultaneous deficiencies of selenium and vitamin E. These deficiencies can be prevented or cured by supplementation with either nutrient alone," Dr. Levander says. (In animals, vitamin E can also protect the heart against cardiomyopathy caused by magnesium deficiency.)

Like selenium, vitamin E has antiviral and antioxidant properties, so it may help protect the heart against infection and toxins. It may also help prevent the development of atherosclerosis, or clogged arteries, which could make a failing heart even weaker, says Peter Langsjoen, M.D., a cardiologist in private practice in Tyler, Texas, with a special interest in nutrition. He recommends 400 international units daily. That high amount is available only from supplements.

Magnesium May Aid Weakened Hearts

In animals, the evidence is clear. When put on a low-magnesium diet, young animals develop heart muscle damage that leads to heart failure.

"In humans, the picture isn't so clear," says William Weglicki, M.D., professor of medicine and physiology at George Washington University Medical Center in Washington, D.C. "For people, there's no good proof that magnesium deficiency causes cardiomyopathy."

Magnesium is so intimately involved in heart function, however, that getting enough may help a compromised heart work better for a number of reasons, says Carla Sueta, M.D., Ph.D., assistant professor of medicine and cardiology at the University of North Carolina at Chapel Hill School of Medicine.

"Magnesium affects heart muscle contraction, and magnesium deficiency can cause abnormal heart rhythms and/or irregular beats," Dr. Sueta says. "Adequate amounts can help prevent constriction of isolated blood vessels, which can affect the blood supply to the heart muscle."

Apparently, magnesium also offers protection during a heart attack. "Magnesium-deficient animals have greater tissue damage after heart attacks than animals getting enough magnesium," Dr. Weglicki says.

If you are a heart patient concerned about magnesium, have your doctor monitor levels in your red blood cells, Dr. Sueta suggests. "If your levels are low, you know for sure you're low in magnesium. And if your levels are borderline, you still are probably low in magnesium," she says. You can have normal levels of magnesium, however, and still be low enough to have magnesium deficiency–related heart problems, she adds.

If you have kidney problems or heart disease, it's important to take magnesium supplements only under medical supervision.

If you're simply concerned about heart health, experts suggest that you make sure to get the Daily Value of 400 milligrams. Nuts, beans and whole grains are your best food sources, and green vegetables also provide a fair amount. Studies show that most people fall short of the Daily Value.

Carpal Tunnel Syndrome

Opening Up to Relief

They were awkward, all right. But Richard Comstock wasn't about to part with his doctor-prescribed wrist splints, weapons in the fight against his painful, hand-numbing case of carpal tunnel syndrome (CTS).

He wasn't about to abandon hope for a vitamin cure, either. So when the Scotia, New York, resident read that vitamin B_6 might be the light at the end of his CTS pain, he combined treatments.

That was more than a decade ago. He's still taking his trusty vitamin B_6, but Comstock's severe carpal tunnel pain is long gone. And so are the wrist splints. "Every once in a while, I'll have a little problem, but it doesn't keep me awake at night like it used to," says the retired utility supervisor.

Comstock may have been way ahead of his time. Even though over 100,000 carpal tunnel surgeries are performed each year, doctors who prefer a less drastic solution are slowly beginning to add vitamin B_6 to their treatment regimens. "For those people who don't seem to have serious problems, I normally recommend they wear splints at night, take an anti-inflammatory and use B_6 for at least two weeks," says Gary Tunell, M.D., chief of neurology at Baylor University Medical Center in Dallas. Dr. Tunell estimates that 40 to 50 percent of people with CTS could experience some improvement using this therapy.

Some doctors are even more enthusiastic about the use of vitamin B_6 for CTS. "Somewhere around 90 percent of carpal tunnel cases can be cured by B_6," says John Marion Ellis, M.D., a retired Mount Pleasant, Texas, family practitioner who has conducted studies and written papers about B_6 and who has been researching the link between B_6 deficiency and CTS for more than 30 years.

Touring the Tunnel

Just inside your wrist is a narrow, bony passage called the carpal tunnel. Anything but empty, this tunnel contains nine tendons as well as a nerve called the median nerve, all of which are encased, sausagelike, in a slippery sheath called the synovium. When the synovium and tendons become inflamed and swollen, they squeeze the median nerve, which runs to the fingers.

Ever watch a live electrical wire rub metal? The pinched median nerve can send angry sparks of pain, numbness and tingling from your fingertips to your shoulder. More often the pain is in the thumb and the index and middle fingers. Sometimes the ring finger is also involved. Many people who suffer from CTS say it feels like their hands have fallen asleep; others complain of weak grips and stiff fingers.

Women seem to suffer from CTS more often than men. Changes in female hormones caused by pregnancy, taking birth control pills and menopause somehow make the synovium swell. And because women generally have small wrists, just a little swelling is enough to cause carpal tunnel pain, experts say.

Surgeons agree that CTS should not be treated with surgery during pregnancy. Studies by Dr. Ellis found that vitamin B_6 helped relieve CTS in 11 percent of the pregnant women with severe CTS signs and symptoms during their pregnancies. These women were treated with 50 to 300 milligrams of B_6 daily for at least 60 to 90 days before giving birth. And there was no harm to either the mother or the child. If you'd like to try this therapy, you should discuss it with your doctor.

Obesity creates a similar situation. "There is about a fivefold increase in CTS in people who are obese and couch potatoes. So we encourage them to be in better shape and lose weight," says Morton Kasdan, M.D., clinical professor of plastic surgery at the University of Louisville in Kentucky and clinical professor of preventive medicine and environmental health at the University of Kentucky in Lexington.

Food Factors

The pain hits your wrist, your hand and sometimes even your shoulder. But carpal tunnel syndrome can start in your stomach. Here are some things to consider.

Hold the reins on cocktails. Alcohol is known to deplete the body of nutrients, especially the B vitamins, which are vital for preventing carpal tunnel syndrome.

Drop those pounds. Many doctors have noted that people who lose weight sometimes also lose their symptoms of carpal tunnel syndrome. If you're on a weight-reducing diet, be sure to eat foods that contain vitamin B_6, such as bananas and avocados.

Prescriptions for Healing

Many doctors recommend B vitamins for carpal tunnel syndrome. Because even the foods richest in vitamin B_6, such as bananas, avocados, brewer's yeast and beef, provide barely a single milligram of B_6, you'll probably need to take a supplement. B-complex capsules often include all of the recommended vitamins.

Nutrient	Daily Amount
Biotin	300 micrograms
Riboflavin	25 milligrams
Vitamin B_6	50–200 milligrams

MEDICAL ALERT: *Take vitamin B_6 in amounts above 100 milligrams only under the supervision of your doctor.*

CTS has also become the unofficial health complaint of the modern age, the result of an increase in cases among people in manufacturing jobs.

Officials at the U.S. Bureau of Labor Statistics don't keep records of the number of CTS cases reported each year. Between 1986 and 1992, cases of "repetitive trauma disorders" (a category that includes CTS and similar conditions) zoomed from 50,000 to 282,000.

Another common culprit is working on a computer, which doesn't require you to take frequent breaks, as changing paper in a typewriter would. "The repetitive activity produces inflammation, and this leads to swelling," explains Dr. Tunell. "That's a major contributor for the patients I see."

The Benefits of B_6

Doctors are divided on why vitamin B_6 seems to provide relief from CTS.

The author of five published studies that demonstrate the benefits of vitamin B_6 for CTS, Dr. Ellis contends that synovium swelling and inelasticity are caused by a B_6 deficiency.

Dr. Ellis and Karl Folkers, D.Sc., Ph.D., professor and director of the Institute for Biomedical Research at the University of Texas at Austin, once healed 22 of 23 people with CTS just by giving them 50 to 300 milligrams of vitamin B_6 daily for at least 12 weeks. And a number of them had already undergone surgery without experiencing relief. "Vitamin B_6 is as important to your body as oxygen and water, only it takes a little longer to show the benefits," says Dr. Ellis.

The average diet, Dr. Ellis says, provides only about 1.4 milligrams of vitamin B_6 a day, in part because the nutrient is lost in processing, so many people are just not getting enough. "Raw foods are the best sources, because heat destroys it," he says. Foods containing B_6 include potatoes, bananas, chicken breast, top round of beef, fish, brown rice and avocados.

Other doctors believe vitamin B_6 acts as a diuretic, helping the body to eliminate excess fluid. "During pregnancy, your feet swell, your hands swell, rings don't fit anymore. You're retaining fluid, especially in the wrists," says Dr. Tunell. For some women, the problem worsens when they lie down, as fluid that makes the ankles swell during the day is redistributed throughout the body, including to the wrists, he says. "B_6 helps you get rid of the extra water gain that's causing carpal tunnel," he says.

Another theory, backed up by two European studies, suggests that vitamin B_6 somehow short-circuits an angry nerve's ability to transmit pain signals. "We don't know the mechanism, but we do know B_6 reduces the amount of pain that animals feel, and that may be what's happening here," says Allan L. Bernstein, M.D., chief of neurology at Kaiser Permanente Medical Center in Hayward, California.

Medical experts do agree on one thing: No matter how vitamin B_6 gets the job done, you have to be careful not to take too much. In studies using laboratory animals, researchers found that excess B_6 can harm your central nervous system.

Researchers at the U.S. Department of Agriculture Western Human Nutrition Research Center in San Francisco fed 12 experimental animals 1, 10, 100, 200 or 300 times their requirement of vitamin B_6 for seven weeks. At the three highest levels of B_6 intake, the animals' reaction time to a loud noise was reduced. Signs of a B_6 overdose also include an oversensitivity to sunlight, which produces a skin rash and numbness.

"Vitamin B_6 toxicity symptoms are rarely seen in healthy individuals. Moderate supplementation of B_6 will not cause that kind of thing," says Robert A. Jacob, Ph.D., research chemist in micronutrients at the Western Human Nutrition Research Center. "You'd have to megadose on it. So I don't think that would happen if you take just a multivitamin/mineral supplement with B_6 or even a 50- or 100-milligram B_6 supplement. It appears only when you chronically take massive amounts."

Doctors recommend 50 to 200 milligrams of vitamin B_6 daily to treat carpal tunnel.

Some Recommend Riboflavin and Biotin

There's some evidence that vitamin B_6 won't work properly unless you're getting adequate amounts of riboflavin and biotin, other B vitamins. "Each one of these vitamins is synergistic; each works in concert with the other," says Flora Pettit, Ph.D., a research scientist at the Biochemical Institute at the University of Texas at Austin. Doctors suggest aiming for 300 micrograms of biotin and 25 milligrams of riboflavin daily.

By law, most cereals, flours and other grain products are fortified with riboflavin; milk, yogurt and cheeses are good sources, too. Biotin is found in brewer's yeast, soy flour, cereals, egg yolks, milk, nuts and vegetables.

Older adults, alcoholics and those with nutritionally poor diets are at particular risk for deficiencies in these vitamins, says Dr. Tunell. "Generally, the elderly have poor diets, and they have trouble absorbing B vitamins anyway," says Dr. Tunell. "So they couldn't go wrong with a B-complex supplement unless they have Parkinson's disease. In that case, vitamin B_6 may interfere with the absorption of their levodopa medication."

"My patients are getting between 50 and 100 milligrams of vitamin B_6 and riboflavin a day, using a B-complex supplement," says Dr. Kasdan. "And 60 percent of them have gotten better."

Most doctors agree that catching CTS early is a key to successful treatment. "If you have severe carpal tunnel, the vitamin B_6 isn't really going to reverse it," says Dr. Bernstein. "But if you catch it early, when you're just starting to have pain and tingling, and if there's no weakness and it bothers you at night but not during the day, you'll do extremely well."

Cataracts

Chasing Away the Clouds

Crack open an egg and drop it into a hot frying pan. You'll see the egg white turn cloudy, then white, as normally clear proteins in the egg are irreversibly altered by the heat.

Well, something similar to that happens when you get cataracts. Proteins in the lens of the eye lose their crystal-clear properties, becoming yellowish, cloudy and about as easy to see through as a fried egg. Of course, cataracts take not seconds but many years to form. And it's not heat but cigarette smoking, a buildup of sugar in the lens (usually associated with diabetes) and especially years of exposure to sunlight that eventually pull the shades on vision for many people.

Many doctors now think that the main cause of cataracts is oxidative damage to cells in the eye's lens. Oxidative damage is the same chemical process that rusts iron and makes cooking oil turn rancid. In the lens, the oxidative process can occur as part of normal metabolism as well as in the presence of light, which creates harmful unstable molecules called free radicals. These free radicals grab electrons from your body's healthy molecules to balance themselves, causing an ever-escalating molecular free-for-all that ends up hurting perfectly innocent cells.

Nutrients Shield the Lens

The lens can partially protect itself from this free radical damage, and it relies on certain nutrients to keep its defense system strong. Vitamins C and E, beta-carotene (a precursor of vitamin A) and minerals such as selenium, zinc and copper—all components of antioxidant enzymes found in the lens—may all play roles in protection. Even B vitamins such as riboflavin and B_{12} as well as an amino acid called cysteine may be involved, but evidence for these nutrients is very slim, says Randall Olson, M.D., professor and chairman of the Department of Ophthalmology at the University of Utah School of Medicine and director of the John A. Moran Eye Center, both in Salt Lake City.

"Not all of the facts are in, but the evidence to date is mostly positive that nutrients such as vitamins C and E and beta-carotene are helpful," Dr. Olson says. "And the evidence seems to indicate that these nutrients are synergistic, that they work best together."

In fact, several small studies suggest that people who take multivitamin/mineral supplements are less likely to develop cataracts than those who do not. A Harvard University study, for instance, found that doctors who regularly took multivitamin/mineral supplements cut by about one-fourth their risk of developing cataracts compared with those not taking supplements. And a study by Canadian researchers found that supplements reduced cataract formation by about 40 percent.

Food Factors

Doctors may recommend these additional dietary tips to people concerned about cataracts.

Save alcohol for special occasions. Daily drinkers up their odds for cataracts by about one-third compared with people who rarely drink.

Pretend you're Popeye. A Harvard University study found that women who ate spinach more than five times a week had a 47 percent decrease in risk of cataract surgery compared with those who ate spinach less than once a month. (Yes, eating spinach five times a week adds up to a whole lot of spinach, but some women in the study were apparently eating it that often.) Spinach may beat out carrots when it comes to cataract protection. In fact, it's always a good idea to eat a variety of fruits and vegetables.

A ten-year nationwide study now in progress called the Age-Related Eye Disease Study is evaluating whether a mix of vitamins, including E, C and beta-carotene, really does help keep eyes crystal-clear. "Until the results of that study are in, we can't say for sure whether these nutrients are really helpful," says Emily Chew, M.D., medical officer in the Division of Biometry and Epidemiology at the National Eye Institute in Bethesda, Maryland.

In the meantime, here's what research shows may help slow the development of cataracts.

Take C and See

Researchers have known for some time that the lens of the eye can concentrate vitamin C. Concentrations of vitamin C in the lens and in the aqueous humor, the watery fluid surrounding the lens, are about 10 to 30 times the concentrations in other parts of the body.

"We're very interested in a possible protective effect, especially since vitamin C is a water-soluble antioxidant and the lens is composed mostly of water and proteins," says Allen Taylor, Ph.D., director of the Laboratory for Nutrition and Vision Research at the Jean Mayer USDA Human Nutrition Research Center on Aging at Tufts University in Boston.

In studies using laboratory animals, vitamin C seems to help protect the lens from oxidative damage from light, sugar and certain drugs, Dr. Taylor says.

And what about people? "It's possible that people are not getting enough vitamin C in their diets to make a difference when it comes to preventing cataracts," says Susan E. Hankinson, Sc.D., associate epidemiologist in the Channing Laboratory at Brigham and Women's Hospital in Boston. And there are a couple of studies that suggest vitamin C supplements can help protect against cataracts.

When Dr. Hankinson and researchers at the Harvard School of Public Health crunched numbers on nutrient intakes for 50,828 nurses, they found that women who had taken vitamin C supplements for ten years or more (average intake: 250 to 500 milligrams daily) fared better. Compared with women who never took supplements, the supplement takers had 45 percent less chance of developing cataracts bad enough to require surgery.

In another study, people taking 300 to 600 milligrams of supplemental vitamin C a day experienced a 70 percent decrease in risk compared with people who were not taking that much vitamin C.

"Our finding makes sense, because cataracts generally form over a long period of time," Dr. Hankinson explains. "It's reasonable to think that long-term use of preventive agents such as vitamin C would result in lowered risk."

Doctors who recommend vitamin C to people at risk for cataracts suggest from 500 to 3,000 milligrams a day. (Some people may experience diarrhea when taking more than 1,200 milligrams of vitamin C daily.) "Research has yet to determine an optimum amount of vitamin C to take to prevent cataracts, but studies do show that the concentration of vitamin C in the lens continues to increase as people move into the 500-milligram range," says Dr. Taylor.

It's true that many doctors believe vitamin C is harmless even in high amounts. But when it comes to the eyes, one researcher contends that it's best to stay below 3,000 milligrams.

"I've found that intakes of 3,000 milligrams or more of vitamin C are associated with retinal macular puckering and sometimes with increased risk of retinal detachment," says Ben C. Lane, O.D., director of the Nutritional Optometry Institute in Lake Hiawatha, New Jersey. High doses of vitamin C seem to make the gelatinous material inside the eyeball watery, which reduces pressure against the retina, allowing it to more easily pull away from the back of the eyeball, Dr. Lane says. (The retina is a light-sensitive area at the back of the eyeball that receives images.)

It may be wise to get at least some of your daily vitamin C from citrus fruits. That's because chemical compounds called bioflavonoids, which are closely related to vitamin C and are found in the white membranes of oranges

Prescriptions for Healing

Doctors sometimes recommend these nutrients to help delay the development of cataracts.

Nutrient	Daily Amount
Beta-carotene	25,000 international units
Copper	1 milligram for every 10 milligrams of zinc, but no more than 2 milligrams
Selenium	50–200 micrograms
Vitamin C	500–3,000 milligrams
Vitamin E	400 international units
Zinc	15–50 milligrams

MEDICAL ALERT: *If you have cataracts, you should be under a doctor's care.*

Don't take more than 100 micrograms of selenium daily without medical supervision.

Some people may experience diarrhea when taking more than 1,200 milligrams of vitamin C daily.

If you are taking anticoagulant drugs, you should not take vitamin E supplements.

Don't take more than 15 milligrams of zinc daily without medical supervision.

and grapefruit, also seem to offer antioxidant protection and, Dr. Lane adds, may even be more important.

14-Carrot Eye Protection

We know. It's an old, old line, but the point is well-taken: The reason (well, maybe one reason) you've never seen a rabbit with glasses may indeed stem from this long-eared critter's penchant for carrots and perhaps spinach.

When it comes to cataracts, beta-carotene and plain old vitamin A may offer protection. At least that's what Harvard School of Public Health researchers found when, once again, they picked apart the diets of their much-studied nurses. They found that women with the highest beta-carotene and vitamin A intakes had a 39 percent lower risk of cataracts severe enough to require surgery than women getting the least beta-carotene and vitamin A.

It is possible that both beta-carotene and vitamin A may help prevent oxidative damage to the lens. Vitamin A itself is not an antioxidant. But, explains Dr. Hankinson, "it's possible that people who get enough preformed vitamin A in their diets have more beta-carotene and other carotenoids available to act as antioxidants, since these compounds may be converted to vitamin A only as the body needs them." In other words, if you're taking in enough vitamin A, your body won't need to use up beta-carotene to make the vitamin for you. Doctors who recommend vitamins suggest about 25,000 international units of beta-carotene daily.

Many doctors, including Dr. Hankinson, warn that it's too early in the research game to place your bets on any one supplement, such as beta-carotene, to prevent cataracts. Vitamin-rich foods seem to be important, too. "Even though we found that carrots offer protection, we found a stronger protective effect from spinach, which doesn't contain as much beta-carotene but has antioxidant compounds such as lutein and zeaxanthin," says Dr. Hankinson.

Best advice to date: Keep packing in those leafy greens as well as orange and yellow fruits and vegetables.

E Is for Eyes

What do wheat germ and sunflower oil have to do with healthy eyes? Both are good sources of vitamin E, an antioxidant nutrient that works its way into cell membranes and disarms free radicals before they have a chance to attack cells.

"Research in animals and test tube studies indicate that vitamin E may help protect the lens from oxidative damage from light, sugar and cigarette smoke," Dr. Olson explains.

In humans, the story seems to be the same. In one study, people taking 400 international units of vitamin E a day had half of the risk of developing cataracts compared with people who did not take vitamin E. In another, people whose blood levels of vitamin E were high had about half of the risk of developing cataracts compared with people with low blood levels.

"Vitamin E is a powerful antioxidant," Dr. Olson explains. "There's reason to believe that combined with other nutrients, it may help slow the progress of lens clouding."

You'd have to plow your way through bowls and bowls of wheat germ to get 400 international units of vitamin E, the amount found in some capsules. So supplementation is in order. "I recommend 400 international units a day," Dr. Olson says. The Daily Value for vitamin E is 30 international units, but most people get only about 10 international units a day from their diets.

The Case for Zinc

Doctors sometimes add a bit of zinc, an essential mineral, to their anti-cataract formulas. There's evidence that zinc is important for the function of the retina and that it may help prevent deterioration of the retina as we age. Plus the body needs zinc to make several antioxidant enzymes found in the eye, including superoxide dismutase and catalase.

Doctors who recommend zinc to prevent or slow cataracts call for a wide range, from 15 milligrams a day (the Daily Value) to 50 milligrams a day, the amount Dr. Olson recommends. Dr. Lane bases his initial dosage on an individual's zinc status, determined by testing. "It may be necessary to start a person at a fairly high amount, then cut back as his status returns to normal," he says.

One thing is for sure with zinc: More is not necessarily better, and doses exceeding 15 milligrams should be taken only under medical supervision. Too much zinc can deplete your body of copper, an essential trace mineral. You should get about 1 milligram of copper for every 10 milligrams of zinc. Even in fairly small amounts, copper can be toxic. Don't use long-term copper supplementation above the Daily Value of 2 milligrams without medical supervision, Dr. Lane cautions.

Selenium Adds Antioxidant Power

Doctors sometimes round out their antioxidant prescriptions with selenium, a mineral involved in the body's production of glutathione peroxidase, another protective enzyme found in the eye and other parts of the body.

Dr. Lane recommends selenium supplements only to people who have been found to be deficient in glutathione peroxidase activity or in red blood cell selenium or who have been subject to mercury poisoning. Dr. Olson does not recommend individual selenium supplements but does sometimes recommend multivitamin/mineral products that contain selenium, such as Icaps and Ocuvite (available in health food stores).

Doctors who recommend selenium supplements suggest 50 to 200 micrograms a day, no more. In even small amounts, selenium can be toxic, so don't take more than 100 micrograms daily without medical supervision.

If you're a fan of garlic, you'll be getting a healthy amount of selenium with each bite. Other selenium-rich foods include onions, mushrooms, cabbage, grains and fish.

Celiac Disease

Fighting to Absorb Enough Nutrition

Weak and pale from fatigue, a woman waits patiently in the examination room for her doctor to return. She thinks she's just tired. But he has seen these symptoms before, and he knows better. His diagnosis: iron-deficiency anemia caused by celiac disease.

Triggered by a sensitivity to wheat, rye, barley and oats, celiac disease also often causes gastrointestinal problems such as gas and diarrhea. The culprit: gluten, an ingredient of these grains that damages the small intestine, causing inflammation and impaired absorption of nutrients, explains Jerry S. Trier, M.D., professor of medicine at Harvard Medical School and senior physician at Brigham and Women's Hospital in Boston.

Although researchers are still figuring out the chemistry, some experts believe an enzyme deficiency results in the incomplete digestion of gluten, allowing the buildup of a toxic substance. This toxin then damages the mucosal lining of the small intestine, says Jean Guest, R.D., former dietary adviser to the Celiac Sprue Association and former pediatric clinical dietitian for the Medical Center at the University of Nebraska at Omaha.

Like a sponge that no longer absorbs, the damaged mucosal lining can't soak up key nutrients, including iron, zinc, folate (the naturally occurring form of folic acid), magnesium and calcium, triggering diarrhea and fatigue, explains Guest. Even fat and fat-soluble vitamins such as A, D, E and K are passed through the body with only a portion of them being used, she says. In someone who has had celiac disease for a long time without the problem being diagnosed, calcium deficiency can result in the bone-thinning disease osteoporosis, she adds.

Food Factors

Because celiac disease is caused by a substance found in most grains, avoiding the offender is the top priority. Here is how it's done.

Go on a grain watch. Tossing out your sandwich bread and pasta is a big step toward becoming gluten-free. But maintaining your independence from wheat, rye, barley and oats also requires careful reading of food labels. Many processed foods use wheat for a variety of purposes, such as for filler and flavoring. It may appear on the label as "hydrolyzed vegetable flavoring" or "textured vegetable protein," explains Jerry S. Trier, M.D., professor of medicine at Harvard Medical School and senior physician at Brigham and Women's Hospital in Boston.

Sometimes the label won't give you even that much of a clue, says Jean Guest, R.D., former dietary adviser to the Celiac Sprue Association and former pediatric clinical dietitian for the Medical Center at the University of Nebraska at Omaha. Without any warning, flour is applied to chewing gum and corn tortillas to keep them from sticking to foil wrappers and conveyor belts during manufacturing. Even foods that have been cooked in restaurant deep fryers and grills that have been used to cook other foods with wheat-containing breadings and coatings can provoke a reaction, she says.

"For these reasons, it's a diet that is hard to maintain," says Dr. Trier. "Even some pharmaceutical drugs contain wheat used as an extender."

Mind your moo. Many people with celiac have yet another food sensitivity: They are unable to digest a sugar in milk called lactose. For this reason, some doctors suggest going easy on dairy products until your recovery is complete, says Dr. Trier. "You can have cream in your coffee, even milk on your rice- or corn-based cereal, but it's a good idea not to overdo with dairy products for a while," he says. Once you've healed, you should be able to eat as much dairy as you like, provided you don't have lactose intolerance. (You'll know that you have this problem if dairy products give you gas.)

Prescriptions for Healing

The key treatment for anyone with celiac disease involves eliminating problem foods. Many experts also advise taking these nutrients.

Nutrient	Daily Amount
Calcium	1,000–2,000 milligrams

Plus a multivitamin/mineral supplement containing the Daily Values of all essential vitamins and minerals

MEDICAL ALERT: *If you have celiac disease, you should be under a doctor's care.*

Dietary Detective Work Pays Off

In most cases, treatment involves avoiding gluten, which isn't always easy. Even the glue on some envelopes contains gluten. "Some people are exquisitely sensitive to gluten, and even a minute amount such as envelope glue can cause a reaction, although that's not usually the case," says Dr. Trier.

But the effort needed to avoid gluten can be worthwhile. Once gluten is no longer included in the diet, nutrient absorption problems quickly disappear. In a yearlong study that looked at whether a gluten-free diet could help children with celiac, researchers found that the bone growth of those on a gluten-free diet was faster than that of healthy children. Since the children with celiac were behind their counterparts in bone growth, the exclusion of certain grains prompted their bodies to play catch-up.

Since a gluten-free diet is strict, it's wise to take a multivitamin/mineral supplement to make sure you get all of the nutrients you need, says Guest.

The Case for Extra Calcium

And since calcium absorption can be dramatically reduced by celiac disease, Dr. Trier recommends calcium supplements for many of his patients.

"It's a good idea," says Dr. Trier. "People are often calcium-depleted when they're diagnosed." In most cases, Dr. Trier says, 1,000 to 2,000 milligrams a day is enough to rebuild calcium stores. The Daily Value for calcium is 1,000 milligrams.

Cervical Dysplasia

Getting Your Cells in Line

It gets scraped during a Pap test, bumped during intercourse, stretched open during childbirth and occasionally covered with latex or squirted with foam when you're trying to avoid pregnancy. But other than that, your cervix is not really a focal point of your life. Out of sight, out of mind, right?

Right. Until your gynecologist says that something is wrong.

For somewhere between 250,000 and 1 million women every year, that something is cervical dysplasia, a condition in which cells lining the cervix stop organizing themselves into nice, neat, horizontal layers that reflect their maturity from youngest to oldest.

Instead, a few older cells apparently decide to hang out with the younger crowd, then become disruptive when their increasing growth no longer allows them to neatly fit in among their younger siblings. They push the other cells around, which eventually disrupts the rows.

Fortunately, the fact that these cells are out of line signals itself on a Pap test. Depending on how many of these juvenile delinquents there are, a lab technician will label the test either "low-grade squamous intraepithelial lesion" for the minor disruptions of mild dysplasia or "high-grade squamous intraepithelial lesion" for the more significant disruptions of moderate and severe dysplasia. Carcinoma in situ, which is also a high-grade squamous intraepithelial lesion, is not a form of cancer, despite its name. Dysplasia becomes cancer when the delinquent cells quit jostling their brothers and sisters and invade the cervix itself.

And that, of course, is what most women who find out they have cervical dysplasia are afraid of. Although not all dysplasia progresses to cervical cancer, most doctors surgically remove or otherwise destroy the cells involved because they feel that dysplasia is the first step down the road to cancer.

But that thinking is beginning to change.

"Researchers are studying both the progression of cervical dysplasia toward cancer and its regression back to the normal state (which is far more common)," says Nancy Potischman, Ph.D., a senior staff fellow at the National Cancer Institute in Rockville, Maryland. So instead of just asking themselves "Why are these cervical changes evolving into cancer?" researchers are also asking "What blocks the cervix's return to normal?"

"Human papillomavirus (HPV), in combination with other genetic and environmental factors such as cigarette smoke, is believed to be the main cause of cervical cancer," says Dr. Potischman. But there may also be nutritional factors that affect whether dysplastic cells return to normal. Based on what she has seen so far, says Dr. Potischman, "it may be that vitamin C, vitamin E, beta-carotene and other carotenoids play parts in whether your cervix returns to normal."

What vitamins C and E and beta-carotene have in common is that they enhance immune function. They are also antioxidants, which means that they protect your body's healthy molecules by neutralizing naturally occurring unstable molecules called free radicals, which cause cellular damage by stealing electrons to balance themselves.

Antioxidant Power

Evidence that antioxidant vitamins can reverse dysplasia is impressive.

In a study at Albert Einstein College of Medicine in New York City, for example, researchers took blood samples from 43 women with cervical dysplasia and compared them with blood samples taken from women who did not have the condition. The comparison revealed that lower levels of beta-carotene and vitamin E corresponded to a significantly increased risk of cervical dysplasia.

And what really knocked the socks off the researchers was a direct correlation between the amounts of beta-carotene and vitamin E in the blood and the stage of cervical abnormality.

In other words, says study leader Prabhudas R. Palan, Ph.D., assistant professor of obstetrics and gynecology at Albert Einstein, the less beta-carotene and vitamin E in a blood sample, the more dysplasia in the cervix.

An older study of vitamin C, also done at Albert Einstein, showed similar results. In that study, researchers figured out the amount of vitamin C in the diets of 87 women with dysplasia, then compared it with the amount of vitamin C in the diets of women without dysplasia. They found that women who consumed less than 30 milligrams of vitamin C a day were ten times more likely to develop dysplasia than women who consumed more.

But will increasing your intake of antioxidants help heal dysplasia?

Perhaps, says Dr. Palan, who is conducting a study to find out. In this study, women with the condition are being given 30 milligrams (about 50,000 international units) of pure beta-carotene every day for nine months.

Food Factors

Beta-carotene, a precursor of vitamin A, is important in the prevention and treatment of cervical dysplasia. But it's not the whole story. There are other members of the carotenoid family—lycopene, lutein, zeaxanthin, beta-cryptoxanthin and alpha-carotene, for example—that may be equally important. Medical researchers say that many of these carotenoids, which are responsible for the yellow and red pigments found in foods, may have healing properties.

Advances in technology have given scientists the tools to measure these carotenoids individually. Here are some carotenoid-rich foods that may be beneficial.

Eat tomatoes. In a study conducted at Albert Einstein College of Medicine in New York City, researchers found that lycopene, a carotenoid found in tomatoes, has a direct effect on the development of cervical dysplasia. Studies are ongoing, says Prabhudas R. Palan, Ph.D., assistant professor of obstetrics and gynecology at Albert Einstein, who is leading the study. But right now it looks as though the more tomatoes you eat, the less cervical dysplasia you get.

Reach for the leafy greens. Kale, raw spinach and fresh parsley are good sources of the carotenoids lutein and zeaxanthin.

Get more fruits. Fresh papaya, tangerines and dried peaches are good sources of the carotenoid beta-cryptoxanthin.

Eat deep orange vegetables. Carrots and pumpkin are good sources of alpha-carotene.

In any event, the signs are good, since other studies have already demonstrated that a diet rich in beta-carotene, vitamin C and vitamin E can prevent cervical cancer.

In a study in four Latin American countries of 748 women with cervical cancer, for example, researchers found that women who got more than 300 milligrams of vitamin C and 6,000 micrograms (about 10,000 international units) of beta-carotene a day from fruits and fruit juices were roughly 30 percent less likely to develop cervical cancer than women who got less of these nutrients.

How beta-carotene, vitamin C and vitamin E might keep cervical dysplasia in check is still unknown, says Dr. Palan. Some researchers suspect

Prescriptions for Healing

A broad array of nutrients found in fruits, fruit juices, green, leafy vegetables and orange and red vegetables have been shown to reduce the risk of cervical dysplasia.

Some experts also recommend that you get the following nutrients from foods or supplements on a daily basis to protect your cervix.

Nutrient	Daily Amount
Beta-carotene	50,000 international units
Folic acid	400 micrograms Up to 800 micrograms for pregnant women
Vitamin C	500 milligrams
Vitamin E	100 international units

MEDICAL ALERT: *If you have been diagnosed with cervical dysplasia, you should be under a doctor's care.*

If you are taking anticoagulant drugs, you should not take vitamin E supplements.

that these nutrients enhance the ability of your immune system to fight off attackers such as HPV, which is known to increase your risk of dysplasia. Others feel that the nutrients work by increasing the amount of vitamin A available to your cells.

"We've found that the antioxidant properties are important," says Dr. Palan.

Depending on supplements alone is not the best way to guard against cervical dysplasia, says Dr. Palan. That's because the fresh fruits and vegetables rich in cervix-protecting vitamins, particularly beta-carotene, may contain other beneficial substances.

But supplements can provide added benefits to a diet that already gets five servings of fruits and vegetables a day. Many nutrition experts do recommend taking daily supplements that include 50,000 international units of beta-carotene, 500 milligrams of vitamin C and 100 international units of vitamin E.

Folic Acid Fixes

Although antioxidants such as beta-carotene, vitamin C and vitamin E clearly play pivotal roles in protecting your cervix from dysplasia, folate (the naturally occurring form of folic acid) may actually be more important.

Researchers have been studying the effects of folate on cervical dysplasia for years, yet the relationship between folate levels and dysplasia is so complex that study results have been equivocal. Some studies indicated that a low level of folate in the body increases the risk of dysplasia; others indicated that it doesn't.

But researchers have begun to suspect that these inconsistencies, frustrating as they may be, are the smoking gun that is actually pointing them in the right direction. So instead of looking just at how many women with low levels of folate have dysplasia versus how many women with high levels of folate have the condition, researchers are looking at the relationship between folate levels and risk factors such as smoking, oral contraceptives, pregnancy and HPV infection. All of these things are known to be associated with dysplasia.

In a study at the University of Alabama in Birmingham, researchers compared the amount of folate in the red blood cells of 294 women with cervical dysplasia with that of women without the condition. Then they checked with the women to see whether they smoked, used oral contraceptives, had given birth or had an HPV infection. And in each case, they found that the risk factor was more likely to be associated with dysplasia if the women had low levels of folate. Women with low levels of folate who were infected with HPV, for example, were five times more likely to develop dysplasia than women who were loaded with folate.

"Micronutrients such as folate are involved in nucleic acid synthesis and repair. And folate deficiency is a cause of chromosomal breaks," explains Tom Becker, M.D., associate professor of medicine at the University of New Mexico in Albuquerque, who is studying the nutrient. It's possible that cervical cells that have had DNA damage related to low folate levels could be further damaged by cigarette smoke by-products or an HPV infection, could become dysplastic and may not be able to repair themselves. As a result, they may very well be blocked from returning to normal and instead progress to cervical cancer.

Given that possibility, it may be more risky to be low in folate than to be low in antioxidants, says Dr. Becker. "Research suggests that a diet with plenty of cereals, fruits and green, leafy vegetables, as well as orange and red vegetables, will help prevent cervical dysplasia," he said. So there's yet another reason to learn to love those colorful veggies.

The recommended Daily Value for folic acid is 400 micrograms a day, although pregnant women should get up to twice that amount. Unfortunately, most American women get only about 236 micrograms a day.

Chronic Fatigue Syndrome

Building Energy with Nutrients

Everyone gets tired. But not everyone gets chronic fatigue syndrome (CFS).

People with this disease aren't just tired. They're constantly exhausted, not just for a few days but day in and day out for six months or longer.

And the fatigue is only the beginning. Many people with CFS also have flulike symptoms, such as sore throat, painful lymph nodes and aching muscles. Others have problems concentrating and bouts of confusion and forgetfulness. And many people with CFS have no tolerance for exercise: Imagine a woman who used to run several miles a day being so exhausted by a walk around the block that she stays in bed for the next couple of days. That's CFS.

While children and older people aren't immune, CFS is most common in younger adults. "About 90 percent of my CFS patients are between ages 25 and 50," says Paul Cheney, M.D., a CFS specialist and director of the Cheney Clinic in Charlotte, North Carolina.

Once it hits, CFS is hard to get rid of. Doctors don't know what causes CFS or how to cure it. And while many people recover on their own within a year or two, some never fully recover.

The Illness behind the Headlines

While CFS has probably been around for a long time, it wasn't until the mid-1980s that a mysterious flulike illness that hit mostly young professional women made headlines. Nicknamed the yuppie flu, it was often written off as burnout or depression. Many people who had CFS looked so healthy that they were told that their symptoms were "all in their heads."

Today most doctors are familiar with CFS, but they still have a hard time diagnosing it. Symptoms vary widely from person to person and often resemble the flu, mononucleosis or depression. And because no one knows what causes CFS, medical science has not yet developed a definitive test that can prove whether a person has it. In the 1980s, some researchers believed CFS, like mononucleosis, was caused by the Epstein-Barr virus; while that theory has been rejected, some experts still suspect that a virus may play a role.

These days, most experts consider CFS an immune activation (autoimmune) disorder similar in some respects to lupus and rheumatoid arthritis. In immune activation disorders, the immune system is so cranked up to defend the body against invaders that it actually attacks the body's own tissues. Doctors also see a high incidence of allergies among people with CFS, another sign that their immune systems tend to overreact.

CFS resembles other immune activation disorders in another way: A disproportionate share of people with CFS—probably around 75 percent—are women, says Dr. Cheney. "It could be that women's immune systems are just stronger than men's," he says. "This is an advantage early in life, when girl infants die less often of infections than boys do. But that strong immune system makes a woman more likely to suffer from immune activation disorders in adulthood."

Like most aspects of this mysterious disease, the reasons that women are more susceptible are subject to much debate. But one thing doctors do agree on is that CFS isn't all in the patient's head. Today CFS is widely regarded as a physical illness, not a mental one.

Getting the Big Picture

No one knows for sure how many people have CFS. The Centers for Disease Control and Prevention (CDC) in Atlanta estimates that 100,000 to 250,000 Americans have seen their doctors for it. But since the CDC uses a very strict definition of the disease in gathering these statistics—unless an individual has the right number and combination of symptoms, the case isn't reported as CFS—many researchers believe the disease is far more common than the figures indicate.

A study of 3,400 nurses from around the country found that while only 11 met the CDC criteria, 23 believed they had CFS. "We chose nurses because presumably they would be more familiar with CFS than the general population and better able to judge whether they have it," says Leonard

Food Factors

When it comes to battling chronic fatigue syndrome (CFS), supplements are only part of the picture. Medical experts agree that the overall quality of your diet also makes a big difference in how you feel. Here are a few dietary changes that might prove helpful.

Go easy on sugar. "Eating too much refined sugar weakens the immune system and may inhibit the ability of white blood cells to stay active," says Allan Magaziner, D.O., director of the Magaziner Medical Center in Cherry Hill, New Jersey. "Both of those factors play roles in CFS."

Some research suggests that people with CFS are deficient in an enzyme needed to metabolize sugar, says Paul Cheney, M.D., a CFS specialist and director of the Cheney Clinic in Charlotte, North Carolina. The result is a buildup of lactic acid in the bloodstream, which can lead to muscle pain, vascular headaches and neuropsychiatric disorders such as panic attacks, all of which are associated with CFS.

"We recommend avoiding sugar as much as possible, but if you're going to have an indiscretion, have dessert after a meal instead of eating something sweet on an empty stomach," says Dr. Cheney. "That slows down the absorption of the sugar, so you don't get a sharp elevation in lactic acid."

Don't depend on caffeine. When you're exhausted all of the time, there's a great temptation to depend on caffeine to make you more alert. "But it's also important to avoid or cut back on foods that may cause loss of minerals. Caffeine is one example," says Dr. Magaziner.

Jason, Ph.D., professor of psychology at DePaul University in Chicago, who conducted the study.

In another study of the general population, 0.2 percent were found to have CFS. Based on these results, Dr. Jason estimates that about 387,000 American adults have CFS.

While no one has found a cure for CFS, dietary changes and nutritional supplements can help to strengthen the immune system, improve energy levels and ease some of the symptoms of CFS, says Allan Magaziner, D.O., director of the Magaziner Medical Center in Cherry Hill, New Jersey. Dr.

Trim the fat. By now just about everyone has gotten the message that a low-fat diet is essential for overall health. This advice takes on new importance for the person with CFS, since fatty foods are difficult to digest and can cause a general sluggish feeling, the last thing a person with CFS needs. "There's also some evidence that too much fat in the diet can have an adverse effect on immunity," says Dr. Magaziner.

Eat healthy. The optimum diet for a person with CFS is the same as for anyone who's aiming for optimum health: high in fiber and complex carbohydrates, with lots of fruits, vegetables, beans and whole grains. Dr. Magaziner also tells people with CFS to avoid processed foods, which are often full of additives, preservatives and artificial colorings and flavorings.

Get tested for food allergies. People with CFS are particularly prone to food allergies and often improve significantly when the allergies are detected and treated, says Dr. Cheney. "It seems to be a combination of difficulty digesting protein and increased gut permeability," he says. In other words, he explains, often the intestines of a person with CFS absorb substances from foods that would pass right through the digestive tract in a healthy person.

Dr. Cheney treats the problem with enzymes to improve protein digestion and, in extreme cases, by eliminating the foods that cause the most problems. "Generally speaking, red meat, wheat and dairy seem to be the most problematic," says Dr. Cheney.

If you suspect that food allergies are making your symptoms worse, discuss the problem with your physician.

Magaziner has been treating people with CFS for more than ten years.

"Of course, taking a supplement isn't going to cure CFS," he cautions. "People need to understand that they also have to eat right, exercise appropriately and work with a physician who's knowledgeable about CFS."

Muscling Up with Magnesium

Some people with CFS have benefited from taking supplements of magnesium, a mineral that is involved in the cells' energy production.

One British study found that people with CFS had below-normal blood levels of magnesium. After receiving injections of magnesium, 80 percent reported improvement in their symptoms.

But even if their blood tests don't show magnesium deficiencies, people can still benefit from extra doses of the mineral, according to Dr. Cheney. "Their blood levels of magnesium may be normal, but that doesn't tell the whole story," he says. "Magnesium, like potassium, is pumped into the cell, so normally there's a higher concentration inside the cell than there is in the blood. And that pump mechanism may not work very well in people with CFS, so their magnesium levels can be normal in the blood and low in the cell."

Dr. Magaziner also finds that most people with CFS notice improvement in their symptoms after starting magnesium supplements. "It doesn't work for everyone," he says. "But many of my patients find it eases their muscle aches and makes them feel less fatigued."

This is probably because people with CFS have enzyme deficiencies that hamper the cells' ability to convert food into energy, according to Dr. Cheney. And extra magnesium improves enzyme function, which results in greater energy production on the cellular level.

If you're interested in trying magnesium, Dr. Magaziner recommends starting with 500 milligrams a day. "This level is perfectly safe, although occasionally a person will develop loose bowels or diarrhea," he says. "If that happens, I would simply reduce the dose to the point where the diarrhea goes away." If you have heart or kidney problems, however, you should check with your doctor before taking magnesium supplements.

Dr. Cheney recommends a chelated form of magnesium called magnesium glycinate. "It's rapidly absorbed in the gastrointestinal tract, so it doesn't cause digestive problems," he explains. "And it tends to be drawn into the cell, where it's needed."

And because taking more magnesium increases the body's need for calcium, Dr. Magaziner suggests taking calcium supplements as well. "I usually recommend taking them in a two-to-one ratio—1,000 milligrams of calcium if you're taking 500 milligrams of magnesium," he advises.

A Boost from B-Complex

The B-complex vitamins help support the adrenal glands, which are among the major organs in the body connected with stress, says Dr. Magaziner. "B vitamins also support the central nervous system, to help us cope with stress in general," he explains. "We lose a lot of B vitamins when we're

Fighting Back with Coenzyme Q_{10}

Coenzyme Q_{10} sounds like something that might be prescribed in sick bay on *Star Trek*. But for those doing daily battle with chronic fatigue syndrome (CFS), they just might hear about it from their doctors, according to Paul Cheney, M.D., a CFS specialist and director of the Cheney Clinic in Charlotte, North Carolina.

Coenzyme Q_{10} is available in supplement form in drugstores and health food stores. This little-known nutrient isn't exactly a vitamin, although its chemical makeup is similar to that of vitamins E and K. Experts believe that like vitamin K, coenzyme Q_{10} can be manufactured by the body, though it's also found in soybeans, vegetable oils and many meats.

Like vitamins C and E and beta-carotene, coenzyme Q_{10} is a member of the antioxidant family, a group of nutrients that protect your body's tissues from everyday wear and tear by disarming destructive free radicals. Free radicals are unstable molecules that wreak havoc at the cellular level by stealing electrons from your body's healthy molecules to balance themselves.

Besides being a potent antioxidant, coenzyme Q_{10} has an important function in energy production: It reacts with another enzyme to let cells convert protein, fat and carbohydrates into energy.

While people with CFS aren't deficient in coenzyme Q_{10}, they seem to have functional shortages of the enzyme it reacts with, explains Dr. Cheney. Taking extra coenzyme Q_{10} prompts the body to improve the function of this partner enzyme. And the better the partner enzyme works, the better the body's ability to convert food into energy.

Dr. Cheney prescribes large doses of coenzyme Q_{10} for his patients, who are under his close medical supervision. For people with CFS who'd like to try coenzyme Q_{10} on their own, he recommends a daily dose of 200 milligrams, taken in divided doses under the tongue. And since this nutrient is fat-soluble, it should be taken with a little bit of fat or oil (although some supplements are in an oil base, similar to vitamin E capsules).

stressed, so we need to replenish them." These nutrients are also involved in energy production, which makes them essential for people with CFS.

Dr. Magaziner recommends a supplement containing the entire B-complex. Thiamin, pantothenic acid and vitamins B_6 and B_{12} are especially important for people with CFS, he says.

You can get the B-complex vitamins in most multivitamin/mineral supplements, says Dr. Cheney. Check the label to make sure the supplement contains at least 50 milligrams each of thiamin, pantothenic acid and vitamin B_6 and 50 micrograms of vitamin B_{12}. He also recommends taking a separate B-complex supplement whenever you're under stress.

Higher doses of vitamin B_{12}, given through injection by a physician, can also be helpful in cases of enzyme deficiency, says Dr. Cheney. Injected B_{12} doses may be 1,000 times higher than the normal daily dose.

Arm Yourself with Antioxidants

Also helpful in treating CFS are the so-called antioxidant nutrients, which include vitamin C, vitamin E, beta-carotene and the mineral selenium.

These nutrients form a veritable SWAT team that helps defend your cells against free radicals, unstable molecules that occur naturally in the body and that are also produced by bad habits such as smoking, sunbathing and drinking alcohol. Free radicals steal electrons from your body's healthy molecules to balance themselves, damaging cells in the process. Antioxidants neutralize free radicals by offering their own electrons, protecting healthy molecules from harm.

"Antioxidants protect the body from deterioration, degeneration and environmental stresses," says Dr. Magaziner. "And since many people with CFS are unusually sensitive to environmental factors such as household chemicals, food additives and artificial fragrances, taking antioxidants makes sense."

Damage from free radicals is such an important factor in CFS that some researchers consider CFS a free radical–generated disease, says Dr. Cheney. "I don't think it's caused by free radical damage, but that seems to be one of the factors that maintains it," he says.

To help bolster the immune system and improve stamina, both doctors recommend an antioxidant-complex supplement, available in most drugstores and health food stores. Because dosage varies widely from brand to brand, read the label to make sure you're getting at least 500 milligrams of vitamin C, 25,000 international units of beta-carotene, 400 international units of vitamin E and 50 micrograms of selenium.

People with CFS may also want to try a vitamin C supplement in the form of ester-C, says Dr. Cheney. "Ester-C is much more bioavailable than

Prescriptions for Healing

Nutrients can play roles in treating chronic fatigue syndrome. Here's what some doctors recommend.

Nutrient	Daily Amount
Antioxidant-complex supplement containing . . .	
Beta-carotene	25,000 international units
Selenium	50 micrograms
Vitamin C	500 milligrams
Vitamin E	400 international units
B-complex supplement containing . . .	
Pantothenic acid	50 milligrams
Thiamin	50 milligrams
Vitamin B_6	50 milligrams
Vitamin B_{12}	50 micrograms
Calcium	1,000 milligrams (2 milligrams for every 1 milligram of magnesium)
Magnesium	500 milligrams (magnesium glycinate)
Vitamin C	4,000 milligrams (ester-C), taken as 2 divided doses

MEDICAL ALERT: *If you have been diagnosed with chronic fatigue syndrome, you should be under a doctor's care.*

If you are taking anticoagulants, you should not take vitamin E supplements.

If you have heart or kidney problems, you should always check with your doctor before taking magnesium supplements.

Doses of vitamin C in excess of 1,200 milligrams a day can cause diarrhea in some people, so it's a good idea to check with your doctor before taking more than that amount.

regular vitamin C," he explains. "Your body absorbs twice as much. People with CFS can take 2,000 milligrams of ester-C twice a day; it's very safe." Taking more than 1,200 milligrams of vitamin C can cause diarrhea in some people, however, so it's a good idea to check with your doctor before exceeding that amount. Ester-C is available in health food stores.

Colds

Common Nutrients for a Common Condition

A phlegm-filled cough. Nose blowing that rivals any air horn blast. Sneezes so severe that even good china in the next room isn't safe.

All of these, of course, are cold symptoms. But experts think that they're also cold senders, launching tiny droplets of mucus into the air with every wheeze, hack and honk.

Inside these specks of mucus are soccer ball–shaped organisms called rhinoviruses, so tiny that 15,000 lined up side by side would barely span the space between two words on this page. Whether carried on a finger as you scratch your nose or inhaled through your nose or mouth, some of these malevolent microbes may eventually get the break they're looking for: the chance to get inside your body.

It's all downhill from there, literally. The wavelike downward motion of the tiny hairlike projections that line your throat pushes the virus as well as your normal throat mucus toward your esophagus. If you're fortunate, powerful digestive acids destroy the virus before it can do any harm.

When you do become infected, however, the virus's cold-producing plan begins to unfold. Finding a warm spot in your throat where your own mucus layer is thin and offers little protection, a single virus attaches itself to a cell and commandeers the cell's own replicating capability. Office copiers should work so well: Within a few hours, over 100,000 viruses are created. "That's the reason therapy is so difficult," says Elliot Dick, Ph.D., professor of preventive medicine and chief of the respiratory virus research laboratory at the University of Wisconsin–Madison and one of the country's leading cold researchers. "Viruses essentially become part of us, part of our cells."

And all of that awful sneezing, snorting and coughing? That's called the host response, your body's way of fighting this unwanted guest from within. Before long, white blood cells, the avenging angels of your immune system,

Food Factors

These dietary tips may help you keep your cold under control.

Get souped up. Chalk up another one for Dr. Mom. Researchers at Mount Sinai Medical Center in Miami Beach have found that hot chicken soup apparently increases the flow of mucus. Although researchers aren't sure whether it's the aroma or the taste, they say chicken soup helps make your nose run, which shortens the amount of time cold germs spend inside your nose. In a test, hot chicken soup worked better than hot water alone.

Historians say chicken soup was first recommended for colds 800 years ago by Maimonides, court physician to Saladin, the caliph of Egypt.

Drink plenty of fluids. The next time you come down with a cold, you can help banish that pesky virus to a digestive grave by drinking lots of liquids. When the mucus that lines your throat is moist, it traps viruses and sends them down to the stomach, where powerful digestive acids destroy them. Normally six to eight cups of water, milk, juice, lemonade or soup a day is enough to meet your liquid quota, but you can easily lose a quart or more of fluids a day when you're sick. The recommendation: Double your fluids. And avoid alcohol, which depletes your body of immune-boosting nutrients and causes dehydration.

Grab some garlic. Long championed by garlic-lovers for fighting off colds, the odorous bulb is gaining new respect in, of all places, the laboratory. Studies with laboratory animals showed that garlic actually helps protect them from flu viruses while boosting their production of immune system antibodies. And preliminary studies showed that people who ate garlic for three weeks had enhanced immune system activity.

Turn up the heat. Spicy foods containing hot peppers, curry and chili powder get your mucus flowing, which can help unplug your nose and make your cough more productive, experts say.

are rushed to the scene of the infection to kill the cells containing the virus. That influx of blood causes swelling in the sinuses. Stepped-up mucus production designed to trap the virus makes for a running nose and eventually a hacking cough.

Chances are, though, that the battle won't be won for another seven days, the average length of the dreaded common cold. Is there anything you can do to put a stop to all of this mayhem? You could take vitamin C.

What Research Says about Vitamin C

Taking vitamin C to treat a cold is about as common as . . . well, the common cold.

And yet the controversy over its effectiveness continues, with the general public serving as its strongest advocate.

Ever since the late Linus Pauling, Ph.D., shocked the medical community with his book *Vitamin C and the Common Cold*, doctors have debated the merits of his recommendations. Among them: taking 500 to 1,000 milligrams of vitamin C every hour for several hours to reduce the length and severity of a cold. Dr. Pauling certainly walked his talk: For six years prior to his death at age 93, the two-time winner of the Nobel prize reportedly took 12,000 milligrams of vitamin C a day.

Dozens of studies of varying professionalism and reliability followed Dr. Pauling's pronouncements, with mixed results. At last count, roughly half supported his megadose claim. The others, testing much lower doses, showed that vitamin C is of little help in ending a cold in progress.

And that is precisely what vitamin C advocates have claimed all along: If

Prescriptions for Healing

Some doctors recommend taking these nutrients to help banish cold symptoms.

Nutrient	Daily Amount
Vitamin C	2,000 milligrams, taken as 4 divided doses
Zinc gluconate	24 milligrams, dissolved in your mouth every 2 hours (up to 8 lozenges a day)

MEDICAL ALERT: *Doses of vitamin C larger than 1,200 milligrams a day can cause diarrhea in some people.*

you're going to take vitamin C for a cold, you have to take a lot. In fact, a review conducted by a British researcher found that all of the studies done since 1970 in which people were taking 1,000 milligrams or more of vitamin C a day to reduce the symptoms of their colds showed positive results, including a 72 percent reduction in the duration of cold symptoms.

Vitamin C Primes Your Defenses

One study, conducted by Dr. Dick and his colleagues at the University of Wisconsin–Madison, even showed that taking vitamin C before you get a cold can be helpful.

His research team found a way to study the spread of the common cold up close. They gathered a roomful of male volunteers, placed tiny amounts of cold virus directly in the nostrils of 8 and then watched the contagion spread to the other 12 as the men sneezed, coughed and blew their noses. Along with poker chips and playing cards, they passed cold viruses to each other. Within a week, almost without fail, Dr. Dick says, every man in the virus-filled, windowless room had a cold.

In three separate studies, Dr. Dick didn't just try to get the men sick. He also experimented with vitamin C to see if it offered any protection.

In each study, half of the men were given 500-milligram doses of vitamin C at breakfast, lunch and dinner and before bed each day, for a total of 2,000 milligrams of vitamin C a day. The rest got placebos (look-alike dummy pills). "Unlike other studies, we didn't have to trust whether they were going to take the vitamin C," says Dr. Dick. "We actually gave it to them. Either they came up to the lab or we went around to where they were housed and gave it to them with a little glass of water."

The pretreatment continued for 3½ weeks; then the poker games began. All of the men caught colds even though they maintained their 2,000-milligram-a-day vitamin C intakes. The study results, however, showed that vitamin C was helpful in weakening their colds' effects.

"We found during those experiments that the vitamin C greatly reduced symptoms of a cold," says Dr. Dick. "The length was a little shorter, but that wasn't the main thing. The main thing was that those who took vitamin C just weren't very ill, while some of the others got real humdingers of a cold."

In fact, only 1 person in the entire vitamin C–taking group came down with a full-fledged cold, while 16 in the placebo group had moderate or severe colds, Dr. Dick says.

So what is it about vitamin C that seems to make it useful for fighting colds?

Your immune system contains a number of natural defenders that spring into action at the first sign of an invading microorganism such as a cold virus. Among them are white blood cells. When your vitamin C levels are high, your white blood cells are apparently reinvigorated, giving them more of the energy they need to neutralize the virus, explains Dr. Dick. "The best experimentation that I've seen suggests vitamin C is in some way or another stimulating the white blood cells to function better," he says. "They attack the infected cell, gather around it, destroy it and then clean up."

And what about the skeptics? "Our results are nice and positive, and a lot of other people's results aren't nice and positive," says Dr. Dick. "But nobody has looked at it in the fashion that we have."

Once a skeptic himself, Dr. Dick now takes 2,000 milligrams of vitamin C an hour for three hours at the first sign of cold symptoms. "Usually the cold is gone by then, but if not, I'll take 1,000 milligrams an hour until it is," says Dr. Dick. "I thought it was a bunch of foolishness, too. Not anymore."

The Daily Value for vitamin C is only 60 milligrams. Doses larger than 1,200 milligrams a day can cause diarrhea in some people.

Zinc: Another Cold Controversy

Long appreciated for its immune-boosting power, zinc attracted considerable attention in the 1980s as a cold remedy, and in a remarkable way.

George Eby of Austin, Texas, observed a three-year-old girl who suffered repeated severe colds. He reported giving her a 50-milligram zinc gluconate tablet at the start of one of her colds in a bid to boost her immune system.

But she refused to swallow the tablet, instead dissolving it in her mouth. Her symptoms were gone within a few hours, far faster than usual. After observing zinc's cold-stopping effect several more times, Eby wondered whether sucking, not swallowing, zinc might actually be the long-sought cure for the common cold.

Eby conducted a scientific study to see if he was on to something. Published in a medical journal, the results of the study were promising. Those who took plain, awful-tasting zinc gluconate tablets reported that their symptoms were gone after an average of 4 days, while those taking better-tasting placebos said that their colds lasted an average of 11 days.

"The results seemed very significant. But the problem was that the zinc gluconate tasted so bad, there was some concern that people had reported their colds were over just because they didn't want to take this awful-tasting stuff anymore," says John C. Godfrey, Ph.D., a medicinal chemist and president of Godfrey Science and Design, a food supplement consulting service based in Huntingdon Valley, Pennsylvania.

In their haste to develop a tastier zinc gluconate cold lozenge, some researchers mixed in additives that apparently rendered the cold-stopping merits of zinc gluconate inactive. "You can take zinc gluconate and add citric acid to it, which is what one pharmaceutical company did, to make something that tastes acceptable. It really does wipe out the nauseating flavor of zinc, but it also inactivates the zinc," says Dr. Godfrey.

Tinkering in his own kitchen with ingredients that he had purchased in a local health food store, Dr. Godfrey combined zinc gluconate and glycine into a lozenge that tasted pretty good to his family—and also seemed to knock out their colds.

"I noticed, and my family reported to me, that when they had colds, as soon as they put one of these lozenges in their mouths, their symptoms disappeared," he says. "It was very dramatic. You would be all stuffed up and sneezing, with a sore throat, and you would put one of these in your mouth, and then you'd actually be getting relief. You could actually hear little crackling noises in your sinuses as they opened up. The postnasal drip is rapidly reduced. Sneezing is not totally wiped out, but it goes way down."

Watching your family get better hardly constitutes a scientific study. Dr. Godfrey followed up his observations, however, with a study conducted at the Dartmouth College Health Service in Lebanon, New Hampshire. Researchers divided 73 college students into two groups: those who were given zinc gluconate and glycine lozenges and those who took similar-tasting placebos. The students were told to suck on the lozenges at two-hour intervals and to take up to eight lozenges a day. Each lozenge contained roughly 24 milligrams of zinc. (The Daily Value for zinc is 15 milligrams.)

Researchers discovered that those students who started taking the zinc gluconate lozenges 1 day after they first felt ill suffered from their colds for only 4.3 days. Those who took placebos suffered for 9.2 days. "Cough, nasal drainage and congestion were the symptoms most improved," says Dr. Godfrey. "That was an indication that the earlier and more vigorously you treat a cold, the better the result will be. That's where our research since then has been focused."

And what is it about zinc gluconate that causes the improvement? There are at least two theories. The unique shape of the rhinovirus that helps it hook into your cells also fits the active ingredient in zinc perfectly, almost like a bag over a bowling ball. "The geometry fits very neatly," says Dr. Godfrey.

Another possibility: Zinc gluconate concentrations in your mouth may literally short-circuit the nerve in your nose that's responsible for sneezes and other symptoms, says Dr. Godfrey.

Will Dr. Godfrey's results end the great zinc debate? Maybe not. Plain zinc gluconate tastes awful, and just swallowing it isn't enough to treat a cold. You have to suck on zinc gluconate to get its symptom-banishing effects. Stomach discomfort is an occasional side effect that can usually be avoided by eating something first; even a cracker will do, says Dr. Godfrey.

If you're looking for zinc lozenges in a pharmacy or health food store, here's what you need to know: Steer clear of zinc lozenges that are combined with citrate, tartrate, orotate or mannitol/sorbitol. They may taste good, but the cold-stopping capabilities of the zinc are completely inactivated, according to Dr. Godfrey. In addition to its bad taste, plain zinc gluconate can cause mouth soreness, but it will do the job. The pleasant-tasting, clinically proven zinc gluconate with glycine is available through the Quigley Corporation, P.O. Box, 1349, Doylestown, PA 18901. No matter which form you choose, a general treatment regimen is one 24-milligram lozenge dissolved in your mouth every two hours (up to eight lozenges a day) to help relieve cold symptoms.

Are zinc lozenges worth taking? "I guess it depends on how you look at a cold," says John H. Turco, Ph.D., director of the Dartmouth College Health Service. "Some people feel like a cold isn't a tremendous setback. But obviously, if you can get rid of some of the symptoms, it's probably worth it."

Cold Sores

Restoring Kissable Lips

Rumor has it that when Michelle Pfeiffer got one during the filming of *The Witches of Eastwick*, the directors didn't stop filming or have it covered up, because it added depth to her character. Unfortunately, for those of us not playing a distressed beauty on the silver screen, the only thing cold sores add to our character is dismay.

They may also make us cranky, of course, because cold sores aren't only unsightly, they're also downright painful. A cold sore announces its arrival with a burning and tingling sensation. Then come the blisters, little pus-filled bumps that often run together to form one big blister that oozes, itches, burns and crusts over before disappearing seven to ten days later. It's hardly glamorous.

To make matters worse, a cold sore (also called a fever blister) is rarely a once-and-done occurrence. Cold sores are usually caused by the herpes sim-

Food Factors

Since the herpes simplex virus often waits until you're stressed out or falling ill to strike, doctors say that keeping your cool and eating a nutritious diet to stay healthy are always good deterrents. Also, some experts have found that certain foods may actually prevent or trigger outbreaks. Here's what they recommend.

Love lysine. Lysine is an amino acid that suppresses the growth of the herpes simplex virus and therefore limits the number of outbreaks, says Craig Zunka, D.D.S., past president of the Holistic Dental Association and a dentist in Front Royal, Virginia.

You can boost your lysine intake by eating potatoes, milk, brewer's yeast, fish, chicken and beans. Since the optimum dose to prevent herpes outbreaks may be higher than the amount you can get from foods, however, some doctors also recommend supplements.

"I recommend taking one or two 500-milligram supplements a day, depending on the severity of the case," says Dr. Zunka. Lysine supplements are available in health food stores.

Go easy on arginine. The flip side of lysine is arginine, an amino acid found in foods such as chocolate, peas, cereals, peanuts, beer, gelatin and raisins. The herpes virus apparently needs a certain amount of arginine to grow. You might try limiting these foods in general and eliminating them during an outbreak, suggests Dr. Zunka.

plex virus. Once you've been exposed to the virus, you have a "friend" for life. Luckily, it keeps a low profile most of the time, but various activating factors, such as stress, fever, trauma and exposure to sunlight, can make it rear its ugly head. It also doesn't limit itself to your lips. Herpes type 1 blisters (type 2 blisters are the ones that affect the genitals) can strike inside the mouth as well as the nostrils, the fingers and even the eyelids.

Fortunately, as bad as the cold sore virus can be, you don't have to be completely at the mercy of this blistering beast. By controlling stress and using sunscreen, you can help prevent cold sores, says Craig Zunka, D.D.S., past president of the Holistic Dental Association and a dentist in Front Royal, Virginia. And, say doctors, over-the-counter ointments containing zinc oxide can speed the healing of the cold sores that do occur.

Some doctors have also found nutritional strategies that, though they

Prescriptions for Healing

If recurrent cold sores have your lips in their grip, some oral health experts suggest that you might find relief from these nutrients.

Nutrient	Daily Amount/Application
Oral	
Vitamin C	1,000 milligrams, taken at the first sign of an outbreak; then 1,500 milligrams, taken as 3 divided doses for 1 or 2 days
Topical	
Vitamin E	Oil from 1 capsule, applied directly to the sore
Zinc oxide	As an ingredient in an over-the-counter ointment

MEDICAL ALERT: *Some people may experience diarrhea when taking more than 1,200 milligrams of vitamin C a day.*

aren't clinically proven, may ward off herpes outbreaks as well as speed up their departure. Here's what these doctors recommend.

Nip 'Em with Vitamin C

You may be able to stop a cold sore before it appears by zapping it with a high dose of vitamin C at the first tingle, say the experts.

"As soon as you start to feel the burning and tingling of a cold sore coming on, take vitamin C with bioflavonoids. The two together inhibit the progression of the virus," says Dr. Zunka. He recommends taking 1,000 milligrams of both vitamin C and bioflavonoids as soon as you feel the tingling, then 500 milligrams of each three times a day for the next day or two. (Bioflavonoids are chemical compounds related to vitamin C. Some vitamin C supplements contain them, but bioflavonoids are also available as a supplement alone.)

"I've also seen people have dramatic reductions in the number of cold sores they get each year just by substituting vitamin C with bioflavonoids for the vitamin C supplements they usually take," adds Dr. Zunka. "Then if you still start to get a cold sore, just take the high-dose regimen in addition to your regular supplement." Some people may experience diarrhea when taking more than 1,200 milligrams of vitamin C a day.

You can also introduce more vitamin C and bioflavonoids into your daily diet by eating fruits (especially citrus), vegetables, nuts and seeds.

Zap It with Zinc

Once a cold sore has made its not-so-grand appearance, you can dry it up and heal it more quickly by applying a dollop of an ointment containing zinc oxide directly to the sore, suggest some experts.

If a cold sore is really getting under your skin, you might consider asking your doctor or dentist about getting a shot of protamine zinc, a protein-zinc compound, says Dr. Zunka.

"I use it all the time for healing lesions in the mouth," he says. "You just inject a small amount at the site of the herpes sore, and it clears up the sore very quickly. Zinc is known for reducing healing time up to 30 or 40 percent."

Add a Dash of Vitamin E

Finally, some doctors have found that the topical application of vitamin E can also take the bite out of a painful cold sore. To try this treatment, just crack open a vitamin E capsule and apply the oil directly to the blister, says Dr. Zunka.

Note: If the cold sore is on or around your eyes, see a doctor before applying any topical treatment.

Cystic Fibrosis

Nutrition Makes the Difference

When jubilant researchers announced at a news conference that they had found the gene responsible for cystic fibrosis, an inherited disease that begins to clog the lungs with a thick, life-threatening mucus in early childhood, the news sent a shock wave of excitement throughout the dozens of cystic fibrosis centers across the nation.

Food Factors

Some of the dietary recommendations suitable for the general population may be downright harmful for people with cystic fibrosis.

"Everything is reversed," explains Donna Mueller, R.D., Ph.D., associate professor of nutrition and foods at Drexel University in Philadelphia. "Good nutrition in cystic fibrosis can sometimes appear to be the antithesis of how we were taught."

In fact, says Dr. Mueller, "we tell patients that going to fast-food restaurants is great, because the food is high-fat, high-sodium and high-protein!"

Here are some other "radical" recommendations for those with cystic fibrosis.

Pig out. "Eat lots of calories," says Dr. Mueller. Cystic fibrosis demands a lot of metabolic energy. And the only way to get it is to fill yourself with high-calorie foods. Go light on salads, which have few calories, and instead reach for calorie-dense foods such as hamburgers, milk shakes and cheesecake.

Eat foods with fat. "People with cystic fibrosis need fat," says Dr. Mueller. "It would be great if instead of trying to eat 30 percent or less of calories from fat, people with cystic fibrosis would eat 30 percent or more of calories from fat."

Put an extra dollop of butter or margarine on breads, vegetables, pastas, potatoes and rice. Add whipped cream to desserts, coffee and hot chocolate. Top fruit and baked potatoes with sour cream. Use meat gravies and fat-based sauces. On those salads, use real oils, not

It might take another decade of work to figure out how to repair the gene, the researchers concluded, but clearly, a cure is at hand.

"Everybody who is working with cystic fibrosis children and their families today does it with a different sense of hope than we had a few years ago," says Virginia Stallings, M.D., nutrition chief at the University of Pennsylvania's Children's Hospital of Philadelphia. "This used to be thought of as a fatal disease. Now we know that the more years we can add to the window of excellent health, the better the chance at one of the new therapies."

And some experts believe that nutrition is a big part of getting that opportunity.

the low-fat dressings; oils have more vitamin E, too. And there's no need to avoid pizza!

Avoid fried foods. Even though high-fat foods are great, don't try to get more fat into your diet by eating greasy fried foods, says Dr. Mueller. Fried foods require more bile, which helps keep that extra fat isolated so that digestive enzymes can work on the food. And bile is in short supply in those with cystic fibrosis.

Salt foods. "When people have cystic fibrosis, the sweat glands are also impaired," says Dr. Mueller. "Instead of being reabsorbed, which is what happens for most of us when we sweat, the sodium and chloride just come out and stay on the skin. That's why people with cystic fibrosis have to supplement their diets with salty foods or salt. Never use salt tablets, though. They are much too concentrated."

The amount? "About one-quarter to one teaspoon (1,375 to 5,500 milligrams) a day, depending on what kinds of foods are eaten," replies Dr. Mueller.

That means babies, too, she adds. "When parents are advised 'Add salt to the baby food,' they just stare at us. Again, it appears to be the antithesis of good nutrition. But each person truly has individual needs, and baby foods no longer have salt added to them."

Drink lots of water. "People with cystic fibrosis should be taking in around two quarts of water daily, plus what's in the foods they eat," says Dr. Mueller. The excess loss of salt as they sweat causes them to dehydrate easily, particularly in hot weather.

Starving in a Land of Plenty

Fifteen years ago, most children born with cystic fibrosis never made it to adulthood. The thick mucus produced by their secretion glands blocked their airways, clogged their digestive tracts and encouraged the growth of bacteria that led to frequent life-threatening infections in their lungs.

Today at least half of these children grow up and make it into their thirties and beyond. And as women with the disease begin to live longer, healthier lives, some are even becoming pregnant, a landmark that is sending waves of both ecstasy and concern into a medical community that must now learn how to help them.

The problem is that anyone who has cystic fibrosis has a lot of trouble getting just the basic nutrients to sustain herself, much less enough to provide for another life.

In healthy people, mucus in the digestive tract is slippery and light, so food can easily slide along the digestive tract and nutrients can pass from digested food through the intestinal wall, into the bloodstream and on to the rest of the body, explains Donna Mueller, R.D., Ph.D., associate professor of nutrition and foods at Drexel University in Philadelphia. But in people with cystic fibrosis, the digestive tract is covered with such thick mucus that many, if not most, nutrients can't get through the intestinal wall and into the bloodstream. That's why people with cystic fibrosis are frequently at risk for malnutrition. They are literally starving in a land of plenty.

Complicating the situation is the fact that the pancreas, which produces enzymes that help your body digest protein, fat and carbohydrates, is also affected by the thick mucus. "The enzymes produced in the pancreas's cells leave the pancreas through little canals that empty out into the small intestine," explains Dr. Mueller. But the canals get so clogged with mucus that most enzymes never reach the food. So most of the food eaten by someone with cystic fibrosis is simply not digested.

"Some nutrients are going to get through," says Dr. Mueller. "But this condition is a walking textbook on nutrition, because every nutrient is affected: protein, fat, carbohydrates, vitamins and minerals."

Meeting the Body's Increasing Demands

Unfortunately, just as the body is least likely to get the nutrients it requires, its need for those nutrients will increase by 20 percent or more.

This is a chronic, progressive disease that hits the airways particularly hard, explains Dr. Mueller. The lungs degenerate. People get sicker and sicker while their bodies work harder and harder. That's why nutrition is always important. As the lungs become more involved, the body is working harder, and energy requirements increase.

"Unfortunately, when someone doesn't feel well, one doesn't feel like eating, either," says Dr. Mueller. "So just when there are greater body needs, there's less of an appetite."

But tough as it is for adults with cystic fibrosis to meet their daily nutritional needs, children with cystic fibrosis also have to meet the demands of growing bodies.

"You know the growth charts doctors use?" asks Dr. Stallings. Children

Prescriptions for Healing

To keep the body as strong as possible while new gene therapies are under development, a person with cystic fibrosis is encouraged to eat a well-balanced diet and to take specially prepared supplemental pancreatic digestive enzymes (these break down food so nutrients can be better absorbed) and an over-the-counter balanced multivitamin/mineral supplement that provides the Recommended Dietary Allowances plus other vitamin and mineral supplements based on individualized blood tests and in consultation with a cystic fibrosis nutrition specialist, says Donna Mueller, R.D., Ph.D., associate professor of nutrition and foods at Drexel University in Philadelphia. For example, vitamin K may be added if someone is also on antibiotics or has liver disease.

MEDICAL ALERT: *Anyone who has cystic fibrosis should be taking vitamin and mineral supplements only after discussing it with his physician.*

with cystic fibrosis are often at the bottom, somewhere around the tenth percentile, she says. That means that 90 percent of everybody else their age is bigger. That's why the goal of most doctors, including Dr. Stallings, is to give kids the nutritional support they need to grow as big as their brothers and sisters and to get them through these growth phases so they go into adulthood as strong and as well-nourished as possible.

On average, Dr. Stallings is successful. "We have a little trouble with adolescent girls because of the body image issues in our society," says Dr. Stallings. With all of the cultural emphasis on thinness as an ideal, "they don't mind being the skinniest kids in class," she says. "But of course, that may be harmful to their health."

Winning with Prevention Power

Once children have completed their adolescent growth spurts, doctors and nutritionists generally breathe a sigh of relief. But only for a moment. They still need to help the adults with cystic fibrosis store up enough nutritional support to withstand the frequent infections associated with the disease without losing ground.

To help meet the nutritional demands of their bodies, most people with cystic fibrosis are encouraged to eat a well-balanced diet and—after very careful personal evaluation by their doctors and nutritionists—to take specially prepared supplemental pancreatic digestive enzymes and a general multivitamin/mineral supplement plus other vitamins and minerals prescribed just for them as their conditions indicate at that time, says Dr. Mueller.

"The major issue is calories," adds Dr. Stallings. "If anything affects growth, energy, quality of life and being able to fight off infection, the big thing is absorbing adequate calories. If you can get enough calories to keep up your body weight, then almost everything else that you can do nutritionally follows."

In fact, she adds, "if someone with cystic fibrosis is consuming adequate calories and has maintained normal body weight, I try to not prescribe any extra supplements besides what has been determined to be absolutely necessary. Since these are people who may be taking 60 pills a day, they don't need to be taking another pill if they don't have to."

Dr. Mueller agrees with the need to keep the food and pill regimens as simple as possible. But she also feels that "even with a well-balanced diet and pancreatic enzyme replacements, most people with cystic fibrosis need extra vitamins and minerals."

Her reasoning is based on the hit-and-miss effectiveness of the enzymes. "There's no good way of knowing exactly how much of these enzymes is necessary at any particular time," she explains. Pancreatic enzyme prescriptions are based on general guidelines, and the enzymes are not 100 percent effective. The thickness of the mucus constantly varies—thicker one day, thinner the next—and people eat different things on different days. With that much variability, how much of the nutrients gets through can vary a lot.

That is also why it's important to have blood levels of target nutrients checked at least once a year, says Dr. Mueller. People with cystic fibrosis have changing needs, and what was fine last year may not be so this year. Some vitamins and minerals might need to be decreased, and some might need to be increased. And because deficiencies of these nutrients may make the body even more vulnerable to infection and disease, "vitamin and mineral levels are as important as drug level tests," says Dr. Mueller.

It is important to remember that anyone with cystic fibrosis should be under a doctor's care. Only a doctor or nutritionist can recommend the right types and amounts of vitamin and mineral supplements for each person. To locate a cystic fibrosis center near you, contact the Cystic Fibrosis Foundation at 6931 Arlington Road, Bethesda, MD 20814 (1-800-FIGHTCF).

Depression

Dispelling the Darkness

Of course you've been depressed. Hasn't everybody?

The answer is, in a word, no.

The word *depression* is thrown around so much in casual conversation that many people don't realize how serious it can be, says Harold Bloomfield, M.D., a psychiatrist in Del Mar, California, and co-author of *How to Heal Depression* and *The Power of Five: Hundreds of Five-Second to Five-Minute Scientific Shortcuts to Ignite Your Energy, Burn Fat, Stop Aging and Revitalize Your Love Life*.

"Depression isn't the same as being sad or discouraged," says Dr. Bloomfield. "Those feelings are just part of being alive. Depression is an illness, one that can be controlled with proper treatment or that can ruin your life if you don't get the help you need."

Are You at Risk?

Depression may look and sound like the blues, but it lasts longer and has a more profound impact on a person's life. If you're clinically depressed, you live in a state of sadness and hopelessness so severe that it makes normal activities seem impossible. You may lose interest in friends or hobbies, have suicidal thoughts or feel overwhelming guilt because you can't "snap out of it." Depression can kill your appetite or make you want to eat all of the time. Sleeping more or less than usual and problems concentrating can also be warning signs.

Depression can happen to anyone. It is estimated that about 15 percent of us will have at least one bout of depression in our lifetimes that's severe enough to require medical attention. Sometimes it's triggered by an emotional blow such as a divorce or the death of a loved one, but it can also appear out of nowhere.

A family history of depression can also put you at risk. "We see depression running in families just as diabetes and high blood pressure run in families," says Dr. Bloomfield. "That doesn't mean there aren't other causes, but a family history of depression makes a person more prone to it."

Depression often surfaces during times of transition, such as the teenage

Food Factors

When it comes to healing depression, individual nutrients are only part of the story. Some experts feel that what you're eating and drinking also plays an important role. Here are some tips from Larry Christensen, Ph.D., chairman of the Department of Psychology at the University of South Alabama in Mobile and author of *The Food-Mood Connection.*

Cut back on sugar. While a sweet treat may temporarily boost your mood, the lift doesn't last. Some people notice a rebound effect and feel a little tired an hour or more after eating something sweet. This slump is especially pronounced in people who are depressed to begin with, says Dr. Christensen. He estimates that up to 30 percent of his depressed patients show some sensitivity to sugar. To find out if sugar is contributing to your depression, cut out sweets and added sugars for a few weeks, says Dr. Christensen. Artificial sweeteners are okay, he adds.

If the thought of never eating another Oreo only contributes to your depression, take heart. While a minority of people are so sensitive to sugar that they shouldn't have it at all, others can handle a little bit, according to Dr. Christensen. Gradually reintroduce sweets to your diet to find out how much you can tolerate.

Avoid the caffeine crash. Studies show that depressed people

years, midlife and retirement. The elderly are particularly vulnerable: Dr. Bloomfield estimates that people over age 60 are four times as likely to be depressed as younger people.

Hormones can also play a role. Some women who take birth control pills or hormone replacement therapy may experience depression as an effect of their pills and should see their doctors for guidance. Premenstrual and postpartum depression are also common.

Feed Your Head

Nutritional deficiencies are common in depressed people, according to Dr. Bloomfield, though which comes first—deficiency or depression—isn't entirely clear. "If people haven't been eating right their whole lives, it can

who depend on caffeine to get them through the day may be setting themselves up for a fall. Dr. Christensen advises his patients to eliminate coffee, tea, cola and chocolate as well as pain relievers containing caffeine. "Depressed people who are sensitive to caffeine generally notice improvement after about four days without caffeine," he says.

If you do find that you're sensitive to caffeine, he adds, it usually isn't an all-or-nothing proposition. "There are some people who can tolerate a cup of tea a day, but not more than that. People need to experiment to find their own limits."

Go low-fat. Some research suggests that besides improving your overall health, a low-fat diet may help stabilize your mood. In a five-year study at the State University of New York at Stony Brook, 305 men and women followed a diet that got only between 20 and 30 percent of its calories from fat. The diet didn't just lower their cholesterol. They actually showed less depression and hostility after adopting the leaner diet.

Cutting the fat from your diet isn't complicated. Avoid fried foods, switch to leaner cuts of meat and remove the skin from poultry. Swap whole milk for 1 percent or skim, and choose low-fat or nonfat cheeses and yogurt. And if you make an effort to eat more fruits, vegetables and whole-grain cereals, you'll be less likely to fill up on fatty fare.

start to catch up with them in their forties or fifties. And if they have a tendency toward depression, it often shows up around the same time."

While poor nutrition probably doesn't cause depression, correcting a deficiency can be beneficial if you're battling it, says Dr. Bloomfield. But nutritional supplements are no substitute for professional evaluation. "If you think you're depressed," he advises, "it's crucial that you see a physician or psychiatrist for help."

A Boost from the B Vitamins

A healthy intake of the B-complex vitamins is important for anyone who wants to keep depression at bay, says Dr. Bloomfield. While the whole B-complex apparently plays a role in keeping you emotionally and physically healthy, a few members of the family seem to have particularly strong effects on depression.

"There has been lots of evidence that if you're deficient in thiamin or riboflavin, over time it's going to lead to a depression of the whole functioning of the body, both physically and emotionally," says Dr. Bloomfield.

Symptoms of thiamin deficiency include fear, uneasiness, confusion and mood changes, which can be signs of depression. A study at the University of California, Davis, found that thiamin supplements improved sleep, appetite and mood in older women who were only slightly deficient in the nutrient.

Another B vitamin that has been linked to depression is folate (the naturally occurring form of folic acid). Researchers know that people who have low levels of folate are more likely to be depressed than those who have normal levels. And in a study at the University of Toronto, depressed people with higher levels of folate in their systems got over their depression faster than those with lower levels.

Experts advise that it's also important to make sure you're getting enough vitamin B_6. People with depression often don't, according to a study of 101 depressed men and women evaluated by the New York State Psychiatric Institute in New York City. Your body needs B_6 in order to manufacture the hormone serotonin, which seems to play a role in regulating your mood.

Many drugs, including those containing estrogen, can interfere with the absorption of vitamin B_6. This may be why some women experience depression after starting oral contraceptives or hormone replacement therapy. Vitamin B_6 may be particularly helpful for women on the Pill or for those who grapple with premenstrual depression, says Dr. Bloomfield.

Some researchers suggest that the B vitamins are even more effective when taken as a group. One study found that elderly people with depression who took supplements of thiamin, riboflavin and vitamin B_6 along with antidepressant medication showed more improvement than those taking medication alone.

The safest, most convenient way to get all of your Bs is to invest in a B-complex supplement, says Dr. Bloomfield. Look for a supplement that contains at least ten milligrams each of thiamin, riboflavin and vitamin B_6 and 100 micrograms of folic acid, he suggests, and take it twice a day.

Staying Up with Vitamin C

If your diet fails to supply all of the vitamin C you need, doctors know that your mental as well as physical health may be at stake. Depression is a

Prescriptions for Healing

To make sure your body is getting the nutrients it needs to combat depression, Harold Bloomfield, M.D., a psychiatrist in Del Mar, California, and co-author of *How to Heal Depression* and *The Power of Five: Hundreds of Five-Second to Five-Minute Scientific Shortcuts to Ignite Your Energy, Burn Fat, Stop Aging and Revitalize Your Love Life*, recommends this daily supplement program.

Nutrient	Daily Amount
B-complex supplement, taken twice a day, containing . . .	
Folic acid	100 micrograms
Riboflavin	10 milligrams
Thiamin	10 milligrams
Vitamin B_6	10 milligrams
Vitamin C	1,000–4,000 milligrams
Selenium	70 micrograms for men

MEDICAL ALERT: If you have symptoms of depression, you should see your doctor for proper diagnosis and treatment.

Doses of vitamin C exceeding 1,200 milligrams a day can cause diarrhea in some people, so it's a good idea to check with your doctor before taking more than that amount. Also, since vitamin C can interfere with the absorption of tricyclic antidepressants, you should discuss vitamin C supplementation with your doctor if you are taking this type of medication.

well-documented symptom of scurvy, a disease that results from severe deficiency of vitamin C. And while scurvy is relatively rare in developed countries, there's reason to believe that even a minor deficiency of vitamin C can affect your mental health.

Vitamin C is important for strengthening the immune system, which isn't in top form in depressed people. "We know that depressed people are more vulnerable to illness, so anything that strengthens the immune system is beneficial," says Dr. Bloomfield. He recommends vitamin C supplements in generous doses, up to 4,000 milligrams a day. This amount is many times the Daily Value, but since excess vitamin C is excreted in the urine, Dr. Bloomfield says that this large dose is safe.

Some people may experience diarrhea from this much vitamin C, however, so experts say it's a good idea to check with your doctor before taking more than 1,200 milligrams a day. Also, since vitamin C can interfere with the absorption of tricyclic antidepressants, you should discuss vitamin C supplementation with your doctor if you are taking this type of medication.

Dr. Bloomfield recommends that vitamin C supplements be taken early, first thing in the morning or at lunch, because some people might have difficulty falling asleep if they take the supplements later in the day.

Mind Your Minerals

Evidence is sketchy, but at least one study suggests that the mineral selenium may play a role in depression. Researchers at the University College of Swansea in Wales found that people who took supplements of 100 micrograms of selenium daily felt less fatigue, anxiety and depression than those who didn't.

Since it's too soon to tell whether selenium is of any benefit in the fight against depression, the best advice is to shoot for getting the Daily Value of this mineral, which is 70 micrograms. Eat a balanced diet and check to see that your multivitamin/mineral supplement contains selenium; that way you can be sure that you're covering all the bases, says Dr. Bloomfield.

Dermatitis

Ending the Irritation

When a husband or wife overreacts at home, the pot roast can end up in the petunias. When your immune system overreacts to an irritant, you get dermatitis.

Dermatitis is simply your immune system flashing its message—"I'm irritated"—on your skin in the form of an itchy red rash. And it doesn't take much to irritate some folks' skin. Culprits include things such as nickel and latex and even certain foods. And such outbursts occur fairly often: 10 percent of all children suffer from dermatitis at one time or another.

Doctors are now aware, however, that immune system irritation and allergy are not the only causes of dermatitis. In rare cases, vitamin and mineral deficiencies can also help launch dermatological tirades. Deplete your body of vitamin A, biotin or any of the other B vitamins, vitamin E or zinc, and it won't be long before a skin rash appears.

"We have known for years that minor deficiencies of certain vitamins and minerals could produce skin, hair and nail problems in both children and adults," says Wilma Bergfeld, M.D., dermatologist and director of the Section of Dermatopathology (the study of the causes and effects of skin diseases and abnormalities) and Dermatological Research at the Cleveland Clinic. "What's far less clear is just how they cause them."

Zero In on Zinc

Perhaps the best-understood deficiency-dermatitis connection is the link to zinc. Imagine your roof without shingles to protect against the elements, and you get a picture of your skin without zinc.

Take in less than the Daily Value of 15 milligrams of zinc for a few weeks, and the shingles of your skin—your top layer of skin cells—begin to dissolve, says Dr. Bergfeld. Without this protective layer, your skin becomes rough and crusted, opening up opportunities for bacteria, yeast and other infections to take hold, she says.

"In a zinc deficiency, your skin simply does not perform the normal barrier function that it otherwise would," says Thomas Helm, M.D., assistant clinical professor of dermatology at the State University of New York at Buffalo and director of the Buffalo Medical Group. "Zinc is important in regulating the production of proteins, fatty acids and DNA. Zinc deficiency causes skin rash, loss of appetite, loss of taste and impaired immunity."

As a result, zinc deficiency can cause dermatitis around the mouths and rectums of young children. Such deficiencies aren't exactly common, but they occur more frequently than other nutrient-related skin problems, says Jon Hanifin, M.D., professor of dermatology at Oregon Health Sciences University in Portland.

Other people who are most susceptible to this kind of dermatitis: those with irritable bowel syndrome (a distressing digestive disorder), those under-

Food Factors

It's rare that a food will cause a case of dermatitis, but experts say certain foods are more likely than others to do so. Here are the most common culprits.

Consider your moo. A great source of protein for young bodies, milk can occasionally worsen atopic dermatitis in allergic children, says Jon Hanifin, M.D., professor of dermatology at Oregon Health Sciences University in Portland.

"This allergy to milk and dairy products seems to subside as the individuals grow older," he says.

If you suspect that an allergy is the culprit behind your dermatitis and you want to try eliminating milk and dairy products from your diet, you have to learn to read food labels carefully. Milk can appear as an ingredient where you least expect it, says Dr. Hanifin.

Go easy on the eggs. During a Japanese study of 27 people with dermatitis, researchers found that 11 had outbreaks within two hours of eating eggs. If you think eggs are causing your dermatitis or eczema, avoid them, and when your skin is clear, test yourself by eating eggs again. If your dermatitis returns, then it would be a good idea to avoid eggs, says Dr. Hanifin.

Say good-bye to wheat. For an unfortunate few, an ingredient in wheat called gluten is enough to give them itchy red rashes on the arms, the legs and sometimes the scalp. But in this case at least, knowing the source of the problem is only part of the solution. "They have their work cut out for them. It's very hard to avoid wheat products," says

going chemotherapy, alcohol-dependent people and some moms-to-be. "In all of these cases, their zinc levels may actually go below the normal range even if they are eating enough zinc," says Dr. Helm. "It's just not being absorbed properly."

Fortunately, alleviating problems caused by a zinc deficiency is as simple as adding more zinc to your diet; you should aim for the Daily Value of 15 milligrams. Even when there is a problem with zinc absorption, zinc deficiency can usually be overcome by increasing dietary zinc, Dr. Helm says.

"When zinc replacement is given, most of these rashes clear right up," agrees Dr. Bergfeld.

Stephen Schleicher, M.D., co-director of the Dermatology Center in Philadelphia. Fortunately, more and more companies are making gluten-free products for people who are sensitive to wheat, he says. (Gluten is also found in rye, barley and oats, but in much smaller amounts.)

Shy away from shellfish. Shrimp and squid provoke dermatitis in some people that's bad enough to scare Davy Jones back to his locker. Don't be surprised if lobster, clams, mussels and other shellfish also bring on the itchies, experts say. These often contain the same dermatitis-causing chemicals.

Search out soy. This inexpensive protein source, which pops up in all kinds of prepared foods, is another trigger for atopic dermatitis in some people, says Dr. Hanifin.

Note those nuts. Peanuts round out the list of foods that most often cause dermatitis or eczema, says Dr. Hanifin.

Go fishing for fish oil. The scientific jury is still out, but some doctors have reported less itching and scaling in people with eczema after they took fish oil capsules containing omega-3 fatty acids. Some experts believe that fatty acids help regulate inflammation and the immune response responsible for dermatitis in some. The recommended dose is five grams twice daily, according to Melvyn Werbach, M.D., author of *Healing through Nutrition*, but it's important to check with your doctor before taking these supplements. You can also try eating more fatty fish such as salmon, sardines and tuna.

Give Vitamin E a Go

You probably won't find a scientific study to confirm it, but clinical reports seem to show vitamin E's effectiveness against some kinds of dermatitis.

One such case, published in the British medical journal *Lancet*, described an otherwise healthy 38-year-old man who suffered from dermatitis on his hands for four years. Under the supervision of his doctor, he tried all kinds of approaches to get rid of it, including changing soaps, watchbands and the wrap on his steering wheel, as well as wearing gloves to the gym and taking a multivitamin/mineral supplement. Then he began taking 400 international units of vitamin E a day.

Nine days after he started the supplement, the man's dermatitis cleared, says Commander Patrick Olson, M.D., an epidemiologist and preventive medicine specialist at the Naval Medical Center in San Diego. Dr. Olson is the one who treated the man. Since writing about the case, Dr. Olson says, he has received no fewer than ten letters from people as far away as Britain reporting the same kind of success with vitamin E.

Although all of the letters sound credible, Dr. Olson says he was most intrigued by one from an infectious disease specialist in Florida who read the article and urged his sister to give it a try. "She started taking 400 international units of vitamin E a day in soft gel form, and it resolved her condition completely for the first time in the six or eight years that it had been diagnosed," says Dr. Olson. "It was very gratifying to hear that."

Dr. Olson theorizes that the antioxidant action of vitamin E prevents damage from free radicals; in this case, the damage is manifested as dermatitis. Free radicals, normal by-products of cell life, are unstable molecules that steal electrons from your body's healthy molecules to balance themselves, damaging cells in the process. Antioxidants neutralize free radicals by offering their own electrons and so protect healthy molecules from harm.

"It's just a theory, but since vitamin E seems completely benign at these

Prescriptions for Healing

Finding out what is irritating your skin and avoiding it are, of course, the keys to dealing with dermatitis. There are also a few nutrients that can help some people. Here's what some doctors recommend.

Nutrient	Daily Amount
Vitamin C	3,500–5,000 milligrams
Vitamin E	400 international units
Zinc	15 milligrams

MEDICAL ALERT: *Some people may experience diarrhea when taking doses of vitamin C exceeding 1,200 milligrams daily.*

If you are taking anticoagulant drugs, you should not take vitamin E supplements.

doses, there's no reason why this area shouldn't be explored further," says Dr. Olson.

While the Daily Value for vitamin E is only 30 international units, doses of up to 400 international units daily are considered safe. To get that amount from food, you'd have to eat a pound of sunflower seeds, five pounds of wheat germ or two quarts of corn oil.

Vitamin C Might Help

It's no secret that a vitamin C deficiency can damage gums and skin. And at least one study showed that taking supplements helps people with severe eczema, according to Melvyn Werbach, M.D., author of *Healing through Nutrition*. (Eczema is a type of dermatitis characterized by weeping breaks in the skin that eventually form scales.) Dr. Werbach recommends taking 3,500 to 5,000 milligrams of vitamin C each day for three months. This is a lot of vitamin C, as some people experience diarrhea from only 1,200 milligrams. If you'd like to try this treatment, you should discuss it with your physician.

Most dermatologists don't suggest vitamin C for dermatitis, but there are reasons that it might work, says Dr. Helm. For one thing, doctors are just learning that vitamin C seems to protect the skin from sun damage. Vitamin C speeds wound healing and prevents ultraviolet-induced free radical damage to the skin. Studies show decreased photoaging and susceptibility to sunburn in animals given vitamin C supplementation, Dr. Helm reports. "It's not unreasonable to suspect that vitamin C can help the skin stay healthy when exposed to harmful stresses other than ultraviolet light," he says.

Diabetes

Helping the Body to Handle Sugar

When she finally went to the doctor, three months after she first noticed her symptoms, Allene Harris of Valley Mills, Texas, was surprised to learn she has diabetes. It doesn't run in her family.

"I just didn't feel right," she recalls. "I was very tired, and I thought it was because of the stress I'd gone through when my mother died. But I was happy to hear it could be controlled by diet. My doctor said that as long as I was willing to make some changes, I probably wouldn't need to take insulin."

Her diet—a careful balance of carbohydrates, protein and fat that's heavy on fiber and light on saturated fat and sugar, with just enough calories to maintain her weight—perked her up as fast as it dropped her blood sugar. She was feeling better in a matter of days.

"I knew this was something that wouldn't get better on its own, so I found out as much as I could about taking care of it and started doing it," she says. Much of her nutrition information comes from a diabetes support group that includes a nutritionist.

This sort of take-charge approach can make the difference between living a long, healthy life despite diabetes and suffering the potential consequences: heart disease, blindness, nerve and kidney damage and poor circulation in the hands and feet.

"There's absolutely no doubt that diet is the cornerstone of diabetes care," says Mary Dan Eades, M.D., medical director of the Arkansas Center for Health and Weight Control in Little Rock. "The change in a person's condition as a result of proper nutritional guidance can be dramatic."

Double Trouble with Sugar

Most of us know that people with diabetes have problems with too much sugar in their bodies. But there's a bit more to be aware of in understanding this complex disease. For one thing, diabetes comes in two different forms.

Type I diabetes, formerly called juvenile diabetes, results from a lack of insulin, the hormone that allows cells to take up glucose circulating in the bloodstream. Glucose is the simple sugar that the body uses for fuel. Type I diabetes is also called insulin-dependent diabetes mellitus. (*Mellitus* means "honeyed" in Latin.) The lack of insulin comes about because of damage to insulin-secreting cells in the pancreas. The damage may be caused by a virus or by an autoimmune reaction, in which the body's immune system attacks cells in the body.

Type II diabetes, or non-insulin-dependent diabetes mellitus (formerly called adult-onset diabetes), results because sugar can't get inside cells, a condition called insulin resistance. Most people with Type II diabetes have plenty of insulin, at least in the beginning stages of the condition. But receptor sites, or portals, on the membranes of the cells don't work properly to allow sugar inside. Exactly why that happens nobody knows, but research indicates that the defect in the receptors probably occurs from damage brought about by chronic exposure to high levels of insulin.

In both types, the end result is too much sugar in the blood. "Excess sugar causes tremendous oxidative stress in the body, which leads to all sorts of problems," explains Joe Vinson, Ph.D., professor of chemistry and nutrition at the University of Scranton in Pennsylvania. That simply means sugar molecules react with oxygen to form unstable molecules called free radicals, which cause havoc by stealing electrons from your body's healthy molecules to balance themselves.

This electron pilfering damages cells and sets the stage for heart disease as well as for kidney, eye and nerve damage. "Oxidative damage is thought to be associated with all of the complications of diabetes," Dr. Vinson says.

Excess sugar also sticks to proteins, causing their structural and functional properties to be significantly changed. "This is another major cause of diabetes complications," Dr. Vinson explains. "It's one reason people with diabetes often have a hard time healing from wounds or surgery. They have trouble making quality collagen, the connective tissue that is the major structural protein in the body."

Nutritional therapy for diabetes covers all the bases. It helps lower blood sugar and blood fats, restores nutrients in people whose diabetes is not well-controlled and protects against oxidative damage.

Changes in eating habits are considered standard treatment for diabetes, especially for Type II. And individual nutrients appear to play important roles. Here's what research shows may be helpful.

Vitamin C Saves Cells

Diabetes itself doesn't kill people. But those nasty complications, such as heart disease and blindness, can make things rough. And that's where vitamin C comes in.

Studies show that vitamin C helps prevent the sugar inside cells from converting to sorbitol, a sugar alcohol that cells can neither burn for energy nor move out. Vitamin C may also be effective in diminishing the damage to proteins caused by free radicals.

"Sorbitol buildup has been implicated in diabetes-related eye, nerve and kidney damage," says John J. Cunningham, Ph.D., professor of nutrition at the University of Massachusetts at Amherst. "It accumulates in cells and disrupts a large spectrum of biochemical reactions." In other words, it really gunks up the works.

In a study by researchers at the University of Massachusetts at Amherst, the red blood cell levels of sorbitol in people with Type I diabetes dropped

(continued on page 216)

Food Factors

Diet is considered the cornerstone of treatment when it comes to diabetes. But don't count on your doctor to fill you in on all of the details.

"I suggest that you ask your doctor for a referral to a dietitian, because I believe dietitians know more about dietary recommendations than most doctors and have more time to explain things," says Kathleen Wishner, M.D., Ph.D., past president of the American Diabetes Association.

Here, then, are the top dietary measures.

Count down calories. If you're overweight, you'll do best if you lose some girth. But you don't necessarily have to get down to bantam weight to gain the advantage. "For some people, simply losing 10 to 15 pounds can make a big difference," says Dr. Wishner.

If your blood sugar is high, it will drop within a day or two of your starting a reduced-calorie diet. (So if you're using insulin, your doctor will need to adjust your dose downward.) In fact, in the days before insulin was available, people were sometimes treated with low-calorie, low-carbohydrate diets or intermittent fasting, after doctors observed that their diabetes patients did better during times of relative famine.

Most doctors recommend that their patients with diabetes cut back on fat to lose weight. But for some people with diabetes, trimming carbohydrates works better, says Mary Dan Eades, M.D., medical director of the Arkansas Center for Health and Weight Control in Little Rock.

Eat beans and barley. Both are packed with fiber, and most experts recommend that people with diabetes double their fiber intakes to 30 grams a day. Dr. Eades recommends up to 50 grams a day, using psyllium, the kind of gelatinous fiber found in Metamucil.

Fiber slows intestinal absorption of sugar and so smooths out blood sugar levels. Many people with diabetes can eliminate the need for insulin with a high-fiber, high-carbohydrate diet, says James W. Anderson, M.D., professor of medicine and clinical nutrition at the University of Kentucky College of Medicine in Lexington and a pioneer in fiber research. In one study, people with diabetes who ate 6.8 grams (about two rounded tablespoons) of psyllium fiber before both breakfast and dinner had 14 to 20 percent drops in postmeal blood sugar.

You can get more fiber by eating whole grains, beans, fruits and vegetables. Top fiber sources: dried pears (11.5 grams in five halves), corn bran (7.9 grams in two tablespoons), blackberries (7.2 grams in one cup) and chick-peas (7 grams in a half-cup).

Make it mono. Some research suggests that certain people with Type II (non-insulin-dependent) diabetes do better on a diet fairly high in monounsaturated fat, the kind found in olive oil and canola oil, than on the standard high-carbohydrate, low-fat (30 percent) diet.

Researchers at the University of Texas Southwestern Medical Center at Dallas found that a diet with 45 percent of calories from fat (a mix of 25 percent monos and 10 percent each of saturated and polyunsaturated fats) produced lower blood levels of triglycerides (a heart disease–promoting fat), glucose and insulin than a typical high-carbohydrate diet. People with diabetes who benefited most from this dietary switch: those with high triglycerides and low levels of HDL cholesterol, the "good" cholesterol.

"It seems apparent that a diet rich in monounsaturated fat improves glucose control in some people, although we don't yet understand exactly why," says Abhimanyu Garg, M.D., the study's main researcher.

If you want to try this diet, start by replacing saturated fats (hard at room temperature) and polyunsaturated fats (oils such as corn, soybean, sunflower and safflower) with olive oil or canola oil, Dr. Garg suggests. Avocados and some nuts are also rich sources of monounsaturated fat. It's best to work with a nutritionist to plan a menu that doesn't add extra calories.

Go extra-easy on the hard stuff. People with diabetes used to be told not to drink at all, period. After all, alcohol is empty calories that most folks with this disease don't need.

But since there is no convincing evidence to show that moderate drinking causes significantly higher blood sugar, and since many people with diabetes are at least occasional social drinkers, the American Diabetes Association offers these guidelines.

- Don't drink more than two drinks two times a week. One drink equals 1½ ounces of distilled spirits, 4 ounces of dry wine, 2 ounces of dry sherry or 12 ounces of beer.
- Drink only when you're also eating food.
- Avoid sugared drinks such as liqueurs, sweet wines and sweet mixes.
- Sip slowly. Make your drink last a long time.

from double the normal amount to normal after they took 100 or 600 milligrams of vitamin C a day for 58 days.

"That's important, because it could mean that over time, people with diabetes who get plenty of vitamin C will have fewer complications," Dr. Cunningham explains. "Given its ability to permeate all tissues in the body and its low toxicity, we believe vitamin C is a superior choice over drugs that do the same thing."

Sorbitol, by the way, is used as a sweetener in some dietetic foods. But that doesn't pose a danger for people with diabetes, says Dr. Cunningham. "Dietary sorbitol is poorly absorbed, for one thing," he says. "And it's not transported inside cells, the only place it does harm."

Doctors who recommend vitamin C for diabetes suggest anywhere from 100 to 8,000 milligrams a day. In his study, Dr. Cunningham found that 100 milligrams of supplemental vitamin C a day works just as well as 600 milligrams a day in people already getting at least the Daily Value (60 milligrams) from foods. Dr. Cunningham suggests that you work with your health care team, including a nutritionist, to determine the right amount for you. For some people, doses exceeding 1,200 milligrams a day can cause diarrhea.

Citrus fruits are tops for vitamin C delivery. Or thrill your taste buds by blending orange juice with a cup of cubed guava or papaya. That tasty concoction packs close to 200 milligrams of vitamin C.

Vitamin E Saves Hearts

Vitamin E gets lots of good press for its role in helping to prevent heart disease. That's important for people with diabetes, whose risk of heart disease is two to four times normal.

That high risk results mostly from free radical damage to fats found in the bloodstream, explains Sushil Jain, Ph.D., professor of pediatrics, physiology and biochemistry in the Department of Pediatrics at Louisiana State University Medical Center in Shreveport.

The damage, called lipid peroxidation, leads to clogging in the miles of tiny capillaries found in the body, to the reduced life span of red blood cells and to something called platelet aggregation, in which blood cells tend to stick to each other and to blood vessel walls, causing serious traffic jams.

"People with diabetes may need more antioxidant protection than is available in a normal diet," Dr. Jain says. In his studies, people with diabetes who took supplements of 100 international units of vitamin E a day had 25 to 30 percent lower blood levels of harmful triglycerides, which are blood fats

Prescriptions for Healing

Doctors agree that good nutrition is important for people with diabetes. What they consider good nutrition varies, however. Doctors who do recommend nutritional supplements suggest these amounts.

Nutrient	Daily Amount
B-complex	100 milligrams
Biotin	15,000 micrograms
Calcium	1,000 milligrams
Chromium	200 milligrams (niacin-bound chromium or chromium picolinate)
Magnesium	500 milligrams
Vitamin C	100–8,000 milligrams
Vitamin E	100–800 international units

Plus a multivitamin/mineral supplement containing the Daily Values of all essential vitamins and minerals

MEDICAL ALERT: *It's best to work with a doctor knowledgeable in nutrition when you're adding nutritional supplements to your diabetes treatment program. Your blood sugar and drug dosage need to be carefully monitored.*

If you have diabetes and you want to try chromium supplementation, you should do so only under your doctor's supervision. He may need to adjust your insulin dosage as your blood sugar level drops.

People who have heart or kidney problems should talk to their doctors before beginning magnesium supplementation.

Doses of vitamin C exceeding 1,200 milligrams a day can cause diarrhea in some people.

It's a good idea to talk to your doctor before taking more than 600 international units of vitamin E daily. If you are taking anticoagulants, you should not take vitamin E supplements.

made of sugar. Vitamin E also reduced the tendency for sugar to stick to proteins in the blood, Dr. Jain says.

Doctors who prescribe vitamin E for their patients with diabetes recommend from 100 to 800 international units a day. "I begin with 100 international units and may go as high as 800 international units," Dr. Eades says. It's important to work with your doctor as you increase levels, she adds. "If you're taking insulin, your doctor may need to drop your insulin dose with each increase in vitamin E. And you should monitor your blood pressure, as there is speculation that vitamin E might increase blood pressure in some people."

The large amounts of vitamin E used for diabetes are not available from even the best food sources: wheat germ and nut and seed oils. Only supplements can provide these large amounts. Doses exceeding 600 international units a day should be taken only under medical supervision.

Magnesium: For Eyes and More

It may be the world's most underappreciated mineral. Magnesium is not a trace mineral but a nutrient necessary for every major biological function in your body. And it offers a long list of potential benefits for diabetes. Low levels have been linked to degeneration of the eye's retina, high blood sugar, high blood pressure and clotting problems that can lead to heart disease.

Although studies have yet to be done that look at whether supplemental magnesium can prevent diabetic complications such as retinal damage, some research indicates that it could be helpful.

In Italy, for instance, doctors found that people with Type II diabetes who took 450 milligrams of supplemental magnesium a day produced more insulin and cleared sugar from their bloodstreams better than before they started taking magnesium supplements.

People with diabetes, especially those taking insulin or whose blood sugar is not well-controlled, tend to come up short on magnesium, studies show. One in four may have the kind of marginal deficiency that often goes undetected, even when they're eating enough. "People with diabetes tend to lose magnesium through their urine," Dr. Eades explains.

"I have people take 1,000 milligrams of magnesium twice a day for four weeks to assess their responses," Dr. Eades says. (She also has people take 1,500 milligrams of calcium a day during this period.) But she cautions against taking these amounts unless you discuss it with your doctor first. This is especially important if you have heart or kidney problems. During this therapy, most people experience some improvement in blood sugar and blood pressure and have less fatigue. After four weeks, she reduces the dose to 500 milligrams a day (100 milligrams more than the Daily Value), taken along with 1,000 milligrams of calcium.

Foods rich in magnesium include whole grains, almonds, cashews, spinach, beans and halibut.

Chromium Helps Insulin Work Better

Chromium is a trace mineral. The very same mineral used to put a shine on car bumpers, it is a key player in the body's use of sugar. It hooks up with insulin to help escort sugar through the cell membrane and into the cell. Deficiencies of chromium make cells resistant to insulin and lead to high blood sugar levels. Of 15 studies that have looked at the effects of chromium supplementation on the body's ability to use sugar, 12 show positive results.

In one study, people with diabetes who took 200 micrograms of chromium or nine grams of high-chromium brewer's yeast a day had lower blood levels of sugar, insulin, triglycerides and total cholesterol and higher levels of heart-healthy HDL cholesterol than before they started taking chromium.

"Deficiency of chromium not only worsens sugar metabolism but also may contribute to development of the numbness, pain and tingling in your feet, legs and hands that diabetes causes," Dr. Eades says. She recommends daily doses of 200 micrograms of either niacin-bound chromium or chromium picolinate, an easily absorbed form of the mineral, or nine grams (two teaspoons) of chromium-rich brewer's yeast.

It's true that chromium improves glucose tolerance, which is the body's ability to maintain normal levels of blood sugar after eating, only in people who are low in this trace mineral. But plenty of people fit that category, says Richard Anderson, Ph.D., lead scientist in the nutrient requirements and functions laboratory at the U.S. Department of Agriculture Beltsville Human Nutrition Research Center in Maryland and a leading chromium researcher. He found that most people get only 25 to 30 micrograms a day, which is much less than the Daily Value of 120 micrograms. You'd need to eat at least 3,000 calories a day to get 50 micrograms of chromium and 7,200 calories a day to get 120 micrograms, Dr. Anderson figures.

"No one knows how many people with diabetes are low in chromium, and there's no good way to assess chromium status," admits Kathleen Wishner, M.D., Ph.D., past president of the American Diabetes Association. Foods high in chromium include broccoli, bran cereals, whole-grain cereals and breads, green beans and various fruits. Eating sugar uses up the body's chromium supply.

If you have diabetes and you want to try chromium supplementation, you should do so only under your doctor's supervision. He may need to adjust your insulin dosage as your blood sugar level drops.

B-Complex May Help Nerves

It's old news that the B-complex vitamins—niacin, thiamin, folic acid, vitamin B_6 and others—are essential for your body to convert sugar and starches to energy. These vitamins are involved in many of the chemical reactions necessary for this process, which is known as carbohydrate metabolism.

A shortage of any one of the B-complex vitamins can cause problems. Vitamin B_6 deficiency, for instance, has been linked to something called glucose intolerance, which is an abnormally high rise in blood sugar after eating. This deficiency has also been linked to impaired secretion of insulin and glucagon. Both of these hormones are essential in regulating blood sugar levels.

Shortages of B vitamins can also lead to nerve damage in the hands and feet. Some studies indicate that people with diabetes experience less of the numbness and tingling of diabetes-caused nerve damage if they get supplemental amounts of B vitamins such as B_6 and B_{12}.

People with diabetes tend to be low in B vitamins, perhaps in part because the diabetes itself uses up B vitamins and because poorly controlled diabetes causes these nutrients to be excreted in the urine.

"In general, my recommendation is 100 milligrams of a B-complex vitamin daily," Dr. Eades says. "Then I'll determine whether someone may need bigger doses of particular B vitamins, such as thiamin, B_6 and B_{12} if there are symptoms of diabetic nerve damage."

In such cases, she may prescribe up to several hundred milligrams a day, or injections in the case of vitamin B_{12}, until symptoms wane, then cut back.

For vitamin B_{12}, she prescribes injections of 300 to 500 micrograms weekly until symptoms respond, then monthly doses of 500 micrograms indefinitely. (If you can't get B_{12} injections, she suggests 500 to 1,000 micrograms taken under the tongue. These supplements are available over the counter.)

Check with your doctor before taking an amount above the Daily Value of any B vitamin, since high dosages may lead to side effects. Doses of 200 milligrams or more of vitamin B_6 a day, for example, have caused nerve damage.

Some people may also benefit from taking biotin, another B vitamin, in amounts of up to 15 milligrams (15,000 micrograms) a day, Dr. Eades adds. A study by Japanese researchers found that this vitamin helps cells in muscle tissue use sugar more effectively.

Covering All the Bases

In addition to these particular vitamins, doctors may also recommend that people with diabetes take a multivitamin/mineral supplement that contains the Daily Value of every essential nutrient. That might not be such a bad idea. Research suggests that a multitude of nutrients—zinc, copper, manganese, selenium, calcium, vitamin D and vitamin A—may be in short supply in people with diabetes.

Diarrhea

Nutrition on the Skids

Your co-workers must think you're nuts, because here you come again, running down the hall, tearing around the corner and blasting into the bathroom. It's your third trip this morning. And as you dash past the sinks and screech to a halt in front of the nearest stall, you wonder what on earth has caused such explosive diarrhea. Leftover bacteria from last night's pork lo mein? Viral invaders from the flu that has hit your office? Alien plankton from a swim at the beach?

You may never know.

"There are a million and one causes of diarrhea," says Joel B. Mason, M.D., assistant professor of medicine and nutrition at Tufts University in Medford, Massachusetts. But fortunately, most short-term cases of diarrhea—those lasting for a day or two or three—will not deplete your body's nutritional reserves enough to harm you, which can be a major health effect of diarrhea.

"Acute infectious diarrhea, what people call gastrointestinal flu, is usually related to a viral or bacterial infection," says Dr. Mason. "It is self-limiting and usually runs its course in several days to a week. The only immediate danger is the loss of fluid and electrolytes, including salt, magnesium, potassium and calcium."

These are the nutrients that regulate many of the body's essential processes: blood pressure, heart rate, nerve conduction and muscle movement. Without them, you run the risk of an irregular heart rhythm, low blood pressure and weak or crampy limbs.

Food Factors

Acute diarrhea may last for only a couple of days, but it can make you feel as weak and vulnerable as a kitten. Here are a few tips to get you back on your paws and in roaring good health.

Listen to your body. Diarrhea should begin to slow 24 hours after you start sipping liquids, says William B. Ruderman, M.D., practicing physician at Gastroenterology Associates of Central Florida in Orlando. When it does, start paying attention to what your body is telling you. When your body says . . . well, maybe it's a little hungry, that's the time to reintroduce food.

Go for the bland. The first foods you should reach for are bland complex carbohydrates such as noodles, white bread and applesauce, says Dr. Ruderman. Start with one-fourth of what would be a normal serving for you, then see how it goes down. If your abdomen feels comfortable and diarrhea does not resume, then increase the amount of food at your next meal.

Go easy on yourself. Gradually increase food until you're back to full portions, says Dr. Ruderman. If your abdomen feels uncomfortable at any point or if diarrhea resumes, go back to the previous levels.

Reintroduce your normal diet after you're able to consume normal kinds of foods such as whole grains, says Dr. Ruderman.

When to Seek Help

"It's not of great concern if you can't absorb this or that nutrient for a few days," says Dr. Mason. But there are two prominent exceptions: the very young and the very old. Both groups—preschoolers, for example, and those over age 70—tend to feel the effects of electrolyte and fluid loss very quickly.

"Remember that between 500 and 1,000 children in the United States still die of acute diarrhea every year," adds Dr. Mason. "And that's largely because small children, preschool children, are very susceptible to dehydration."

"Whenever diarrhea lasts more than 6 to 8 hours in the very young or the very old or more than 12 hours in healthy adults, you should add fluids and electrolytes to the diet," says William B. Ruderman, M.D., practicing physician at Gastroenterology Associates of Central Florida in Orlando. The same goes for anyone who develops signs of dehydration, such as dry mouth, dry skin, decreased urination and skin that tents when pinched.

"When these symptoms occur, you can assume that levels of electrolytes and fluid need to be supplemented," says Dr. Ruderman.

Fortunately, electrolytes are easily replaced. "Sodium and potassium losses are the most important, so you want to get sodium, potassium, fluids and a simple sugar in first," says Dr. Ruderman. "The sugar helps your body absorb the fluids and nutrients. The easiest way to get these in our busy lives is to go to the store and buy one of those sports drinks, such as Gatorade."

"If there's nausea or vomiting with the diarrhea, wait until it clears," says Dr. Ruderman. "Then begin rehydration. Start with a small amount: four ounces every hour for as long as the diarrhea lasts." That should combat the nutritional effects of most short-term cases of diarrhea, he adds.

If diarrhea lasts for more than 12 to 24 hours in an infant or an older person, you should seek medical attention. Signals to see your doctor if you're an otherwise healthy adult: if the diarrhea lasts for more than three days, if it is accompanied by fever or lethargy, if there is blood or pus in the stool or if any signs of dehydration continue despite efforts to replace fluid.

Prescriptions for Healing

For most people, a bout of diarrhea is not harmful. The exceptions are preschoolers and people over age 70. As a general rule, medical experts say, diarrhea lasting more than 8 hours in the very young or the very old or more than 12 hours in an otherwise healthy adult requires replacement of fluid as well as of essential nutrients known as electrolytes. Here's what these experts recommend.

Nutrient	Daily Amount
Potassium and sodium	4-oz. sports drink, taken every hour for as long as diarrhea lasts (the idea is to sip constantly)

MEDICAL ALERT: *If diarrhea lasts for more than 12 to 24 hours in an infant or an older person, you should seek medical help.*

If you're an otherwise healthy adult, you should see your doctor if diarrhea persists for more than three days, if it is accompanied by fever or lethargy, if there is blood or pus in the stool, or if any signs of dehydration continue despite efforts to replace fluid.

Eating Disorders

Mending the Mind-Body Connection

Lisa thought college would be the perfect opportunity to lose some weight. Typically about five or ten pounds overweight, she had always felt fat and wanted to take advantage of her newfound independence to shed a few pounds.

At first she just restricted her eating: no snacks, no fat, just salads. Then she discovered that if she occasionally wavered, she could "undo the damage" by vomiting. Before long she was planning daily binges and purges that sometimes consisted of a dozen doughnuts, pizza, cookies and candy bars. Weighing herself five or six times a day, she became so afraid of gaining weight once she hit 100 pounds that she could barely eat anything without purging.

Two years later she knew she was in trouble. "I was so weak that I would skip classes because I couldn't make it across campus. I had heart palpitations, my teeth were rotting, I couldn't stand the cold, I had terrible mood swings, I couldn't concentrate, and my hair was breaking off and falling out," she recalls. "It sounds ridiculous in retrospect, but the only thing that made me get help was having too many bad hair days."

Lisa didn't realize then that her "bad hair" was just one sign of what had become severe malnutrition. Though her body could digest some food during a binge, the high-fat foods she binged on didn't stay with her long enough to provide much nutrition.

Diseases of Depletion

Lisa suffered from a combination of related eating disorders: bulimia nervosa and anorexia nervosa. Although these disorders primarily affect females in their teens and twenties, they can also affect men, older women and young children.

Of the two, anorexia is easier to spot. People with this disease have an intense fear of being fat, causing them to starve themselves to emaciation. In women, it also causes amenorrhea, or the cessation of the menstrual cycle. People with bulimia are generally closer to normal weight, but they are also obsessed with body size. Bulimia is characterized by frequent binge-purge episodes, which involve eating a large amount of food in a short period of time and then trying to prevent weight gain by vomiting, using laxatives, dieting, fasting or exercising vigorously. It is common for people to have symptoms of both.

Medical experts don't know exactly why some women dive headlong into this pool of self-destruction, though they generally agree that the cause includes an intricate web of social, psychological and biological factors. They also agree that malnourishment exacerbates the condition, rendering women less receptive to treatment.

"It's a vicious cycle," says Amy Tuttle, R.D., a nutrition therapist at the Renfrew Center in Philadelphia. "Malnutrition creates a physical and emotional shutdown, and the lethargy that results makes reaching out for physical and emotional nourishment even more difficult."

Feeding Your Brain and Your Body

"It's a tragedy how often this disease is treated as a mental illness rather than as one of mind-body," says Joseph D. Beasley, M.D., co-author of *Food for Recovery* and director of Comprehensive Medical Care in Amityville, New York. Dr. Beasley advocates vitamin and mineral supplements for people with eating disorders. "You could have the world's most renowned psychotherapists—Freud, Jung and Adler—talk to most of these patients until the sky turns green, and it won't do any good until you get nourishment to the brain and clear the way for therapy."

Dr. Beasley is not alone in his beliefs. Contrary to the old practice of first putting people in therapy and then slowly reintroducing food, treatment specialists now know that re-establishing proper nutrition is critical before psychological therapy can be effective. Many use vitamin and mineral supplements to help pave the way.

Generally, the supplement of choice is a multivitamin/mineral that provides 100 percent of the Daily Values of all essential nutrients while people are relearning to eat real food. Doctors do not recommend exceeding the Daily Values; they may, however, recommend supplements of certain individual nutrients, particularly potassium, calcium, iron, zinc, vitamin A, vitamin E and the B vitamins.

Note: Experts warn that supplements cannot take the place of food. The body will not properly absorb and use vitamins and minerals without also receiving adequate calories.

"A multivitamin/mineral supplement is disadvantageous for the person

Food Factors

Part of the recovery process for people with eating disorders is making peace with food instead of battling with it. Here are some tips that many experts believe might prove helpful.

Say no to joe and sugar. It's very common for people with eating disorders to use caffeine and sugar to boost blood sugar levels to combat feelings of fatigue and depression, says Joseph D. Beasley, M.D., co-author of *Food for Recovery* and director of Comprehensive Medical Care in Amityville, New York. "It's better to eat a nutritionally balanced meal than to maintain this cycle of dramatic ups and downs, which always leaves you feeling worse," he says.

Go organic. "My patients do better if they stay away from insecticides, pesticides, steroids and all of the other chemicals that are found in refined or processed foods," says Dr. Beasley.

who takes it and then thinks she will be okay," warns dietitian Cheryl Rock, Ph.D., assistant professor in the Program in Human Nutrition at the University of Michigan School of Public Health in Ann Arbor and co-author of *Nutrition and Eating Disorders*. "With that mind-set, the illness could drag on for ten years or more."

Untreated, 10 to 15 percent of people with anorexia die, usually after losing at least half of their body weight. And over the long term, people with bulimia increase their risk of serious complications, such as abnormal heartbeat and stomach rupture. So even if you're taking supplements, it's important to work with a specialist to learn how to eat normally again.

Balancing Electrolytes

It is well-documented that one of the consequences of eating disorders is a potentially life-threatening electrolyte imbalance. Electrolytes are minerals that, when dissolved in the body's fluid, become electrically charged. They are responsible for controlling heart rate and blood pressure.

Potassium and sodium are the body's major electrolytes. Although potassium deficiency is not common, rapid weight loss and dehydration can cause potassium to plummet, leaving you at risk for serious heart problems, including heart attack.

"People with eating disorders need to have these nutrients stabilized as quickly as possible," says Dr. Beasley, who often recommends supplements of potassium as well as magnesium, another electrolyte that can lead to serious heart problems if deficient. "I have never seen an eating disorder patient who didn't have major deficits of these nutrients."

Because too much potassium can make you ill, it is best to get the Daily Value of this mineral (3,500 milligrams) by eating fruits and vegetables such as bananas, oranges, spinach and celery. You can get 885 milligrams just by eating half of a cantaloupe. Magnesium supplements are available in various forms, but eating seafood and green, leafy vegetables can help you easily get your Daily Value of 400 milligrams. People who have heart or kidney problems or diabetes should check with their doctors before supplementing these minerals.

Experts recommend that people with eating disorders have a physician monitor all of their electrolytes: potassium, magnesium and sodium as well as phosphorus and chloride, which can also become dangerously low.

Calcium to Protect Bones

Calcium, an essential mineral in the development and maintenance of bone health, is one of the nutrients most likely to be deficient in people with eating disorders. Those who treat eating disorders say the impact of severe calcium deficiency, especially when combined with amenorrhea, can be devastating.

"We see 28-year-old women with the bones of 80-year-olds," says Tuttle. "They are already in the middle stages of osteoporosis. It's sad, but fortunately, sometimes this serious medical issue is the alarm that helps a woman choose to move forward in her recovery." Tuttle notes that doctors often give women with eating disorders calcium supplements of 1,000 milligrams (the Daily Value) or more while also attending to the amenorrhea.

"Certainly, it's important that these girls get sufficient amounts of calcium in their diets," says Steven A. Abrams, M.D., a research scientist at the U.S. Department of Agriculture Children's Nutrition Research Center and associate professor of pediatrics, both at Baylor College of Medicine in Houston. "But supplements may not be sufficient to resolve osteoporosis if hormonal inadequacy remains present."

Drinking skim milk is a good way to increase your dietary calcium, as just three cups packs more than 1,000 milligrams. Other sources include broccoli, tofu and fortified orange juice.

Prescriptions for Healing

Although eating food is absolutely essential to preventing the damage that eating disorders can do to the body, some doctors believe that vitamin and mineral supplements can expedite the process of recovery and healing.

Nutrient	Daily Amount
Calcium	1,000 milligrams
Iron	18 milligrams
Magnesium	400 milligrams
Niacin	20 milligrams
Potassium	3,500 milligrams
Thiamin	1.5 milligrams
Vitamin A	5,000 international units
Vitamin E	30 international units
Zinc	15 milligrams

Plus a multivitamin/mineral supplement containing the Daily Values of all essential vitamins and minerals

MEDICAL ALERT: *Experts warn that supplements cannot take the place of food in someone who has an eating disorder. The body will not properly absorb and use vitamins and minerals without also receiving adequate calories. It is important to be under a doctor's care when treating this condition.*

People who have heart or kidney problems should check with their doctors before taking magnesium supplements.

People who have kidney problems or diabetes should check with their doctors before taking potassium supplements.

If you are taking anticoagulant drugs, you should not take vitamin E supplements.

Breaking the Cycle with Zinc

Because zinc deficiency causes symptoms that are similar to those seen in people with anorexia and bulimia, including weight loss, depression, stomach bloating and amenorrhea, many researchers believe that low zinc intake, which is common in people with eating disorders, helps to perpetuate the illness.

Fortunately, studies have found that zinc supplementation can help turn the tables. In fact, researchers studying 35 girls with anorexia at St. Paul's Hospital in Vancouver found that those who took just 14 milligrams of zinc a day were able to achieve their target weight gains twice as fast as those not taking zinc.

The Daily Value for zinc is 15 milligrams, an amount you can come close to by eating just one cooked medium-size oyster. You can also find this essential mineral in roast beef, wheat germ and whole grains.

A and E to the Rescue

Because vitamins A and E are fat-soluble, if you don't have fat in your body, you don't have enough of these vitamins. So in people with eating disorders, these important nutrients can be in short supply.

One study, by researchers at Hebrew University in Israel, found that women with anorexia had significantly lower levels of both vitamin A and vitamin E in their bodies than women without anorexia.

"We generally supplement the fat-soluble vitamins in the beginning of treatment, because these women have no fat," says Kathryn J. Zerbe, M.D., vice-president for education and research and staff psychoanalyst at the Menninger Clinic in Topeka, Kansas, and author of *The Body Betrayed: Women, Eating Disorders and Treatment*. "Fortunately, you don't have to get your fat stores up too high before your body is able to store the vitamins again."

If you want to get your Daily Value of 5,000 international units of vitamin A and build your stores of this important vitamin, two of the best food sources are spinach and pumpkin. And you can get plenty of beta-carotene, which turns to vitamin A in the body, by eating carrots, sweet potatoes and other bright orange and yellow fruits and vegetables as well as dark green, leafy vegetables.

The Daily Value for vitamin E is 30 international units, and good dietary sources include whole-grain cereals, eggs and green, leafy vegetables.

Iron against Anemia

Because people with eating disorders generally shun red meat and don't eat enough to get iron elsewhere, they sometimes develop iron-deficiency anemia.

"Anemia is caused by not having the fuel to produce energy, which adds to the fatigue and general lack of interest," says Dr. Zerbe. She prefers that women get iron from foods but notes that supplementation can be helpful for reaching the Daily Value.

Though red meat is one of the best sources of iron, you can also get the Daily Value of 18 milligrams by eating clams, chick-peas, tomato juice, raisins, Cream of Wheat, tofu and soybeans.

Beat Depression with B

Depression is such a common thread in eating disorders that many doctors now use the drug fluoxetine (Prozac) to treat bulimia.

Many experts who prefer a drug-free approach, however, believe that depression is a natural consequence of starvation and that it can be alleviated with proper nutrition.

"If it's a case of serious depression, we'll use antidepressant therapy. But we always try the nutritional route first. Many people are greatly improved just by getting their nutrition stable," says Dr. Beasley. Deficiencies in thiamin and niacin in particular cause psychological symptoms, including depression, he notes.

The Daily Value for thiamin is 1.5 milligrams. The vitamin can be found in virtually all plant and animal foods but especially in brown rice, seafood and beans. Niacin is plentiful in lean meats, fish and poultry, and its Daily Value is 20 milligrams.

Endometriosis

Living without Pain

Picture a puffy white dandelion that has gone to seed blowing in the wind, with all of the tiny parachuted seeds spawning new dandelions across your front lawn. Now picture yourself trying to get rid of all of those deep-rooted weeds that crop up again and again and again, even after being pulled, mowed and sprayed. Think also of how your whole body hurts after a day spent on your knees wrestling with these yellow devils.

By now you have a pretty clear picture of what endometriosis is all about: easily spread, hard as heck to get rid of and downright painful.

Of course, endometriosis is a whole lot harder to live with than a lawn full of dandelions—almost impossible for many women whose menstrual cycles become monthly nightmares of extreme cramping and bleeding. But help may be on the horizon, say the experts, and it may be as close as your local supermarket.

"We've found that adopting a healthy lifestyle goes a long way in preventing and relieving the symptoms of endometriosis," says Susan M. Lark, M.D., author of *Fibroid Tumors and Endometriosis: A Self-Help Program*, director of the PMS and Menopause Self-Help Center in Los Altos, California, and a physician specializing in women's health. As part of her practice, Dr. Lark helps women with endometriosis live pain-free through a wide variety of dietary regimens and herbal and nutritional supplements.

Before you start stocking your pantry, it will help to understand what causes endometriosis and how it affects your body.

Strange Tissue in Strange Places

Endometriosis is simply tissue growing where it doesn't belong. During normal menstruation, cells from the uterine lining, the endometrium, break off and are flushed out through the vagina. In someone with endometriosis, these cells back up into the fallopian tubes. From there, they flow into the pelvic cavity and, like dandelion seeds, implant themselves in places you'd rather they not be, such as the cervix and the bowels. Being uterine tissue, these implants respond to hormone stimulation, swelling and bleeding each month just as they would if they were still inside the uterus. Except this blood doesn't have the vagina for an escape route. It gets trapped in the pelvic cavity, where it can cause pain, inflammation, cysts, scar tissue and even structural damage and infertility.

No one knows why these implants occur in some women but not others. Some researchers believe excessive circulating estrogen may be to blame. Others say that an impaired immune system is likely at fault.

Bad Times Call for Good Nutrition

That's why nutrition is so important, say the experts. Whether estrogen or immunity is to blame, all of your body's systems need to be operating at

Food Factors

The best line of dietary defense for women with endometriosis is a healthful diet full of fruits, grains and vegetables and void of fatty foods, which can aggravate the disease. Here's what many experts recommend.

Lighten up on dairy products. One of the most common recommendations made by endometriosis experts is to eliminate or limit consumption of dairy products.

Dairy products contain saturated fat, which puts stress on the liver and increases circulating estrogen, says Susan M. Lark, M.D., author of *Fibroid Tumors and Endometriosis: A Self-Help Program*, director of the PMS and Menopause Self-Help Center in Los Altos, California, and a physician specializing in women's health. Saturated fat also produces a muscle-contracting component in the body called prostaglandin F_2-alpha, which can make the cramps and inflammation of endometriosis much worse, says Dr. Lark.

Stick to veggies. Because meats also contain saturated fat, experts recommend getting your nutrients from whole-grain and vegetable sources whenever possible.

Go organic. When shopping for veggies, buy organic whenever you can; when you can't, scrub or peel your fruits and vegetables before eating them. Several studies show a direct correlation between exposure to dioxin, a chemical found in pesticides, and the incidence of endometriosis in laboratory animals.

Cut caffeine. Caffeine depletes the body's B vitamin stores and hampers healthy liver function, which can increase estrogen levels and worsen endometriosis symptoms. Women should limit coffee, black tea, chocolate and caffeinated soft drinks, says Dr. Lark.

Banish alcohol. Since optimum liver function is essential for mopping up excess estrogen and controlling endometriosis, imbibing alcohol is a definite no-no, says Dr. Lark. Eliminating alcohol from the body stresses the liver, she explains. Dr. Lark recommends that women with endometriosis avoid alcohol entirely, if possible.

maximum efficiency to properly regulate your hormones, maintain your immunity and keep endometrial implants at bay.

This is not to say that medical treatments such as estrogen-blocking hormones and surgical removal of endometrial growths aren't effective, says Dr.

Lark. They are. But too often endometrial implants recur even after surgical removal.

"Nutritional plans are particularly successful for women who have recently undergone traditional treatment," says Dr. Lark. "I don't suggest that women not use medications, because hormone treatments can really help lessen endometriosis. But to prevent the pain from recurring, nutritional programs work very well."

The following are nutrients that many experts recommend for controlling endometriosis.

Note: Because the required doses are high and vary from woman to woman, be sure to consult your doctor before starting a nutritional regimen. Because getting the Daily Values of all of the essential nutrients is important if you have endometriosis, doctors who use nutritional regimens recommend starting with a general multivitamin/mineral supplement and adding additional supplements as needed.

B Vitamins Lower Estrogen Levels

If you're looking for a natural way to keep your estrogen levels low and thus reduce recurrent episodes of endometriosis, try boosting your intake of B-complex vitamins, say the experts.

"The liver is responsible for breaking down and disposing of excess estrogen," explains Dr. Lark. "The B vitamins are important in regulating estrogen because they promote a healthy liver. Studies dating back to the 1940s show that if you remove B vitamins from animals' food, they can no longer metabolize estrogen." Studies have also shown that B vitamin supplementation helps alleviate other symptoms of excess estrogen, such as premenstrual syndrome and fibrocystic breasts, she says.

Some women apparently find that supplements alone do the trick for them. Dian Mills, for example, a nutrition consultant in London and author of *Female Health: The Nutrition Connection*, became a strong advocate of B vitamin supplements through personal experience.

"I was in absolute crawl-around-the-house agony. And none of the traditional treatments was taking the pain away," recalls Mills. Her doctor even recommended a hysterectomy, advice she flatly refused. "So I went to doctors of nutritional medicine in London, and I've been pain-free ever since."

Mills's supplement regimen included B vitamins, particularly thiamin, riboflavin and vitamin B_6. Not only did her pain disappear, but she was so inspired by her success with the nutrition program that she went on to study clinical nutrition at the Institute of Optimum Nutrition in London and is

Prescriptions for Healing

Increasingly, endometriosis specialists are discovering the power of nutritional healing. But since the necessary doses can be high and vary from woman to woman, they recommend consulting a physician before starting a vitamin and mineral regimen.

Because getting the Daily Values of all of the essential nutrients is important if you have endometriosis, doctors who use nutritional regimens recommend starting with a general multivitamin/mineral supplement and adding other supplements as needed.

Nutrient	Daily Amount
Beta-carotene	25,000–50,000 international units
Biotin	200 micrograms
Folic acid	400 micrograms
Niacin	50 milligrams
Pantothenic acid	50 milligrams
Riboflavin	50 milligrams
Selenium	25 micrograms
Thiamin	50 milligrams
Vitamin B_6	30 milligrams
Vitamin B_{12}	50 micrograms
Vitamin C	1,000–4,000 milligrams
Vitamin E	400–2,000 international units

MEDICAL ALERT: *If you have symptoms of endometriosis, you should see a doctor for proper diagnosis and treatment.*

Doses of vitamin C exceeding 1,200 milligrams a day may cause diarrhea.

Before taking the amount of vitamin E recommended here, you should discuss it with your doctor. Doses of vitamin E exceeding 600 international units a day can cause side effects in some people. If you are taking anticoagulant drugs, you should not take vitamin E supplements.

now pursuing her master's degree in health education at the University of Brighton in England.

Dr. Lark recommends that women with endometriosis take considerably more than the Daily Values of the B vitamins. She suggests approximately 50 milligrams each of thiamin, riboflavin, niacin and pantothenic acid, 30 milligrams of vitamin B_6, 50 micrograms of vitamin B_{12}, 400 micrograms of folic acid and 200 micrograms of biotin.

You can also fortify your diet with B vitamins by eating whole-grain cereals, pastas and rice, fish, legumes and green, leafy vegetables.

Antioxidant Onslaught

Another way to thwart the effects of endometriosis is by upping your intake of these antioxidant nutrients: vitamins C and E, beta-carotene (which converts to vitamin A in the body) and the mineral selenium. Antioxidants are best known for their ability to fight free radicals, the naturally occurring unstable molecules that cause tissue damage in the body by stealing electrons from healthy molecules to balance themselves. Doctors know that antioxidants can also build immunity, lessen cramping and reduce excessive menstrual bleeding. All of these are useful functions in treating endometriosis.

"While you can't just pop these supplements and expect instant relief from acute pain, I've found that doses of antioxidants, along with dietary changes, can treat the chronic problem of endometriosis," says Dr. Lark.

Dr. Lark recommends a daily regimen of 1,000 to 4,000 milligrams of vitamin C, 25,000 to 50,000 international units of beta-carotene, 400 to 2,000 international units of vitamin E and 25 micrograms of selenium. These are dosages at which she has arrived during her many years of treating women's health problems.

Because the recommended doses of vitamin C and vitamin E are many times the Daily Values of these nutrients, you should check with your doctor before trying this therapy. Vitamin C can cause diarrhea when taken in doses exceeding 1,200 milligrams a day.

And just because symptoms improve, that doesn't mean you can stop taking supplements, cautions Dr. Lark.

Antioxidants can have a dramatic effect on the regulation of bleeding as well as on the reduction of pain and cramps that may accompany endometriosis, says Dr. Lark. "Vitamin C is good for controlling excessive bleeding," she explains. "Vitamin A has also been shown to lessen profuse menstrual bleeding. And vitamin E has antispasmodic effects, which help in pain management."

To get more antioxidants in your diet, start by hitting the farmers market. Broccoli, spinach and cantaloupe are excellent sources of vitamin C and beta-carotene; cabbage, celery and cucumbers are great sources of selenium. For more vitamin E, try sautéing these veggies in sunflower oil or safflower oil. Or reach for a handful of almonds, another good source of vitamin E.

Epilepsy

Quieting a Short-Circuited Brain

Like all nerve tissue, our brains rely on electrical impulses to receive and send messages. Electrical currents that enter our brains through the spinal cord or optic nerves allow us to process billions of pieces of information and react to our environment, scratching an itch here, swerving to avoid a confused groundhog there or adding a comma here . . . or is it there?

Normally, electrical currents move through the brain in an orderly and limited fashion. In epilepsy, however, the currents get short-circuited or out of sync for a variety of reasons. The result is a burst of electrical activity that causes a seizure, which can be anything from a staring spell, called an absence seizure, to a full-fledged grand mal, complete with jerking arms and legs and loss of consciousness.

People can become seizure-prone for many different reasons. "An injury to the brain from an accident, a stroke or lack of oxygen during birth, alcohol abuse, poisoning, a severe bacterial or viral infection such as meningitis or encephalitis and high fever may all cause seizures," says James Neubrander, M.D., a doctor in private practice in Hopewell, New Jersey, with a special interest in epilepsy and nutrition.

Nutrients Can Play a Role

Less commonly, seizures are the result of a metabolic disease, an inherited disorder that results in an inability to properly utilize a particular nutrient in the body, such as a vitamin or an amino acid. "Seizures associated with metabolic disorders usually begin soon after birth and rarely start after age six," says Robert J. Gumnit, M.D., president of the Minnesota Comprehensive

Epilepsy Program and director of the Epilepsy Clinical Research Center at the University of Minnesota, both in Minneapolis.

In about half of these cases, the metabolic disorder can be figured out. "A specialist, a pediatric neurologist, may consider 20 to 80 different metabolic disorders that are most commonly associated with seizures," Dr. Gumnit says. Sometimes seizures can be controlled by a diet that restricts certain foods. Children with a condition called phenylketonuria, for instance, need to avoid the amino acid phenylalanine, found in large amounts in aspartame (a sugar substitute).

Adding more of a nutrient may help others. Children who develop seizures because their bodies have a hard time using vitamin B_6, for instance, may take 25 to 50 milligrams of B_6 each day, an amount large enough to overcome metabolic roadblocks.

If you think your child has seizures because of a metabolic disorder, see a specialist for a diagnosis, Dr. Gumnit urges. Don't try to treat a metabolic disorder on your own.

Seizures can also be caused by nutritional deficiency. "Most doctors, however, think that nutritional deficiency is only rarely the cause of repeated seizures," Dr. Gumnit says. Shortages of magnesium, thiamin, vitamin B_6 and zinc have been reported to be associated with seizures in some individuals. These nutrients, among numerous others, are needed for normal chemical reactions in the brain.

Nutritional support for people with seizure disorders, then, involves correcting metabolic problems and nutritional deficiencies. In some cases, it may also involve taking larger amounts of certain nutrients to help protect against drug-related damage and, in theory at least, against damage caused by the seizures themselves.

"There's absolutely no reason that optimum nutritional support can't be combined with traditional treatment," Dr. Neubrander says.

Here's what seems to be helpful.

Vitamin E Helps Prevent Seizures

There is good reason to believe that vitamin E could be helpful for some kinds of seizures. Animals given vitamin E are more resistant to seizures induced by pressurized oxygen, iron and certain chemicals. And clinical studies show that people taking antiseizure drugs have reduced blood levels of vitamin E.

(continued on page 240)

Food Factors

Most cases of epilepsy are not treated with dietary changes, but some are. Here are a few things that might prove helpful.

Ask your doctor about a ketogenic diet. A diet virtually devoid of starches and sugars and high in fat has been used as a treatment for children whose epilepsy cannot be controlled with drugs or who have to take such high doses of drugs that side effects become intolerable.

"The diet makes the body burn fat, not sugar, for energy and produces waste products called ketones that are thought to help suppress seizures," explains John M. Freeman, M.D., professor of pediatric neurology at Johns Hopkins Medical Institutions in Baltimore. Studies suggest that about 30 percent of children who try the diet have their seizures completely controlled; another 40 percent have enough benefit to warrant staying on the diet. Some are able to reduce medication, some have fewer seizures, and some function better.

Most children who benefit stay on this very restrictive diet for two years, then gradually begin to eat more starches and sugars. Often the children eventually stop the diet and find their seizures do not recur.

Vitamin and mineral supplements are necessary during this diet, since it is low in fat-soluble vitamins and calcium. Critics say the diet is too high in fat and is unhealthy for growing children. But, says Dr. Freeman, "we've seen no evidence of heart disease or growth problems."

Avoid aspartame. The official word, from the Food and Drug Administration's Center for Food Safety and Applied Nutrition, is this: Aspartame is not likely to cause seizures. (An important exception: It will cause seizures in people with phenylketonuria, a metabolic disorder that makes it difficult to break down phenylalanine, an amino acid found in aspartame.) Nevertheless, there are scattered reports of seizures associated with this food additive in apparently healthy people.

A report from Ralph G. Walton, M.D., former chief of psychiatry at Jamestown General Hospital in New York, describes a woman who switched from sugar to aspartame to sweeten her iced tea. Since she drank about a gallon of tea a day, she was exposed to large amounts of aspartame. After a few weeks of the artificially sweetened drink, she began having seizures. Doctors could find nothing wrong. The seizures stopped when she switched back to sugared tea.

Use common sense, experts suggest. "If you're getting more than a serving or two of aspartame a day, try eliminating it completely from your diet for at least one week and see if it helps," suggests James Neubrander, M.D., a doctor in private practice in Hopewell, New Jersey, with a special interest in epilepsy and nutrition.

Go easy on alcohol. People who drink too much have three times the normal risk of developing epilepsy, a risk similar to that of people who've had head injuries or central nervous system infections. In adults newly diagnosed with epilepsy, alcohol abuse accounts for symptoms in one in four, report researchers from Columbia University in New York City.

Ease up on coffee. "Although most can tolerate two to three cups of coffee or tea a day without trouble, a small percentage of people with epilepsy are very sensitive to caffeine and shouldn't take it at all," says Robert J. Gumnit, M.D., president of the Minnesota Comprehensive Epilepsy Program and director of the Epilepsy Clinical Research Center at the University of Minnesota, both in Minneapolis.

Check for food triggers. Food sensitivities may cause seizures, especially in people with personal or family histories of food allergies or sensitivities, says Dr. Neubrander. Such people might have additional symptoms such as migraines, recurrent stomach pains, diarrhea and hyperactivity. "Everyone is different, however, and may react to any food to which the body is sensitive," Dr. Neubrander points out.

Pinpointing trouble foods can be difficult, so find a specialist in food allergy testing. It's possible to be sensitive to a food and not know it. It's also very common for a person to eat the very food he is sensitive to on a daily basis, says Dr. Neubrander.

In a study by researchers at the Hospital for Sick Children in London, doctors found that cow's milk, cheeses, citrus fruits, wheat and two food additives, tartrazine and benzoic acid, are mostly likely to cause seizures in children with epilepsy. According to Dr. Neubrander, tartrazine (a food dye known as FD&C Yellow #5) and benzoic acid (a preservative) are found in thousands of foods, and the best way to avoid them is to read food labels. "Though certain foods are more commonly implicated as offenders, it is important to note that everyone is biologically different and therefore reacts differently to any food or food additive," adds Dr. Neubrander.

Prescriptions for Healing

There are a number of nutrients that have proven useful in helping to prevent seizures. But please note: These supplements are meant to provide optimum nutritional support, not to be treatments in and of themselves. It's important to work with a doctor knowledgeable in nutrition, especially if you are giving nutritional supplements to children. These are the nutrients that doctors recommend.

Nutrient	Daily Amount
Folic acid	No more than 2,500 micrograms for children ages 5–15
	400–5,000 micrograms for adults
	1,600 micrograms for women of childbearing age on antiseizure drugs
	3,000 micrograms for women on antiseizure drugs who are planning to become pregnant, taken for 3 months before stopping birth control (requires a prescription)
Selenium	50–150 micrograms for children
	50–200 micrograms for adults

That's why researchers at the University of Toronto decided to test vitamin E in 24 children with epilepsy whose seizures could not be controlled by medication.

They found that the frequency of seizures was reduced by more than 60 percent in 10 of 12 children taking vitamin E supplements. (They took 400 international units a day for three months in addition to their regular medication.) Six of them had a 90 to 100 percent reduction in seizures. By comparison, none of the 12 children who took placebos (inactive substances) along with their medication improved significantly.

What's more, when the children who were taking placebos were switched to vitamin E, seizure frequency was reduced 70 to 100 percent in all of them.

Nutrient	Daily Amount
Vitamin E	400 international units for children ages 3 and over (d-alpha-tocopherol acetate) 400–600 international units for adults (d-alpha-tocopherol acetate)

Plus a multivitamin/mineral supplement containing the Daily Values of all essential vitamins and minerals

MEDICAL ALERT: If you have been diagnosed with epilepsy, you should be under a doctor's care.

Make sure you are under a doctor's supervision when taking more than 400 micrograms of folic acid daily. High amounts can mask the symptoms of vitamin B_{12} *deficiency, also known as pernicious anemia.*

Don't take more than 100 micrograms of selenium daily without medical supervision.

Don't take more than 600 international units of vitamin E daily without medical supervision. Infants under one year of age should not be given more than 50 international units daily. If you are taking anticoagulant drugs, you should not take vitamin E supplements.

The researchers noted that there were no adverse side effects.

"Vitamin E apparently has no direct anti-epileptic action," says Paul A. Hwang, M.D., the study's main researcher, associate professor of neurology in the University of Toronto Department of Pediatrics and Medicine and director of the epilepsy program at the Hospital for Sick Children in Toronto. In other words, once a seizure is taking place, vitamin E can't help. "But it may act as a scavenger of free radicals in some forms of epilepsy, such as post-traumatic seizures, and so help protect the membranes of brain cells."

Free radicals are unstable molecules that are generated by chemical reactions involving oxygen. These molecules are potentially harmful because they grab electrons from the healthy molecules embedded in cell membranes, damaging the protective membranes. Free radical scavengers called antioxidants, such as vitamin E, offer free radicals their own electrons and so save cell membranes from harm, Dr. Hwang explains.

In animals, seizures can be induced by chemicals that produce free radicals (ferrous chloride, for instance). Iron from blood that gets into the brain after a head injury may cause seizures in the same way, Dr. Hwang says. "And the seizure itself generates more free radicals, possibly setting up a cycle that leads to frequent seizures," he adds.

Dr. Hwang and his colleagues continue to use vitamin E with good results in their patients with seizures who don't respond to standard anticonvulsant drugs. "It's not a cure-all, but it can be very helpful," he says. "If someone is going to be helped by vitamin E, the benefits will be apparent in about three months."

He has found that 400 international units daily of d-alpha-tocopherol acetate, the most biologically active form of vitamin E, is safe and effective even in children as young as age three. (Nutrition experts say that infants under age one should not be given more than 50 international units daily.) Most adults can safely take up to 600 international units without problems, but don't take more than this amount daily without medical supervision. These high amounts are not easily available from foods, says Dr. Hwang.

"It's important to work with a doctor on this," Dr. Hwang adds. "In some cases, under medical supervision, it may be possible to reduce the dosages of some seizure drugs."

Selenium May Stop Seizures

The mineral selenium, another nutrient with antioxidant properties, also appears to help control seizures in some children, says Georg Weber, M.D., Ph.D., assistant professor in the Department of Pathology at Harvard Medical School and a researcher at the Dana-Farber Cancer Institute in Boston.

Dr. Weber has found that some children with severe, uncontrollable seizures and repeated infections have low blood levels of glutathione peroxidase, a selenium-dependent antioxidant enzyme.

"We've found that giving these children 50 to 150 micrograms of selenium a day significantly reduces their seizures," Dr. Weber says. "We believe that these children have a metabolic problem that prevents them from using selenium properly and that the problem may be far more frequent than has been believed."

Talk to your doctor if you're thinking about taking selenium supplements yourself and especially if you're considering giving them to your child with epilepsy, Dr. Weber says. Although he has found amounts up to 150 micrograms a day to be safe for children with severe deficiency, children's needs can vary greatly depending on the amount of deficiency they have, and giving too much selenium could be detrimental to their health.

For adults with epilepsy, experts who use nutritional therapy recommend 50 to 200 micrograms of selenium daily to control seizures. But be sure not to take more than 100 micrograms daily without medical supervision. You can get more selenium from foods if you eat lots of garlic, onions, whole grains, mushrooms, broccoli, cabbage and fish.

Fill Up on Folic Acid

Deficiency of folate (the naturally occurring form of folic acid) isn't thought to often play a role in the development of seizures. But some antiseizure drugs deplete this B-complex vitamin, sometimes leading to abnormalities in red blood cell formation.

"Folate deficiency can also lead to serious birth defects called neural tube defects," explains Dr. Gumnit. "These birth defects happen very early in the pregnancy, often before a woman knows she is pregnant." (For more information on birth defects, see page 113.)

That is why any woman of childbearing age who's taking antiseizure drugs should also take 1,600 micrograms of folic acid a day, Dr. Gumnit says. And any woman who's taking antiseizure drugs and planning to become pregnant should also take three milligrams (3,000 micrograms) of folic acid every day for three months before she stops using birth control, he says. (That high amount requires a prescription supplement.)

Other people taking antiseizure drugs should simply take 400 micrograms, the amount of folic acid found in ordinary multivitamin/mineral supplements, Dr. Gumnit says. A few doctors recommend up to 5,000 micrograms a day for adults.

Make sure that you are under a doctor's supervision when taking more than 400 micrograms, because high amounts of folic acid can mask the symptoms of vitamin B_{12} deficiency, also known as pernicious anemia.

Some experts say that children ages 5 to 15 may safely take up to 2,500 micrograms of folic acid daily, but it's best to talk to a doctor about this, Dr. Gumnit says.

Many doctors also recommend a multivitamin/mineral supplement for their patients with epilepsy, and that's probably not a bad idea. Some research suggests that deficiencies of vitamin B_6, zinc and magnesium may also play roles in seizure disorders.

Fatigue

What to Do When You're Running on Empty

What do all doctors' waiting rooms have in common, besides outdated magazines?

Lots of tired people.

Surveys show that fatigue is one of the most common reasons that we consult our family doctors. And that's not surprising when you consider the number of conditions, both major and minor, that have fatigue as a symptom. Stress, depression, thyroid problems, anemia and food allergies can all cause persistent tiredness, says Susan M. Lark, M.D., author of *Chronic Fatigue and Tiredness*, director of the PMS and Menopause Self-Help Center in Los Altos, California, and a physician specializing in women's health. Many women also have premenstrual fatigue or fatigue that's related to menopause.

And while it may seem obvious, many of us simply don't get enough sleep. "While a small minority of people can get by on four or five hours a night, most people need six to nine hours," says Peter Hauri, Ph.D., director of the insomnia program at the Mayo Clinic Sleep Disorders Center in Rochester, Minnesota. The real test of whether you're getting enough sleep is how you feel and function during the day.

And if your fatigue continues for six months or longer and is so severe that you can't function normally, you may have chronic fatigue syndrome, a mysterious illness that causes flulike symptoms, persistent muscle pain and problems remembering or concentrating. Chronic fatigue syndrome hits mostly people between ages 25 and 50 and is relatively rare. Experts estimate that of all of the people who are fatigued enough to see a doctor about it, only 1 in 30 has chronic fatigue syndrome.

Finally, there are a number of vitamins and minerals that play roles in helping to keep you fatigue-free.

Iron: The Usual Suspect

One of the most common causes of fatigue is iron-deficiency anemia, says Dr. Lark. She estimates that 20 percent of women who menstruate are ane-

Food Factors

When it comes to beating fatigue, what you don't eat is just as important as what you do eat.

Keep yourself on the wagon. "Alcohol is a central nervous system depressant, which is the last thing you need if you are feeling chronically tired," says Susan M. Lark, M.D., author of *Chronic Fatigue and Tiredness*, director of the PMS and Menopause Self-Help Center in Los Altos, California, and a physician specializing in women's health.

Don't lean on caffeine. It's tempting to reach for a cup of strong coffee when you can barely keep your eyes open, but if you're mainlining coffee, tea or cola from morning to night, you're doing yourself more harm than good, says Dr. Lark. Caffeine may give you a temporary jolt of energy, but in a few hours, you'll be just as tired as before—if not more tired.

In place of coffee, Dr. Lark recommends a caffeine-free herbal tea containing ginger root. "It tastes good and is mildly stimulating, but there's no rebound effect," she says. You can find herbal ginger teas in your local supermarket.

Master your sugar cravings. Simple sugars, such as those found in cookies, candies and sweet desserts, cause sharp increases in your blood sugar level, which may make you feel temporarily energized. But after the initial rush, blood sugar drops sharply, says Dr. Lark, which can result in an energy crisis.

Lighten up on fat. "Fatty foods, including most meats, are very hard to digest," says Dr. Lark. "Eating meat two or three times a day is like eating Christmas dinner 21 times a week. You're spending all of your energy digesting rich, heavy foods." She recommends a low-fat diet high in whole grains, legumes and fresh fruits and vegetables, the same type of diet that is recommended for preventing heart disease and some types of cancer.

mic because of the blood they lose each month. "Women with heavy menstrual flow have the greatest risk," she adds. Anemia is also common among teenagers, pregnant women and women nearing menopause.

If you suspect that you may be anemic, the first step is to make an appoint-

Prescriptions for Healing

Here's what experts recommend to help you banish fatigue.

Nutrient	Daily Amount
Iron	12–15 milligrams
Magnesium	100–200 milligrams
Potassium	100–200 milligrams
Vitamin C	4,000 milligrams

MEDICAL ALERT: *People with heart or kidney problems should consult their doctors before taking supplemental magnesium.*

People with kidney problems or diabetes should consult their doctors before taking supplemental potassium.

High doses of vitamin C may cause diarrhea in some people.

ment with your doctor, says Dr. Lark. It's the only way to find out for sure.

But even if you're not anemic, a slight iron deficiency can affect your energy level, and you may benefit from getting more iron in your diet, says Dr. Lark. Experts who recommend iron to combat fatigue generally suggest between 12 and 15 milligrams a day. The best source of iron is animal products, so go for lean meats, cooked oysters and clams. Some vegetables such as spinach as well as legumes such as green beans, lima beans and pinto beans are also rich in iron, but the type of iron found in them is not as easy to absorb as the iron found in animal sources.

If you're a vegetarian, drinking some orange juice or taking a vitamin C supplement of at least 75 milligrams along with iron-rich vegetables will help your body absorb more iron from your food, says Dr. Lark. Many commercial breads and breakfast cereals are also fortified with iron.

Potassium and Magnesium: A Potent Combination

Two other minerals that may be beneficial for people with persistent fatigue are potassium and magnesium, says Dr. Lark. "In studies where potassium and magnesium were given together, 90 percent saw improvements in their energy levels," says Dr. Lark. She recommends trying between 100 and 200 milligrams of each mineral for up to six months to see if they alleviate fatigue. It's safe for anyone in good health, she says, although people with heart or kidney problems or diabetes shouldn't take these minerals without consulting a doctor first.

Rev Up with Vitamin C

While more research needs to be done, some older studies suggest that low vitamin C intake can also contribute to fatigue. A 1976 study of 411 dentists and their wives found that those with low vitamin C intakes reported twice as many fatigue symptoms as those who got the most vitamin C. And studies of adolescent boys showed that even those with slight vitamin C deficiencies had more stamina after taking vitamin C supplements for three months.

Dr. Lark recommends about 4,000 milligrams of vitamin C a day for people with persistent fatigue. She warns that this high dose can cause temporary diarrhea in some people. "If this happens," she says, "just cut back on the dose to the point where the diarrhea goes away."

Fibrocystic Breasts

Lessening the Lumps

Debra was 18 years old when she found the first lump in her breast. "Then I noticed I had one in my other breast, almost identical and in the same position. I was terrified," she recalls. "My mother took me to her doctor. He felt the lumps and without a word walked out of the room. He gave me a form to take to radiology. It was an order for a mammogram, and though I couldn't make out the whole word, I could clearly read 'cyst.' I was sure I had cancer.

"When I finally got the courage to ask the doctor what was wrong, he said that I had fibrocystic breast disease and that there was nothing I could do about it except become very familiar with my breasts, so I would know if I

Food Factors

Ever wish that the food you eat would go straight to your bustline instead of your waistline? For women with fibrocystic breasts, that's often what happens, only not in a way they appreciate. Here are some dietary changes that doctors recommend to lessen the pain and lumpiness of fibrocystic breasts.

Cool the coffee habit. Some experts consider reducing caffeine consumption to be the best, most cost-effective treatment for fibrocystic breasts. That's because caffeine apparently stimulates estrogen production and promotes swollen, painful breasts.

According to researchers at Michigan State University College of Human Medicine in East Lansing, women who ingest more than 500 milligrams of caffeine a day, the amount in about four cups of coffee, are at 2.3 times greater risk of fibrocystic breasts than those who abstain. And those who eliminate caffeine from their diets, the researchers say, experience a 60 to 65 percent reduction in symptoms.

Other sources of caffeine include tea, chocolate and cola.

Trim the fat. "Eating too much saturated fat increases estrogen levels and stimulates fibrocystic changes," says Susan M. Lark, M.D., author of *PMS: Self-Help Book* and *Menopause: Self-Help Book*, director of the PMS and Menopause Self-Help Center in Los Altos, California, and a physician specializing in women's health. Dr. Lark recommends that women avoid animal fat whenever possible. That means cutting back on meats and eating nonfat dairy products.

found anything new. He told me not to worry, but I couldn't help but wonder if this 'disease' meant that cancer was next.

"Ten years and many lumps later, I finally understand what I have and that it's not a disease. I also know I can make changes in my diet that will make my breasts less tender and reduce the lumpiness. I finally feel more comfortable about my breasts."

Debra is not alone in her experience, according to Susan M. Lark, M.D., author of *The PMS Self-Help Book* and the *Menopause Self-Help Book*, director of the PMS and Menopause Self-Help Center in Los Altos, California, and a physician specializing in women's health. Dr. Lark frequently treats women who have this frightening and often painful condition. "Being diagnosed with fibrocystic breasts is scary and confusing for a lot of women," says Dr.

Power up with bran. "A good complement to cutting fat is boosting fiber," says David P. Rose, M.D., D.Sc., Ph.D., chief of the Division of Nutrition and Endocrinology at the Naylor Dana Institute of the American Health Foundation in Valhalla, New York.

"Fiber absorbs estrogen and helps excrete it from the body," says Dr. Rose. He recommends that women increase their fiber intakes to 25 to 30 grams a day, roughly double what most women eat. You can increase your fiber intake by eating more whole grains, fruits and vegetables.

Lean toward teetotalism. "The liver is responsible for detoxifying circulating estrogen, and alcohol is toxic to the liver," says Dr. Lark. "I suggest that women with fibrocystic breasts avoid drinking or limit their alcohol intakes."

Lower the sodium. Doctors have found that benign breast cysts are affected by how much fluid you retain. Since sodium makes you hold water, many doctors recommend limiting salt intake to less than 1,500 milligrams a day. (That's not much salt; one teaspoon contains 2,000 milligrams of sodium.)

Eat your diuretics. A diuretic is a substance that helps your body get rid of excess water. As a sodium-cutting complement, Dr. Lark recommends that women increase their intakes of naturally diuretic foods such as parsley, celery and cucumbers, which can help decrease fluid retention.

Lark. In many cases, they can be helped by "natural, gentle treatments" such as nutrition, she adds.

First, however, it helps to understand how breasts become fibrocystic to begin with.

Taking Your Lumps

Fibrocystic breasts is a term for nothing more than lumpy breasts, a condition that affects about 70 percent of women at some time in their lives, usually during their childbearing years. It is very likely that once a woman reaches menopause, her cysts will shrink or even disappear. Some postmenopausal women may experience fibrocystic breasts as a consequence of

Evening Primrose Relief

Want relief from swollen, tender fibrocystic breasts without the side effects of hormone therapy? Evening primrose oil—a rich source of gamma-linolenic acid, which your body uses to regulate its salt and water balance—could be your answer. Welsh researchers who have studied the supplement for nearly 20 years now recommend it as the first line of treatment to relieve the pain of fibrocystic breasts without side effects.

"Evening primrose oil is a common treatment," says Susan M. Lark, M.D., author of *PMS: Self-Help Book* and *Menopause: Self-Help Book*, director of the PMS and Menopause Self-Help Center in Los Altos, California, and a physician specializing in women's health. "It's a good source of essential fatty acids, and it has a diuretic and anti-inflammatory effect on the body."

For relief from breast pain and lumps, some experts recommend taking 1,000 milligrams three times daily for a period of three months. Before you start with supplementation, check with your doctor.

hormone replacement therapy if the dosage of estrogen is too high.

For most women, the condition means lumps ranging from tiny, BB size to larger, egg size. These lumps recur monthly as estrogen stimulates milk glands in the breasts, causing the glands to accumulate fluid and swell. For other women, it means lasting cysts that result from milk ducts that clog and don't drain. Some women even experience a little discharge from their nipples. Though they aren't life-threatening, swollen, fibrocystic breasts can be both physically painful and emotionally stressful.

Unfortunately, there is no cure for this condition, only potential treatments. Because it's hormone-triggered, doctors advise that the best strategy for relieving fibrocystic pain and lumpiness is to decrease the levels of the female hormone estrogen circulating in your blood. Though hormone therapy is one approach, some experts, including Dr. Lark, maintain that nutritional regimens can work just as well without the side effects of hormone therapy. Here's what they recommend.

Note: Even if you have fibrocystic breasts, it's always important to have every new lump or breast change checked by your doctor, says Dr. Lark.

Ease Fibrocystic Breasts with E

Although clinical studies during the past decade have yielded mixed results and no research has been done recently, vitamin E remains a commonly recommended supplement for treating fibrocystic breasts—one that many doctors swear by.

"Honestly, I don't think anyone can tell you exactly why vitamin E works against fibrocystic breasts," says Dr. Lark. "We know just that it relieves symptoms caused by excessive estrogen levels and that it has an anti-inflammatory effect that gives many women relief from their symptoms."

Echoing those sentiments is Bernard Ginsberg, M.D., a physician in private practice in Santa Monica, California, who became interested in the value of vitamin therapy while working at the Research Institute at Sinai Hospital in Baltimore with Robert London, M.D., assistant professor of obstetrics and gynecology at Johns Hopkins University School of Medicine in Baltimore.

"I was doubtful about it in the beginning, but during the past ten years, I've found that vitamin therapy can really make a difference," says Dr. Ginsberg, who has concentrated much of his practice on women's health and natural healing. "Vitamin E, along with vitamin B_6, counteracts the swelling effects of estrogen. It also increases the metabolism of female hormones, getting them out of circulation."

Both Dr. Lark and Dr. Ginsberg recommend that women with fibrocystic breasts take about 600 international units of vitamin E daily, an amount that was used and found to be successful in several studies of vitamin E and fibrocystic breasts, says Dr. Lark.

It is impossible to get such high amounts of vitamin E without supplementation. But adding almonds, wheat germ and sunflower oil or safflower oil to your daily fare can give you a healthy boost of this helpful nutrient.

Extra Help from Vitamin A

Pointing to a promising pilot study of the effects of vitamin A on fibrocystic breasts as well as her own work with her patients, Dr. Lark believes that this potent nutrient may also be effective for soothing sore, lumpy breasts.

In this study, which was conducted at the University of Montreal, 12 women with moderate to severe breast pain were given high doses of vitamin A for three months. Nine of the women experienced significant pain relief, and 5 of the women experienced decreases in breast lumps. The bad news is that the dosage in that study was 150,000 international units a day, an amount 30 times the Daily Value and one with which few experts feel comfortable, since vitamin A is toxic in high doses.

"From my experience, I believe that women who have substantial breast pain from benign breast disease are likely to get relief from vitamin A," says the study's lead researcher, Pierre R. Band, M.D., head of epidemiology at the British Columbia Cancer Agency in Vancouver. "But you are dealing with a potentially toxic compound, so you have to be careful. Researchers have studied the effects of lower doses of vitamin A than what I used and have received good results, so it is promising, but we need more investigation."

"My answer is to use beta-carotene instead," says Dr. Lark. She suggests taking between 25,000 and 50,000 international units of beta-carotene a day for fibrocystic breasts. "Beta-carotene, also called preformed vitamin A, converts to vitamin A in the body, and you don't have to worry about toxicity with large doses," she explains.

While you can buy beta-carotene supplements, it's easy to get all of the beta-carotene you need just by eating plenty of orange and yellow fruits and vegetables, says Dr. Lark. One sweet potato alone, for instance, packs a beta-carotene punch of 10,000 international units.

Better Breasts with B_6

Although scientific tests have yet to be done, some doctors who treat women for fibrocystic breasts also recommend vitamin B_6 because of its known importance in maintaining normal hormone levels.

"The women I treat find that it's useful in reducing swelling," says Dr. Ginsberg. He recommends taking 50 milligrams of vitamin B_6 two or three times a day before breast pain and tenderness occur, which is usually during the week prior to menstruation. But be sure to consult your doctor before exceeding 100 milligrams of B_6 a day, since large doses have resulted in nerve damage.

To increase your vitamin B_6 intake from foods, try slicing a banana on your morning cereal and adding a baked potato to your evening meal.

Iodine on the Horizon

According to researchers, iodine might be the wave of the future for fibrocystic breast relief. Before you reach for the saltshaker, however, you should know that iodized salt will likely not be of much help. The iodine experts are recommending diatomic iodine, and these supplements are still awaiting approval from the Food and Drug Administration.

So far, though, the results of studies using diatomic iodine to treat fibrocystic breasts look promising. In one five-year study at Hotel Dieu Hospital at Queen's University at Kingston in Ontario, more than 1,000 women were supplemented with sodium iodide (that's what is in iodized salt), protein-bound iodide or diatomic iodine. Researchers found that diatomic iodine reduced breast pain in the most women, and with the fewest side effects.

"Sodium iodide is marginally helpful, because about 5 percent of it breaks down into elemental iodine in the body," explains one of the lead researchers, Bernard A. Eskin, M.D., of the Department of Obstetrics and Gynecology at the Medical College of Pennsylvania in Philadelphia. "But you

Prescriptions for Healing

Doctors can't promise that anything will lessen breast pain and lumpiness for sure, but some experts have had some success with these nutrients.

Nutrient	**Daily Amount**
Beta-carotene	25,000–50,000 international units
Iodine	150 micrograms
Vitamin B_6	100–150 milligrams, taken as 2 or 3 divided doses
Vitamin E	600 international units

MEDICAL ALERT: *If you feel any new or unusual lump in your breasts, check with your doctor for a complete diagnosis.*

Iodine supplements are not yet available, and the iodine in your medicine cabinet is poisonous. Until the supplement is available, you must get your iodine from food sources.

Be sure to consult your doctor before exceeding 100 milligrams of vitamin B_6 a day, since large doses have resulted in nerve damage.

If you are taking anticoagulant drugs, you should not take vitamin E supplements.

need much more sodium iodide for the same effects as elemental iodine, and that much causes greater side effects." Plus too much sodium leads to fluid retention, which can aggravate already swollen breasts.

The researchers believe that iodine prevents fibrocystic breast symptoms by making cells in the milk ducts less sensitive to circulating estrogen. They are hopeful that a supplement containing diatomic iodine, Amydine, will be available within a few years.

In the meantime, you may reap a few benefits by eating iodine-rich foods such as seafood and seaweed and by making sure to get the Daily Value of 150 micrograms of iodine, concedes Dr. Eskin. Your best results, he says, will come from the supplement once it is available.

Note: The iodine in your medicine cabinet is poisonous and should not be ingested for any reason.

Fingernail Problems

Beating Brittle Nails

It's true that they are the perfect way to display the latest fashion colors. But don't sell fingernails short. Besides protecting your sensitive fingertips from the abuses of daily life, they can tell you a lot about whether you're eating right.

Like bone health, nail health depends on good nutrition. Brittle nails have been associated with deficiencies of calcium, zinc and iron and with too much selenium. And slow nail growth can result from general malnourishment.

But so far, only one nutrient—biotin, part of the B-complex—has been proven helpful for nail health in people who aren't malnourished. You can thank veterinary science for that bit of information. Biotin has long been used to help harden horses' hooves.

Here are the details.

Biotin Banishes Brittle Nails

A study by Swiss researchers looked at people with apparently normal intakes of biotin: 28 to 42 micrograms a day. Researchers found that people in the study with thin, frail and split nails who took extra amounts of biotin—2.5 milligrams (2,500 micrograms), or roughly 70 times the average daily intake—experienced a 25 percent increase in nail thickness.

Prescriptions for Healing

Only one nutrient, biotin, has been shown in scientific studies to help fingernails.

Nutrient	Daily Amount
Biotin	2,500 micrograms

MEDICAL ALERT: While biotin is considered one of the safest of all nutrients, the dosage recommended here is extremely high and should be taken only under medical supervision.

"Biotin is absorbed into the matrix of the nail, where it may help correct brittle nails," explains Richard K. Scher, M.D., dermatologist and head of the nail section at Columbia Presbyterian Medical Center in New York City. (The matrix is the part embedded in the finger where nail cells are generated.) Dr. Scher recommends biotin supplements to his patients with weak nails. "It seems to help about two-thirds of them," he says.

The amount of biotin used in the Swiss study is very high. This dose should not be taken except under medical supervision.

Top dietary sources of biotin are egg yolks, soybean flour, cereals and yeast. Cauliflower, lentils, milk and peanut butter also provide decent amounts.

Gallstones

Clearing Out the Gravel Pit

The woman was about 20 pounds overweight. Nevertheless, she downed pizza, fries and a milk shake with barely a pause to breathe, then topped it off with cheesecake.

Three hours later, she was in the emergency room, a sharp pain boring into the upper right quarter of her abdomen.

The diagnosis? One nasty little gallstone about the size of a pea, stuck in a duct that connects the gallbladder to the bowel. And it was there to stay until it would somehow squeeze through to the bowel or drop back into the gallbladder or until a surgeon would go in and yank it out—along with her gallbladder.

Eat and Squirt

Whether or not a doctor has ever looked you in the eye and announced the presence of a pea-size pellet wandering through your digestive system, there's a good chance that you have at least one. Close to 30 million Americans do. Most of them are over age 40, most of them are women, and most of them don't even know that the gallstones are there.

The stones are formed when a grain or two of calcium arrives in the gallbladder and hangs around long enough to become coated with either cholesterol or bilirubin, a substance that is part of the hemoglobin in your blood. Eighty to 85 percent of all stones are coated with layer upon layer of waxy-looking cholesterol, although many stones are coated with both substances. A few are made exclusively of yellowish green bilirubin.

Exactly what causes this buildup of cholesterol or bilirubin on the calcium is not totally clear. Normally, the gallbladder is a storage compartment for the somewhat slimy bile that your body needs to digest fat. You eat fat, the stomach sends it through to the bowel, and your gallbladder squirts some bile onto the food to break up the fat. Your body then finishes its digestive process, and everything heads for the exit.

But occasionally, your body screws up. Something breaks down during the eat-squirt-exit process, and the gallbladder's sludgelike contents crystallize. This provides the opportunity to layer thicker and thicker coats of cholesterol or bilirubin around a calcium speck, thus forming a gallstone.

Naturally occurring female reproductive hormones are known to encourage that process by delaying gallbladder emptying, such as during pregnancy and dieting. What's more, birth control implants that contain progesterone may do the same, while birth control pills containing estrogen seem to increase the cholesterol content of bile—not a helpful situation, either.

Blame Your Genes and Diet

All told, hormones, pregnancy, dieting and birth control may help explain why two-thirds of all gallstones belong to women. But aside from being a woman, what else puts you at risk for gallstones? (After all, many men get them, too.)

Food Factors

Dietary strategies are crucial in reducing gallstone formation, according to medical experts. Here's what they recommend.

Can the cholesterol. Stick closely to the American Heart Association's recommendation to consume no more than 300 milligrams of dietary cholesterol a day, advises Henry Pitt, M.D., vice-chairman of surgery at Johns Hopkins University School of Medicine in Baltimore. Reducing the amount of cholesterol in your blood may reduce your body's ability to incorporate it into gallstones.

Dietary cholesterol comes exclusively from animal sources: meats and dairy products. To reduce your cholesterol levels, you need to cut back on these foods as well as on saturated fat. (That's any fat that is solid at room temperature.)

Cut those calories. Studies indicate that women who consume so many calories that they become obese can have up to six times the risk of gallstones of women of normal weight. That's why Dr. Pitt suggests maintaining a healthy weight and following the American Heart Association's recommendation to get less than 30 percent of your calories from fat.

Watch that sweet tooth. A study of 872 men in the Netherlands showed that a high-sugar diet can nearly double the risk of gallstones. No one knows exactly why, but researchers suspect that sugar may increase the amount of cholesterol—the raw material from which most gallstones are built—in your gallbladder.

Eat fish. Animal and human studies at Johns Hopkins University School of Medicine have indicated that fish oil may reduce the formation of gallstones. "We're not saying that we can dissolve gallstones," says Dr. Pitt. "But we can slow the rate at which they form. So people at high risk, such as those who diet frequently and those who are pregnant, might want to incorporate fish as a regular part of their diets."

"Diet and genetics," replies Henry Pitt, M.D., vice-chairman of surgery at Johns Hopkins University School of Medicine in Baltimore. And it's difficult to sort out which is responsible for what. So far, many scientific studies of populations only add to the confusion.

In Chile, for example, 60 percent of people have gallstones by the time they're 80 years of age. Yet in Africa, gallstones affect only 1 to 2 percent of the population.

Is that diet or genetics?

It could be one or the other or both, says Dr. Pitt. Studies of ethnic groups who rarely get gallstones indicate that when they move from a geographic location in which they have consumed a low-fat, low-cholesterol diet to a location in which they consume a high-fat, high-cholesterol diet, they start getting gallstones.

Aside from lowering calories and fat, another dietary factor may have an impact on gallstone formation, and it involves a mineral: calcium.

The Calcium Controversy

A low-fat, low-cholesterol diet may help prevent gallstones, agrees Alan Hofmann, M.D., Ph.D., professor at the University of California, San Diego, but the most important aspect of the diet is that it doesn't have too many calories, so a person stays slender. But Dr. Hofmann also feels there is reason

Prescriptions for Healing

Although reducing dietary fat and cholesterol and keeping your weight down are clearly the two most important strategies that you can choose to prevent gallstones, there is one mineral that may help as well, according to Alan Hofmann, M.D., Ph.D., professor at the University of California, San Diego.

Nutrient	Daily Amount
Calcium	1,000 milligrams

MEDICAL ALERT: *If you have a gallstone, you should be under a doctor's care.*

Dr. Hofmann considers calcium supplementation to be fine for men. Calcium may contribute to the formation of some kinds of gallstones in women, however. He suggests that women discuss supplementation with their physicians.

to believe that supplementing the diet with calcium may act to prevent gallstones.

"In addition to helping your bones, calcium has a good effect on bile acid metabolism," explains Dr. Hofmann. "What has been found is that large doses of oral calcium form calcium phosphate in the gut." This sets off a chain of chemical events that eventually lowers the amount of cholesterol in the gallbladder, thus reducing the possibility that gallstones will form, he explains.

It also seems to explain why a study of 872 Dutchmen between the ages of 40 and 59 found that the more calcium the men consumed over a 25-year period, the fewer gallstones they were likely to have.

In fact, one study in the Netherlands revealed that men who had more than 1,442 milligrams of calcium in their diets every day had a 50 percent lower prevalence of gallstones.

"Since most individuals have stopped drinking much milk by the time they're 45 years old, it makes good sense to take calcium supplements," says Dr. Hofmann. Nonetheless, the view that large doses of supplemental calcium can prevent gallstones has not yet been tested experimentally. Normal doses of calcium do not increase the risk of kidney stones, however, and are likely to be good for both bones and bile. Studies are needed to prove this point as well as to prove that there are no important risks associated with long-term use of oral calcium supplements, says Dr. Hofmann.

Experts who recommend calcium to help prevent gallstones suggest aiming for the Daily Value, which is 1,000 milligrams. But before you race out to the drugstore, Dr. Pitt suggests that you take a moment to check with your physician, especially if you're a woman.

"Calcium may have something to do with the origin of most of the gallstones in this country," says Dr. Pitt. "It's at the center of almost every stone we find. And in our animal studies, diets with high calcium seem to enhance the formation of pigment stones," the stones made of bilirubin.

And keep in mind all of the hormonal factors that affect women, says Dr. Pitt. It may turn out that calcium prevents gallstones in men but actually contributes to their formation in women.

So while men can feel comfortable taking calcium supplements, women should ask their family physicians to help evaluate individual risks and benefits, particularly in light of their family medical histories, says Dr. Pitt.

"If all of the women in your family get gallstones and none of them gets osteoporosis, then I'd stay away from calcium," he advises. But if all of the women get osteoporosis and only an occasional stone rolls down someone's duct, then calcium should be okay, he adds.

Genital Herpes

Heading Off a Return Visit

Safe sex. Everywhere you turn, the message is there: If you're going to have intercourse, even just once, use protection.

Despite the prevalence of that warning, over the years millions of people have ended up with recurring infections, the most common being herpes simplex virus type 2, otherwise known as genital herpes.

Even today, with our vast pool of knowledge, researchers estimate that each year at least 500,000 people in North America contract genital herpes. And once herpes moves in, it becomes a permanent resident. Although dormant most of the time, this infection flares up occasionally to remind you that it's still there. Fortunately, after the initial infection, which causes flulike aches and pains as well a painful crop of blisters on and around the genitals, recurrent outbreaks of genital herpes are usually not as bad. Unfortunately, outbreaks are usually marked by a small cluster of genital blisters that itch, burn, ooze and generally make life miserable for the week or so that they are around.

No one really knows what triggers recurrent outbreaks, but scientists believe that stress may play a role, along with other factors that challenge the immune system, such as menstrual periods, fever and bodily injury.

Nutrition Might Help

Though researchers are testing a vaccine, there is no cure for genital herpes. But one fairly successful medication is the prescription drug acyclovir (Zovirax). Some studies show that if taken during the initial outbreak, it can help reduce the number of recurrences.

Nutritional therapies for genital herpes do exist, but experts have found them to be less than consistent: Some people have considerable success with them, while others have none at all. "None of these treatments is well-researched, and we can't recommend them across the board because the success rates are so random," says Stephen Tyring, M.D., Ph.D., professor of dermatology, of microbiology and immunology, and of internal medicine at the University of Texas Medical School at Galveston. "If it's safe and it

Food Factors

Along with keeping your stress levels under control, there are a number of dietary approaches that many medical experts say can help prevent genital herpes from recurring. Here's what they say helps.

Load up on lysine. Researchers have found that lysine, an amino acid that your body needs in order to function, interferes with reproduction of the herpes virus. And apparently, increasing your intake of lysine just might help reduce your number of outbreaks.

Good sources of lysine include fish, chicken, cheeses, potatoes, milk, brewer's yeast and beans.

Lighten up on arginine. They say that for every force, there's a counterforce. Well, in the case of lysine, that counterforce is arginine, another amino acid that your body needs.

Arginine, which has been linked to herpes outbreaks, is found in abundance in foods such as peanuts and other nuts and seeds as well as chocolate and gelatin. You don't have to eliminate these foods completely, but some doctors suggest that when you're under stress, it might be a good idea to cut back on them.

seems to help a person, however, then I don't discourage it."

That said, here's what some doctors recommend as potential nutritional treatments.

Boost Immunity with Vitamin C

Since herpes tends to become reactivated when your defenses are down, some doctors recommend upping your intake of vitamin C, which is known to help your body's infection-fighting white blood cells do their duty.

"There is strong scientific evidence that vitamin C can boost the immune system, and therefore it should help. But people who take megadoses of vitamin C are sometimes helped and sometimes not," cautions Dr. Tyring. "It'll probably have the biggest effect if you're not getting enough in your diet to begin with."

Doctors who recommend large doses generally call for anywhere from 1,000 to 4,000 milligrams up to 8,000 milligrams, divided throughout the day during the active part of the infection. This is considerably higher than the

Daily Value of vitamin C, which is only 60 milligrams, and unpleasant side effects, especially diarrhea, can show up in some people with as little as 1,200 milligrams. So it would be a good idea to discuss vitamin C with your doctor if you'd like to try a higher dose.

If you suspect that you're among those who don't get enough vitamin C, you can give your diet a boost of this important nutrient by eating more fruits and vegetables, particularly oranges, broccoli and red bell peppers.

Think Zinc for Relief

The mineral zinc acts as a double agent in the fight against herpes, working both from the inside out and from the outside in.

Like vitamin C, zinc is a frontline player in boosting the immune system, especially the production of T lymphocyte cells, which are important body defenses against viral infections. Though they admit that zinc's effect against herpes is speculative, doctors who recommend nutritional regimens for preventing recurrent herpes outbreaks often suggest taking zinc supplements.

How much you should take varies depending on whom you ask, but the recommended range is somewhere between 30 and 60 milligrams a day, well above the Daily Value of 15 milligrams. (You should consult your doctor before exceeding 15 milligrams of zinc a day.) And because zinc can interfere with the absorption of copper, doctors also suggest taking 1 milligram of copper for every 10 milligrams of zinc.

If you want to get more zinc through your diet, then soup up your intake of seafood. Just six steamed medium oysters pack about 76 milligrams of zinc.

Also, if you're a man with genital herpes, some doctors recommend having a topical preparation containing zinc oxide on hand. Applied directly to the blisters, the ointment will ease the burning and dry out the blisters more quickly. Doctors warn women not to use zinc oxide ointments for vaginal herpes, however, because drying agents shouldn't be used on mucous membranes.

"This doesn't work as an antiviral agent," says Dr. Tyring. "But it may numb the pain and itching."

Keep It at Bay with Vitamin A

Although it's not a common treatment, some doctors recommend taking high doses of vitamin A to boost immunity and prevent herpes recurrence.

"Vitamin A helps the immune system fight viruses, so the symptoms are

Prescriptions for Healing

While there are no guarantees when it comes to treating genital herpes, some people experience fewer, less severe outbreaks by boosting their intakes of certain nutrients. Here's what many experts recommend.

Nutrient	Daily Amount/Application
Oral	
Copper	3–6 milligrams (1 milligram for every 10 milligrams of zinc)
Vitamin A	50,000 international units
Vitamin C	1,000–8,000 milligrams, taken as divided doses during the active part of the infection
Zinc	30–60 milligrams
Topical	
Zinc oxide	As an ingredient in ointment, applied directly to the blisters (for men only)

MEDICAL ALERT: *If you have symptoms of genital herpes, you should see your doctor for proper diagnosis and treatment.*

Vitamin A can be toxic in high doses. Consult your doctor before exceeding 15,000 international units a day (or 10,000 international units a day for women of childbearing age). Women who are pregnant should not use this therapy.

Doses of vitamin C above 1,200 milligrams a day can cause diarrhea in some people.

You should not exceed 15 milligrams of zinc a day without first discussing it with your doctor.

less and the number of infections is fewer," explains Jonathan Wright, M.D., a doctor in Kent, Washington, who specializes in nutritional therapy and is the author of *Dr. Wright's Guide to Healing with Nutrition.*

For fighting herpes, Dr. Wright recommends taking 50,000 international units daily, an amount that far exceeds the Daily Value of 5,000 international units, for the duration of the outbreak. If you want to try this, clear it with your doctor first. Vitamin A can be toxic in high doses and can build up in the body.

Taking 10,000 units of vitamin A in early pregnancy has been linked to a high risk of birth defects. If you are pregnant, do not use this therapy. And if you are of childbearing age, be sure to check with your doctor before starting vitamin A supplementation.

Gingivitis

Exploring the Role of Vitamin C

What if you floss and brush until you're blue in the face and you still have bleeding, receding gums?

You're dealing with a stubborn case of what's known as gingivitis. And it is cause for concern. Left for even a short time along your gum line, food particles and bacteria combine to form plaque, which hardens on your teeth and irritates your gums. Irritated gums bleed and eventually start to recede, creating pockets next to your teeth that collect even more junk. Before long, the plaque starts attacking the roots of your teeth and your jawbone; this is the point at which gingivitis turns into a more serious gum problem known as periodontal disease. If periodontal disease progresses too far without proper medical intervention, you might even lose some teeth.

When it comes to healthy gums, most dentists rightly focus on clearing out the crud with frequent flossing and brushing. But there's no doubt that diet also plays a role.

"After all, the mouth is attached to the rest of the body," says Cherilyn Sheets, D.D.S., a spokesperson for the Academy of General Dentistry and a dentist in Newport Beach, California. "Anything that improves health overall and the body's ability to resist disease will affect the mouth positively." Eat badly enough, or indulge in damaging behaviors such as smoking and excessive drinking, and your whole body suffers, including your mouth, says Dr. Sheets.

Food Factors

Keeping these dietary tips in mind may keep your gums in the pink.

Phase out soft drinks. Canned soda contains excess phosphorus, a mineral that could lead to the leaching of calcium from your bones, a potential cause of osteoporosis. Some researchers believe that calcium is first robbed not from your hips or spine but from your jaw, leading to tooth loss, says Ken Wical, D.D.S., professor of restorative dentistry at Loma Linda University in California.

"We see a number of young women in their teens who, I believe because of poor dietary habits such as drinking diet soda and not getting enough calcium, have the jaws of much older women," says Dr. Wical. "And by the time they're in their thirties, they're wearing dentures."

Reduce your sugar. In addition to promoting dental decay, sugar is thought to harm gums. Many dentists believe that sugar feeds the bacteria that cause the infection leading to gingivitis, although there are no definitive studies to prove this.

Take Vitamin C and See Improvement

"Certainly, vitamin C is the one nutrient that has been shown to have quite a positive effect on the mouth when in adequate levels in the body and a negative effect on the mouth when in low levels in the body," says Dr. Sheets. People with vitamin C deficiencies can have some of the worst gum and dental problems that dentists see.

To measure the effect of vitamin C deficiency on gum health, researchers at the University of California, San Francisco, School of Dentistry for 14 weeks fed 11 men rotating diets that purposely excluded fruits and vegetables. Vitamin C, in the form of a supplement dissolved in grape juice, was added to their diets only during certain weeks. At the end of the study, researchers found that as vitamin C levels in the men went down, their gums bled more. When they received more vitamin C, their gums bled less.

Further research with laboratory animals confirmed that vitamin C deficiency causes gum swelling, decreased mineral content of the jawbone and loose teeth.

Prescriptions for Healing

You may see substantial improvement in the health of your gums by making sure you brush, floss and get adequate levels of vitamin C each day, says Mary Dan Eades, M.D., medical director of the Arkansas Center for Health and Weight Control in Little Rock. Here are her recommendations for a healthier mouth.

Nutrient	Daily Amount
Vitamin C	1,000–2,000 milligrams (slow-release capsules), taken as 2 divided doses
	½ teaspoon (crystalline vitamin C), mixed with a sugar-free citrus beverage and used as an oral rinse twice a day (swish in your mouth for 1 minute)

MEDICAL ALERT: *If you have gingivitis, you should be under a dentist's care.*

Chewable and powdered vitamin C have been found to erode tooth enamel, so it's best to use the crystalline form in a mouth rinse. This is a big problem and can also cause tooth sensitivity. Some dentists prefer using the oral rinse for three to five days at a time. Follow the rinse with plenty of fresh water.

Vitamin C can also cause diarrhea in doses exceeding 1,200 milligrams.

Why the damage? As it turns out, vitamin C is vital for production of collagen, the basic protein building block for the fibrous framework of all tissues, including gums, explains Mary Dan Eades, M.D., medical director of the Arkansas Center for Health and Weight Control in Little Rock. "Vitamin C strengthens weak gum tissue and makes the gum lining more resistant to penetration by bacteria," she says.

Dr. Eades recommends using vitamin C in two ways—as a mouthwash and as a supplement—to fight gingivitis. "Mix a half-teaspoon of crystalline vitamin C with a sugar-free citrus beverage, swish the mixture in your mouth for one minute, then swallow, twice daily," she advises. Follow each rinse with plenty of fresh water.

Crystalline vitamin C is also called powdered pure ascorbic acid and is available in health food stores and through vitamin supply houses. Your doctor could help you find a supply. (Chewable or powdered vitamin C can erode tooth enamel. So it's best to stick to the crystalline form if you're using it as a mouth rinse.)

You can also take 500-milligram slow-release vitamin C capsules, one or two in the morning and one or two in the evening, says Dr. Eades. (Some people may experience diarrhea when taking vitamin C in doses exceeding 1,200 milligrams a day.) Meanwhile, keep on brushing and flossing!

Glaucoma

Easing the Pressure

Thomas Goslin had the classic symptoms of glaucoma: a steady buildup of fluid in the eyeballs, creating excessive pressure and some loss of peripheral vision.

At his ophthalmologist's instruction, Goslin, a retired Presbyterian minister from Wildwood Crest, New Jersey, reluctantly began using prescription eyedrops, one of the most common treatments. He was reluctant because he has a history of allergic reaction to medication, and sure enough, by the end of the first day of using the drops, he was ready to try just about anything else.

That's when he was referred to Ben C. Lane, O.D., director of the Nutritional Optometry Institute in Lake Hiawatha, New Jersey. Dr. Lane had done research on nutrition and eye diseases at Columbia University in New York City before founding the institute.

"Dr. Lane told me that over the years, he had been successful in treating normal glaucoma based primarily on nutrition and diet, so I thought I'd give it a try," says Goslin. After doing a thorough eye exam and nutritional analysis, including a blood test and diet history, Dr. Lane made some specific recommendations for Goslin that included taking supplements of vitamin C and the mineral chromium.

It was a year before Goslin saw measurable improvement, but since then he has even regained the peripheral vision that he thought had been lost for-

Food Factors

Try these tips to help knock out glaucoma.

Veer away from vanadium. Vanadium is a commonly occurring trace mineral that can deplete your body of chromium. And chromium is important in normalizing the pressure inside your eyeballs. Vanadium is found in kelp, dulse and other kinds of seaweed as well as in shark, swordfish, tuna, commercially raised chicken and turkey (they're often fed a seafood-based meal), vinegar, mushrooms, pickles, chocolate and carob.

Cut the sugar. Chromium stores that could be used to keep the pressure inside your eyeballs stable are diverted to handle added sugar in the diet, says Ben C. Lane, O.D., director of the Nutritional Optometry Institute in Lake Hiawatha, New Jersey.

ever. "The proof is in the pudding," he says. "I would certainly attribute my improvement to Dr. Lane and his recommendations."

Goslin says he took oral chromium supplements until Dr. Lane discovered that his body wasn't absorbing them properly because of interference from other nutrients that were taken at the same time. He now takes two drops of aqueous chromium every day, under the tongue, either 30 minutes before a meal or more than three hours after a meal but not at the same time as vitamin C.

The Diet Connection

To fight glaucoma, which can cause blindness in its advanced stage, most ophthalmologists prescribe eyedrops or use surgery to relieve pressure inside the eyeballs.

Prescription eyedrops and surgery may be necessary in some glaucoma cases, Dr. Lane says, but nutritional evidence suggests that many people can experience some improvement through measures as simple as changing what they eat.

"It's not going to help everyone," he says. "But if they get the right nutrients over a period of a few years, many people with glaucoma are able to be weaned off medication or to use much less medication."

Taking a Shine to Chromium

Aside from making sure that your reading prescription is up-to-date, one of the best ways to lower pressure inside the eyeballs is with a mineral called chromium, says Dr. Lane.

In a study done at Columbia University, Dr. Lane asked more than 400 people with eye disease to detail the foods they had eaten during the previous two months. Then they took tests to measure the vitamin and mineral content of their blood. Among the findings: Those people who didn't get enough chromium and who ate too many vanadium-containing foods were at higher risk for glaucoma. (Vanadium is another common mineral that occurs naturally in many foods, including kelp, dulse and other seaweed as well as large marine fish.)

"What set of muscles do we use more today than ever before in recorded history? The focusing muscles in our eyes," says Dr. Lane. "And what nutrient helps facilitate the ability of our eye muscles to focus? The bottom line is that most of us need more chromium, especially if we have been eating refined and sugar-supplemented foods." Adequate chromium levels are necessary to help deliver needed energy to your eye-focusing muscles, he says.

And what's the connection between eye muscles and glaucoma? When you perform tasks that require prolonged intense focus, such as reading, too much fluid can be produced inside the eyeballs, Dr. Lane explains. In some people, he says, the fluid doesn't drain properly and pressure builds, contributing to glaucoma.

People who suffer from Type II (non-insulin-dependent) diabetes seem more likely to develop glaucoma, says Dr. Lane. And that's not surprising, he says, because both people with diabetes and those with glaucoma have been found to be low in chromium.

The best sources of chromium include egg yolks, brewer's yeast and most unrefined foods rich in energy content. Consequently, ripe fresh sweet and starchy fruits and vegetables also contain more than adequate chromium, says Dr. Lane.

The Daily Value for chromium is 120 micrograms.

If you want to try chromium supplementation, discuss it with your doctor. This is especially important if you have diabetes, since chromium may cause your blood sugar level to drop and reduce your need for insulin. Your doctor should monitor your insulin level carefully while you're taking supplements.

Dr. Lane also notes that many people make the mistake of taking

Prescriptions for Healing

It's important to be under a doctor's care if you have glaucoma. Uncontrolled, the disease can lead to blindness.

Doctors generally prescribe medication in the form of eyedrops to treat glaucoma. If you'd like to try supplements as an adjunct to your treatment, discuss it with your ophthalmologist.

Some doctors recommend these nutrients to help treat glaucoma.

Nutrient	Daily Amount
Chromium	120 micrograms
Vitamin C	750–1,500 milligrams, taken as 2 divided doses

MEDICAL ALERT: Nutritional therapy for glaucoma is not commonly practiced, nor is it for everyone. It is important to remain under a doctor's care if you have glaucoma and to continue using whatever medication your doctor prescribes.

If you want to try chromium supplements, discuss it with your doctor. This is especially important if you have diabetes, since chromium may affect your blood sugar level. Also, many people make the mistake of taking chromium at the same time that they take vitamin C. Vitamin C interferes with the uptake of chromium.

Taking more than 1,200 milligrams of vitamin C daily can cause diarrhea in some people.

chromium at the same time that they take vitamin C. Vitamin C interferes with the uptake of chromium.

Vitamin C Lets Up on Pressure

Like chromium, vitamin C also seems to reduce intraocular pressure, but by a different method. Studies show that it apparently raises the acidity of the blood, explains Dr. Lane. "That in and of itself seems to help normalize intraocular pressure," he says. (Intraocular pressure is the pressure inside the eyeballs. In people with glaucoma, the pressure is too high, which hinders the blood supply to the eye.)

Vitamin C delivers yet another benefit for your eyes. It increases the efficiency of fuel utilization by the eye muscles, says Dr. Lane. Between 750 and 1,500 milligrams of vitamin C daily seems to work best. Any more than that increases the risk that the jellylike substance in your eye may gradually become more liquefied, causing it to be pulled away from the retina and related structures at the back of the eye, says Dr. Lane. (The retina contains a light-sensitive layer of cells that receives images.) Taking more than 1,200 milligrams of vitamin C daily, however, can cause diarrhea in some people.

Take part of your vitamin C with juice before breakfast in the morning, then allow at least one meal to go by before taking the rest, advises Dr. Lane. Vitamin C has a tendency to block the absorption of other nutrients such as copper and chromium, he says.

Nutritional therapy for glaucoma is not commonly practiced, nor is it for everyone. It is important to remain under a doctor's care if you have glaucoma and to continue using whatever medication your doctor prescribes. But do discuss your concerns with your doctor.

Gout

Counterattack with Dietary Changes

It has been called a disease of overindulgence. But not everyone with gout fits the image of a beer-drinking, beef-eating, overweight middle-aged man with an exquisitely aching toe.

"I simply seem to be sensitive to meats, especially red meat, and to gravies and other fatty, rich foods," says Frances George of Cusick, Washington. She blames bad genes, not bad habits. "My father had gout, and so does my son," she says. In fact, it wasn't until her son was diagnosed with gout as a teenager that she realized that her long-standing ankle pain has the same cause. "I've never had it in my toe, so that misled me for a while," she says.

A form of arthritis, gout causes the same symptoms: joint pain and swelling. Usually, the pain is limited to the first joint of the big toe, other joints in the foot, the knee and sometimes the wrist and elbow.

Prescriptions for Healing

Dietary changes and drugs, not vitamins, are considered the primary strategies for preventing gout attacks. But some experts believe that these vitamins may provide an additional edge.

Nutrient	Daily Amount
Folic acid	10,000–40,000 micrograms
Vitamin E	400–800 international units

Plus a supplement containing the Daily Values of all of the B-complex vitamins

MEDICAL ALERT: *If you have symptoms of gout, you should see a doctor for proper diagnosis and treatment.*

This dosage of folic acid is way beyond the Daily Value of 400 micrograms and is available only by prescription. Take this much folic acid only under medical supervision. Large doses of folic acid can mask symptoms of pernicious anemia, a vitamin B_{12}*–deficiency disease.*

If you are considering taking more than 600 international units of vitamin E, it's a good idea to discuss it with your doctor first. If you are taking anticoagulant drugs, you should not take vitamin E supplements.

The pain occurs when sharp crystals of uric acid form in the fluid surrounding a joint. That happens when blood levels of uric acid become too high—or, paradoxically, drop too quickly. Alcohol, rich foods, drugs that reduce blood pressure, lead poisoning, even inherited metabolic disorders can cause gout. Uric acid can also crystallize in the kidneys and other soft tissues, causing damage. So staving off attacks is important for reasons that go beyond pain prevention.

A gout attack often starts at night, as a joint becomes increasingly hot, swollen and painful. "It can come on fast," George says. "It usually doesn't wake me up at night, but I can go to bed fine and wake up in the morning with a stiff, swollen ankle." For her, that attack might come after eating meat for a few days in a row or chowing down at a favorite local restaurant with an all-you-can-eat buffet that features prime rib. "I don't eat any more than anyone else, but I'm the only one who ends up with gout," she laments.

George knows that if she sticks with low-fat vegetarian fare, her symptoms will subside. So that's what she does when her ankle acts up.

Indeed, most cases of gout respond very nicely to dietary changes, says Joseph Pizzorno, Jr., N.D., a naturopathic physician and president of Bastyr University in Seattle. "Dietary changes are all that many people need to control their symptoms," he says. For some, avoiding alcohol is all that's necessary. Others may need to cut back on both alcohol and certain foods, such as meats. These foods are rich in purines, protein components that are converted to uric acid in the body.

Ironically, gout can also be induced by very low calorie diets—starvation diets, for example—which also increase blood levels of uric acid as the body begins to break down tissues, explains Jeffrey Lisse, M.D., associate professor of medicine and director of the Division of Rheumatology at the University of Texas Medical Branch at Galveston.

Although individual nutrients are not the main dietary treatments for gout, there are a few that can prove helpful.

Folic Acid Dissolves Crystals

Some doctors recommend folic acid, a B vitamin that in large doses inhibits xanthine oxidase, the enzyme responsible for the body's production of uric acid. In fact, one prescription drug used to treat gout, allopurinol (Zyloprim), also inhibits this enzyme.

"I wouldn't use folic acid alone, but it may be helpful to some people as part of a complete package of dietary changes and nutritional supplements," says Dr. Pizzorno. The vitamin won't resolve an acute attack, when uric acid crystals have already formed in a joint. But it may help ward off further attacks.

The recommended dosage, 10,000 to 40,000 micrograms of folic acid a day (25 to 100 times the Daily Value of 400 micrograms), is far more than is available from even the best food sources. "People must take supplements to get this large amount," Dr. Pizzorno says. And supplements in this large amount are available only by prescription. So if you'd like to try folic acid as a preventive, you'll have to discuss it with your physician.

Here's another good reason for taking large doses only under medical supervision: Not all studies find side effects at large doses, but in one that did, people taking 15 milligrams (15,000 micrograms) of folic acid a day complained of nausea, bloating, problems sleeping and irritability. Large doses of

Food Factors

Even if drugs control your gout, some doctors believe that it's wise to change your eating habits to avoid future attacks. That way, you can avoid taking drugs, with their unpleasant side effects. Plus you'll be eating heart-healthy fare.

In most cases, gout responds well to dietary changes. Here's what many doctors recommend.

Purge purines from your platter. Liver, beef, lamb, veal, shellfish, yeast, herring, sardines, mackerel and anchovies are all high in purines, protein components that break down to form uric acid. Doctors recommend avoiding these foods during a gout attack and limiting your intake of them between attacks.

Say good-bye to booze. Drinking alcohol causes a buildup of uric acid in the body because it increases uric acid production at the same time that it reduces uric acid excretion. That's why so many gout sufferers pay the price for a single episode of overindulgence. "Eliminating alcohol is all many people need to do to avoid attacks," says Joseph Pizzorno, Jr., N.D., a naturopathic physician and president of Bastyr University in Seattle. If you do drink occasionally, stick to hard liquor or wine, both of which have fewer purines than beer.

Try cherries. Many people with gout swear that eating cherries helps quickly resolve attacks. Only one study, though, published in

folic acid can also mask symptoms of pernicious anemia, a vitamin B_{12}–deficiency disease.

Since some experts contend that large doses of any one of the B-complex vitamins can cause shortages of others, your doctor probably will also have you take a supplement containing the entire B-complex.

Vitamin E Adds Anti-inflammatory Power

Some doctors add vitamin E to their gout-relieving prescriptions. While there are no studies to show that vitamin E alone can abort or prevent a gout attack, this vitamin has properties that may help dampen inflammation, Dr. Pizzorno says. He suggests 400 to 800 international units daily, both during

1950, found that eating about a half-pound of fresh or canned Royal Ann or black Bing cherries a day helps lower uric acid levels. But it's worth a try.

"Cherries, hawthorn berries, blueberries and other dark red-blue berries are rich sources of anthocyanidins and procyanidins," Dr. Pizzorno explains. These compounds apparently help strengthen and prevent the destruction of the connective tissue that forms joints as well as inhibit tissue-destroying enzymes secreted by immune cells in the course of inflammation, he explains.

Go for the H_2O. Drinking lots of water keeps urine dilute and promotes the excretion of uric acid, says Jeffrey Lisse, M.D., associate professor of medicine and director of the Division of Rheumatology at the University of Texas Medical Branch at Galveston. Drinking lots of nonalcoholic fluids during a bout of gout is particularly important. It prevents your kidneys from forming uric acid crystals, which can lead to damage and kidney stones.

Peel off the pounds. If you're overweight, reducing will lower uric acid levels, Dr. Pizzorno says. "A high-fiber, low-fat diet—fruits, vegetables, whole grains, beans and the like—is the best way to go," he says.

Gradual weight loss is mandatory, however. Losing weight too fast also increases uric acid levels and can trigger an attack, says Dr. Lisse.

and between attacks. (If you are considering taking more than 600 international units of vitamin E daily, it's a good idea to discuss it with your doctor first.)

Vitamins to Banish

Two vitamins that you'll want to avoid in excess during a bout of gout are vitamin C and niacin. "Both increase uric acid levels in the body," Dr. Pizzorno says. By the way, low doses of aspirin, a commonly used anti-inflammatory drug, also increase blood levels of uric acid, says Dr. Lisse. So you'll want to avoid using it to relieve gout pain. "Any other nonsteroidal pain reliever is safe," he adds.

Hair Loss

Keeping What You Have

The big question: Is there any connection between what you put in your mouth and keeping a full head of hair?

For men, the answer is a resounding no. (Sorry, guys. Except in cases of extreme malnutrition, no amount of vitamins or minerals will regrow hair.) But for some women who have experienced hair loss related to physical trauma, crash dieting or heavy menstrual flow, the answer is yes.

Actually, when it comes to hair loss, everyone is a loser—all of the time. Even the owner of the world's most luxurious locks sheds 50 to 150 hairs a day. What separates him from the guy who could double as a billiard ball? In someone with a full head of hair, new hairs constantly grow in, filling all of the empty spaces. Whether you sprout enough new hairs to prevent baldness depends mostly on your parents. Genes are the culprits in what is known as male- or female-pattern baldness.

Researchers have found, however, that certain nutrients often seem to be determining factors in hair regrowth in women.

Iron and the Maiden

When a woman loses iron because of something such as trauma, poor diet or heavy menstruation, several things happen. Among them: Her body literally stops producing hair until she gets more iron.

"I've been practicing medicine for more than 30 years now, and it's my experience that in most females who are menstruating regularly, there is mild to severe iron-deficiency anemia," says Wilma Bergfeld, M.D., a dermatologist and director of the Section of Dermatopathology (the study of the causes and effects of skin diseases and abnormalities) and Dermatological Research at the Cleveland Clinic.

The Daily Value for iron is 18 milligrams. But getting enough iron is only part of the picture, says Alexander Zemtsov, M.D., associate professor of biochemistry and molecular biology at Indiana University School of Medicine in Indianapolis.

Because iron absorption is boosted by vitamin C, he recommends talking

Food Factors

What you eat may well have an effect on how good your hair looks, but there's little you can do in terms of diet that will have an impact on how much hair you have. Here are a couple of things that doctors say you can do for healthier hair.

Steer clear of crash diets. Trimming pounds gradually not only is healthier than crash dieting but also keeps your hair on your head. "Any woman who has lost 20 pounds or more in a period of three months is going to have a problem with hair loss," says Wilma Bergfeld, M.D., a dermatologist and director of the Section of Dermatopathology and Dermatological Research at the Cleveland Clinic. The safe and effective way to lose weight: trimming no more than a pound a week.

Pump up your iron. To boost iron absorption, some doctors also recommend drinking orange juice, which is high in vitamin C, whenever you eat foods high in iron, such as broccoli and red meat, says Alexander Zemtsov, M.D., associate professor of biochemistry and molecular biology at Indiana University School of Medicine in Indianapolis.

to your doctor about a prescription for Niferex with Vitamin C. Each capsule contains 50 milligrams of iron and 100 milligrams of vitamin C. Or you can get over-the-counter Niferex, which has 50 milligrams of iron, and take it with 100 milligrams of vitamin C. "I recommend taking one of these capsules a day until the hair is back to normal, usually in two to three months," says Dr. Zemtsov.

High daily intake of iron can cause iron overload in some people. For this reason, doses exceeding the Daily Value (18 milligrams) should be taken only under medical supervision.

Taking a Little Insurance

Because a broad array of nutrients, including vitamin C, iron, biotin, folate and zinc, seem to play roles in hair growth, some experts recommend taking a multivitamin/mineral supplement to cover all your nutritional bases.

Prescriptions for Healing

Except in cases of starvation, it doesn't seem that vitamins and minerals affect hair growth in men. On the other hand, nutrients may prove helpful for some women who have experienced hair loss. Here's what the experts recommend.

Nutrient	Daily Amount
Iron	50 milligrams (Niferex)
Vitamin C	100 milligrams
Plus a multivitamin/mineral supplement containing the Daily Values of all essential vitamins and minerals	

MEDICAL ALERT: *High daily intake of iron can cause iron overload in some people. For this reason, doses exceeding the Daily Value (18 milligrams) should be taken only under medical supervision.*

"Biotin, for example, appears to enhance hair growth, thicken fibers and diminish shedding. But all of these nutrients sort of do the same thing," says Dr. Bergfeld. "What we're talking about is fitting multiple pieces together. There are just so many factors that it's hard to isolate which one is the most important."

Further strengthening the argument for taking a multivitamin/mineral supplement is that many older people get fewer nutrients, says Dr. Bergfeld. "As women get into their forties and fifties, medical conditions that exaggerate hair loss include reduction of female hormones, thyroid disorders and diabetes. The frequent necessity for drug therapy for medical conditions can also exaggerate hair loss," she says.

Some Promises Don't Wash

What about feeding your hair from the outside? Some ads for shampoos and conditioners that contain nutrients make it sound like your hair needs an infusion of what these products provide to stay lush and healthy.

"These really aren't very helpful," says Dr. Bergfeld. "They can help hair have the appearance of body and fullness by temporarily swelling the hair shafts, but that's about it."

Hair care products can't help hair grow because the hair on your head is dead. The only way nutrients can affect hair growth is if they make it to the scalp, where hair is produced, explains Dr. Zemtsov. "You can put whatever you like on there," he says. "But if it doesn't penetrate about a half-centimeter or deeper into the scalp to reach the hair follicle—and it never will—it doesn't work." Nutrition must come from the inside.

Heart Arrhythmia

Subduing Electrical Storms of the Heart

Day in and day out, our hearts have the seemingly endless task of pumping blood through the 62,000 miles of arteries, veins and capillaries in our bodies. Seventy or so beats a minute, 4,200 beats an hour, 100,800 beats a day—it adds up fast, and most of us never give it a moment's thought.

If your *lub-dub* becomes a *lub-lub-a-dub* or *lub-a-dub-dub*, however, it's going to attract attention—either yours or your doctor's. Such irregular heartbeats, called arrhythmia, occur when nerves that regulate the contraction of the heart go haywire.

Normally, a heartbeat is a highly coordinated event, directed by the sequential firing of nerves that signal each chamber of the heart to contract. When all goes well, the atrial chambers and the ventricular chambers of the heart work in sequence, pumping blood to the lungs and the rest of the body. When things go awry, the nerve signals may be delayed, or the nerves may fire more often than necessary. The chambers may not pump in proper sequence. The end result is that the heart pumps blood less efficiently.

In the case of Joel Levine of Pine Brook, New Jersey, blood flow was so disturbed that he would faint during episodes. "My arrhythmia kept getting worse, despite changes in medication," he says. "Finally, it got so bad that I was having an attack a day." This was inconvenient, to say the least. But it speaks for his skill as a home furnishings salesman that he did not lose his job despite occasionally ending up on the floor. "He would try to lie down if he knew he was going to faint," explains his wife, Anne. "There was no hiding the fact that something was wrong."

Arrhythmia comes in all sorts of variations. Some types, such as atrial fibrillation (chaotic, quivering contractions), the kind Joel Levine had, may be upsetting. But since they rarely cause serious symptoms, they're not likely to kill you. Other types, such as ventricular fibrillation, are deadly.

"People with serious arrhythmia are usually under a doctor's care," says Michael A. Brodsky, M.D., associate professor of medicine at the University of California, Irvine, and director of the Cardiac Electrophysiology/Arrhythmia Service at the University of California, Irvine, Medical Center. Indeed, it's often a doctor who discovers the problem, since arrhythmia frequently has no apparent symptoms, he adds.

What makes the heart get out of sync? In serious cases, disease of the coronary arteries or heart muscle is the most likely cause, Dr. Brodsky says. But in some cases, and often in conjunction with heart disease, mineral imbalances interfere with the heart's normal nerve function.

Nutritional therapy for arrhythmia focuses on two minerals in particular: magnesium and potassium. Nerve cells make use of both to help fire off messages, and a shortage of either one can cause life-threatening problems.

Doctors have known for some time just how vital potassium is for normal heartbeat. Magnesium is an entirely different story, however. "Apparently, many doctors still don't realize how important a role this mineral can play in some heart patients," says Carla Sueta, M.D., Ph.D., assistant professor of medicine and cardiology at the University of North Carolina at Chapel Hill School of Medicine. "We see patients referred by doctors from all over our state, and magnesium levels have not been routinely checked."

Here's what research has to say about these two heart-healthy minerals.

Magnesium Helps Hearts Stay Regular

Several studies have shown that when it comes to certain types of arrhythmia, magnesium can save lives.

One study, by Dr. Sueta and her colleagues at the University of North Carolina at Chapel Hill, found that the risk of developing potentially fatal ventricular arrhythmia was reduced by more than half in people with heart failure who received large intravenous doses of magnesium compared with those who did not receive the mineral.

"This is important, because ventricular arrhythmia can progress to ventricular fibrillation, which can result in sudden death," Dr. Sueta explains. The study showed that magnesium reduced the incidence of several types of ventricular arrhythmia by 53 to 76 percent.

Food Factors

Mineral balance plays an important role in regulating heartbeat. But other dietary factors can also throw your heart out of sync. Here are two items to avoid and one to add to your anti-arrhythmia diet.

Go fish. Arrhythmia is most likely to occur after blood flow to the heart is blocked, which is exactly what happens during a heart attack. Although it hasn't been proven in humans, a study with laboratory animals showed that a diet high in fish oil (omega-3 fatty acids) helps reduce the likelihood of fatal heart arrhythmia sometimes associated with heart attack.

Doctors suggest that you replace the saturated fat in your diet with fish oil by substituting salmon or mackerel for beef, chicken or dairy products several times a week. If you want to take fish oil supplements, discuss amounts with your doctor, suggests Michael A. Brodsky, M.D., associate professor of medicine at the University of California, Irvine, and director of the Cardiac Electrophysiology/Arrhythmia Service at the University of California, Irvine, Medical Center.

Stick to herbal brews. A small amount of caffeine (less than 300 milligrams a day, about three cups of brewed coffee) doesn't seem to cause many problems. But more than this amount may aggravate heartbeat irregularities, some experts say.

Be a party pooper. When it comes to heavy drinking, evidence is firm: People who abuse alcohol not only have a higher than normal risk of heartbeat irregularities but also are more likely to die suddenly and unexpectedly, a fate that may be linked to fatal arrhythmia. Even moderate drinking—no more than a drink or two a day—may increase your risk by depleting body stores of magnesium and potassium.

Not everyone with arrhythmia needs to stop drinking entirely, Dr. Brodsky says. "I tell people to keep diaries of the foods they eat and drink, their activities and their symptoms," he explains. "If we see a trend develop, they may have to make some behavior changes, such as cutting back on alcohol."

Joel Levine, for instance, found that his attacks stopped completely within 24 hours of his first dose of 400 milligrams (the Daily Value).

Intravenous magnesium, says Dr. Sueta, is now considered standard therapy for two types of arrhythmia: torsades de pointes, an unusual type of ventricular arrhythmia, and ventricular arrhythmia induced by digitalis, a commonly prescribed heart drug.

And researchers are doing preliminary work to see if people with heart disease who take oral magnesium supplements can reduce their chances of developing arrhythmia. "Right now we're trying to establish a dosage that raises people's blood levels of magnesium enough to do some good," Dr. Sueta says.

In the meantime, both she and Dr. Brodsky test all of their heart patients for magnesium deficiency. They prescribe oral magnesium supplements or intravenous magnesium when blood levels are low and sometimes oral supplements when blood levels are normal but symptoms suggest it might help. "If blood levels are low, you can be pretty sure someone is deficient," Dr. Brodsky says. "But people can have low tissue stores of magnesium and still have normal blood levels."

One thing on which more doctors than ever apparently agree is that a fair number of people with heart problems can benefit from getting enough magnesium. "I'd say 50 to 60 percent of the people I see have at least mild magnesium deficiencies," Dr. Brodsky says.

Getting Enough Magnesium

Studies have shown that 65 percent of all people in intensive care units and 11 percent of people in general care sections of hospitals are deficient in magnesium, according to Dr. Sueta. So are 20 to 35 percent of people who have heart failure. "This is much more common than most people realize," she adds.

Magnesium deficiency can be induced by the very drugs meant to help heart problems. Some types of diuretics (water pills) cause the body to excrete both magnesium and potassium, as does digitalis. And magnesium deficiency is often at the bottom of what's called refractory potassium deficiency, Dr. Brodsky adds. "The amount of magnesium in the body determines the amount of a particular enzyme that determines the amount of potassium in the body," he explains. "So if you are magnesium-deficient, you may in turn be potassium-deficient, and no amount of potassium is going to correct this unless you are also getting enough magnesium."

If you have arrhythmia, talk to your doctor about the possibility of magnesium supplementation, Dr. Brodsky suggests. Have your blood level of magnesium checked, and if you start taking magnesium supplements, have your blood levels of magnesium and potassium checked regularly, especially if you are taking large amounts of either of these minerals.

"How much magnesium you need to take depends on the results of your blood tests," Dr. Brodsky says. "Not everyone needs to take the same amount."

Both Dr. Brodsky and Dr. Sueta give their patients supplements of magnesium lactate. Both magnesium lactate and magnesium gluconate are easily absorbed and are less likely to cause diarrhea than magnesium oxide and magnesium hydroxide, the other forms of magnesium. (Magnesium hydroxide is found in Phillips' Milk of Magnesia, Mylanta and Maalox.)

"I generally give my patients either Slow-Mag or MagTab, up to about six tablets—about 450 milligrams—a day," Dr. Brodsky says.

He has found that magnesium can help heart medications such as digoxin work better. "Most people won't be able to go off their drugs completely, but they may be able to cut their dosages," Dr. Brodsky says. It's important to cut dosage slowly, over time, with your doctor's supervision, he adds. Stopping abruptly could make your heart problems worse.

Although magnesium is considered to be a fairly safe mineral, even in high doses, don't take supplemental magnesium without medical supervision if you have kidney or heart problems. Your heart or breathing could slow down too much.

Studies have shown that men get about 329 milligrams of magnesium daily, while women average 207 milligrams. The highest concentrations of magnesium are found in whole seeds such as legumes, nuts and unmilled grains. Bananas and green vegetables are also good sources.

Potassium Powers Healthy Hearts

There's no doubt that potassium is just as important as magnesium for regular heartbeat. And doctors know it. In heart patients, low potassium levels are likely to be recognized and quickly corrected. Heartbeat irregularities, along with muscle weakness and confusion, are among the classic signs of potassium deficiency.

"Unlike magnesium, potassium levels are carefully regulated in the kidneys, and the body normally conserves potassium," Dr. Brodsky says. People who have normal kidney function and healthy hearts usually have adequate blood levels of potassium, even if they eat only a serving or two of fruits and vegetables a day.

People run into severe potassium deficiency that causes heart arrhythmia only when something interferes with the kidneys' potassium-hoarding tendency. "People who take thiazide diuretics or digitalis, who have poorly functioning kidneys or who are alcoholics often become low in potassium unless they take supplements," Dr. Brodsky says. Prolonged diarrhea or vomiting and laxative abuse can also cause dangerously low potassium levels.

Here again, the amount of potassium each person should take depends on blood levels of this mineral. Too much potassium is as bad as too little, which is one reason potassium supplements containing more than 99 milligrams per tablet (the amount found in a bite or two of potato) are available only by prescription. Potassium supplements should not be taken by those with diabetes or kidney disease or by those using certain medications, including nonsteroidal anti-inflammatory drugs, potassium-sparing diuretics, ACE inhibitors and heart medications such as heparin.

Prescriptions for Healing

To prevent potential problems with heart arrhythmia, experts recommend aiming for the Daily Values of these two nutrients.

Nutrient	Daily Amount
Magnesium	400 milligrams
Potassium	3,500 milligrams

MEDICAL ALERT: *If you have been diagnosed with a heart arrhythmia, you should be under a doctor's care.*

Mineral balance is important to a beating heart, but people with irregular heartbeats should take mineral supplements only under medical supervision. That's because the amounts of minerals they need to take depend on their blood levels, which must be carefully monitored.

People with kidney problems should check with their doctors before taking supplemental magnesium.

Potassium supplements should not be taken by those with diabetes or kidney disease or by those using certain medications, including nonsteroidal anti-inflammatory drugs, potassium-sparing diuretics, ACE inhibitors and heart medications such as heparin.

"Even though doctors may advise their patients to eat more potassium-containing foods, if they're on high-dose diuretics there's no way they're going to get all of the potassium they need from foods alone," Dr. Sueta says.

The Daily Value for potassium is 3,500 milligrams. Studies show that among the general population, intakes vary widely—anywhere from 1,000 to 3,400 milligrams a day. Eating lots of fruits, vegetables and fresh meats and drinking juices is the way to pack in the most potassium. A medium banana supplies 451 milligrams of potassium; one cup of cubed cantaloupe, 494 milligrams; and one cup of cooked cabbage, 146 milligrams.

Heart Disease

Low Levels of Nutrients Put You at Risk

Your friend Lou has just had a heart attack. He was lining up a shot off the 17th tee—something he does every Saturday morning—when he dropped his driver, stumbled to the golf cart and slumped over the seat.

The pain was overwhelming. But Lou's golf partners got him to the hospital in minutes. And after doctors opened a clogged artery, Lou is doing fine.

Yet the whole experience has left Lou—and you—somewhat shaken. Lou is only 45 years old. He gets lots of exercise, balances work with play and keeps an eye on his cholesterol. He is nobody's fool.

So why did he have a heart attack?

For at least a decade, doctors have known that the most important ways to prevent a heart attack are to avoid tobacco smoke, eat a low-cholesterol diet, keep dietary fat to a minimum, sweat through at least three workouts a week and reduce stress across the board.

But today doctors are also beginning to realize that specific nutrients—particularly vitamin C, vitamin E and beta-carotene—may be just as important.

Nobody knows whether a lack of these nutrients can actually lead to heart disease, but it's certainly starting to look that way. In the ongoing Nurses' Health Study, being conducted at Harvard Medical School and Brigham and Women's Hospital in Boston, researchers compared the diets of more than 73,000 nurses and found that a diet rich in vitamin E reduced

Food Factors

What you eat—and what you don't eat—in large part determines whether you eventually develop heart disease. Here are a few tips to help you keep the number one killer in this country at bay.

Cut the fat. "We need to follow the American Heart Association's Step I guidelines," says Howard N. Hodis, M.D., director of the atherosclerosis research unit at the University of Southern California School of Medicine in Los Angeles. "In general, that means a total cholesterol intake of less than 300 milligrams a day and a total fat intake of less than 30 percent of total calories a day."

Most Americans get approximately 40 percent of their calories from fat. You can lower the amount of fat in your diet by cutting back on fatty meats and whole-fat dairy products, avoiding fast foods, candies and most baked goods and eating more fruits and vegetables.

Get hooked on fish. In a study of several thousand men who smoke, researchers in the Honolulu Heart Program at the University of Hawaii at Manoa found that those who ate fish more than twice a week cut their risk of death from heart disease in half.

"One of the magic bullets against heart disease could be fish," says William Castelli, M.D., former director of the Framingham Heart Study and now medical director of the Framingham Cardiovascular Institute in Massachusetts. "The societies whose diets emphasize fish have the lowest heart attack rates."

Eat your fruits and veggies. A Dutch study of more than 800 men between the ages of 65 and 84 found that the more bioflavonoids these guys consumed (they got them from tea, onions and apples), the less likely they were to die from heart disease.

Bioflavonoids, chemical compounds related to vitamin C that may neutralize "bad" LDL cholesterol and reduce the tendency of red blood cells to stick together and block arteries, are found in nearly all plants, so fruits and vegetables are likely to be good sources.

Dine on soy. Soy products such as tofu contain isoflavones, which are naturally occurring substances that may prevent the formation of plaque on artery walls.

Don't forget the garlic. Several studies indicate that one-half to one clove of garlic, eaten daily, can significantly lower total cholesterol. High cholesterol is a major risk factor for heart disease.

heart attack risk by 52 percent, a diet rich in vitamin C reduced risk by 43 percent, and a diet rich in beta-carotene, one of the nutrients that give orange and yellow vegetables their color, reduced risk by 38 percent. What's more, nurses who got a rich supply of all three nutrients were 63 percent less likely to have heart attacks than those who did not.

How do these nutrients work?

"Nobody really knows," says Howard N. Hodis, M.D., director of the atherosclerosis research unit at the University of Southern California School of Medicine in Los Angeles. At this point, scientists have more theories than answers. But it looks as though these three nutrients might work by actually neutralizing LDL cholesterol, the "bad" kind that damages your arteries, before it can do any harm.

Understanding the Disease

To comprehend just how powerfully these nutrients protect your arteries, you need to take a look at what causes heart disease to begin with.

Most heart disease, including angina and electrical problems that are responsible for sudden cardiac death, is actually caused by atherosclerosis, a condition in which cholesterol and cells roaming your bloodstream build up along the walls of coronary arteries and cause them to narrow. Narrowing reduces the flow of blood to the heart and increases the chance that a bunch of blood cells might clump together and get wedged in the artery. When that happens, or if an artery suddenly spasms, blood flow to the heart is cut off, triggering a heart attack.

Sometimes referred to as hardening of the arteries, atherosclerosis is a silent process that can begin in childhood. It starts when the cells lining an artery are damaged by constant pounding from high blood pressure, by repeated exposure to toxic chemicals such as those in cigarette smoke, by repeated exposure to high concentrations of LDL cholesterol or even by a bacterial or viral infection.

Once the damage occurs, the body tries to repair it. LDL cholesterol and blood cells called monocytes are attracted to the site, where they try to patch the damage. When that fails, cells from other areas of the arterial wall move in and form a protective mat, usually referred to as plaque, over the injury. The plaque hardens as it takes up calcium, and it continues to grow until it protrudes into the artery's hollow interior. Eventually, the plaque can narrow the artery's interior enough to slow the flow of blood to your heart and set you up for a heart attack.

Enter the Three Musketeers

Doctors have tried for years to prevent the development of atherosclerosis by telling people to stop doing those things that damage arteries to begin with: "Stop smoking!" "Stop eating high-cholesterol foods!" "Stop eating high-fat foods!" But over the next few years, doctors may actually be able to go one step further: They may be able to tell people how to interrupt the formation of atherosclerotic plaque, no matter what its cause.

It's a complicated story that scientists are only beginning to untangle. But it seems that LDL cholesterol may not be able to contribute to the formation of atherosclerotic plaque unless the fat in the LDL particle goes rancid when exposed to oxygen in the arterial wall, a process called oxidation, says Balz Frei, Ph.D., associate professor of medicine and biochemistry at Boston University School of Medicine.

Fortunately, laboratory studies indicate that there are at least two nutrients that can prevent the LDL particle from becoming oxidized, which is why the nutrients are called antioxidants, explains Dr. Frei.

The nutrients? Vitamin C and vitamin E, the same nutrients that scientists have found reduce the risk of heart disease when present in your diet. Beta-carotene also was originally thought to protect LDL against oxidation, but studies have shown that this is not the case, says Dr. Frei. "Scientists are now exploring other mechanisms that would explain beta-carotene's beneficial effects against heart disease—perhaps the rejuvenation of vitamin E," he adds.

Vitamin E: Neutralizing Cholesterol

Although all three nutrients seem to have roles in thwarting atherosclerosis, vitamin E may be the most protective.

In a study at the University of Texas Southwestern Medical Center at Dallas, 24 men were given either placebos (blank pills) or supplements combining 800 international units of vitamin E, 1,000 milligrams of vitamin C and 30 milligrams (about 50,000 international units) of beta-carotene. After three months, scientists found that it took twice as long for particles to oxidize in the men taking supplements compared with the men taking placebos. The supplement group also had a 40 percent reduction in the number of LDL particles oxidized compared with the placebo group. These results indicate that the antioxidant regimen used in the study might slow, and perhaps even prevent, atherosclerosis.

Curious as to which nutrient might be doing most of the antioxidant work, researchers went back to the drawing board and compared the group taking the antioxidant "cocktail" with a similar group of men taking 800 international units of vitamin E alone.

The result?

No significant differences.

It's not that vitamin C and beta-carotene weren't doing their jobs, concluded the researchers. But it is possible that their efforts were simply overshadowed by the sheer power of vitamin E.

Scientific studies indicate that vitamin E hops on board the LDL particle when it forms in your liver and then enters your bloodstream. Once part of the LDL particle, vitamin E helps prevent the particle from going rancid and forming artery-clogging plaque, explains Dr. Frei. Instead, the LDL particle and its vitamin E passenger actually pass into the artery wall, where they set up housekeeping. And as long as there's a plentiful supply of vitamin E and other antioxidants to keep replacing the vitamin E that's used up, the LDL particle should remain harmless.

At least that's the theory. Fortunately, vitamin E seems to work just as well at preventing heart disease in real life as it does at preventing plaque in the laboratory.

In the Health Professionals Follow-Up Study of almost 40,000 men, conducted by researchers at Harvard School of Public Health, men who took at least 100 international units of vitamin E a day for at least two years reduced their risk of heart disease by 37 percent. A companion study of more than 87,000 nurses between the ages of 34 and 59 found similar results.

Vitamin E even seems to benefit those who are already suffering from advanced heart disease.

In a study at a hospital in Albuquerque, New Mexico, of 440 people who had undergone angioplasty, a procedure to open blocked arteries, the 57 people who took an average of 574 international units of vitamin E a day had about half of the incidence of reblocked arteries of those who did not.

The same seems to hold true for people who've had bypass surgery. When scientists at the University of Southern California asked 162 men ages 40 to 59 who had undergone heart bypass surgery which vitamins they took, they found that the men who reported taking more than 100 international units of vitamin E daily had significantly slower buildup of plaque clogging their arteries.

What does this mean to us? "Well, we can answer that only partly," replies Dr. Frei. "Several studies have suggested that an increase in vitamin E to a level of about 100 international units or more per day is protective against heart disease. That level cannot be achieved by dietary means, so you have to supplement. But I think it's too early to make a specific recommendation, although I'll tell you that after publication of the results of the Nurses' Health Study and the Health Professionals Follow-Up Study, a lot of doctors started to take vitamin E.

"It's sort of a paradoxical situation, where the evidence appears to be good enough for many doctors to take vitamin E but not good enough for them to recommend it to their patients," Dr. Frei adds.

Although some doctors involved in vitamin E research do not recommend vitamin E supplements, others feel that 100 to 200 international units of vitamin E a day might prove beneficial. While the Daily Value is only 30 international units, this amount is certainly considered safe, says Dr. Frei. If you have heart disease, you should discuss vitamin supplements with your doctor.

Beta-Carotene: Preventing Heart Attacks

Although sometimes overshadowed in the lab by vitamin E, beta-carotene, the nutrient that gives carrots their color, is a champion on the dinner plate when it comes to fighting heart disease.

One study after another touts the heart-healthy benefits of beta-carotene, beginning with the Physicians' Health Study at Harvard Medical School. In this study, a group of 333 men between the ages of 40 and 84 who had severe heart disease were given 50 milligrams (83,000 international units) of beta-carotene every other day. Beta-carotene had no effect on the men's conditions during the first year. But from the second year on, the men's risk of heart attack was literally cut in half.

What's more, other investigators have found that the protective effects of beta-carotene may be even more pronounced among those who have risk factors that predispose them to heart disease, such as smoking and high cholesterol.

In a study at the Johns Hopkins University School of Medicine in Baltimore, for example, researchers compared blood levels of beta-carotene and other carotenoids of 123 people between the ages of 35 and 65 who had had a first heart attack with those of people of similar age who had not had a first heart attack.

"The study found that smokers with the lowest blood levels of beta-carotene had about 3½ times the risk of heart attack of people who had high levels of beta-carotene and did not smoke," says Debra A. Street, Ph.D., who led the research at Johns Hopkins and is now an epidemiologist with the Food and Drug Administration.

People with high cholesterol levels may also find that beta-carotene and its carotenoid cousins protect their hearts. In a 13-year study at the University of North Carolina at Chapel Hill and the University of Tennessee in Memphis, researchers monitored more than 1,800 men between the ages of 40 and 59 who had high cholesterol levels. When comparing the 282 men who subsequently had heart attacks with those who stayed healthy, the researchers found that those who had high levels of beta-carotene and other carotenoids in their blood at the start of the study were 40 percent less likely to have heart attacks than those with lower levels.

It's not that you can go out and smoke cigarettes or load up on high-cholesterol foods, says Dexter Morris, M.D., Ph.D., assistant professor at the University of North Carolina at Chapel Hill School of Medicine, who led the study. But "the higher your carotenoid levels, the lower your risk of getting a heart attack," he says.

Gelcap or Carrot?

Researchers across the board resoundingly recommend eating five or more servings of fruits and vegetables a day, including some servings rich in carotenoids, to protect yourself against heart disease. They are less likely to recommend beta-carotene supplements.

Why would beta-carotene in the diet be better than beta-carotene in a gelcap? "One possibility is that in some of these studies, it's not just the beta-carotene that's good for you, it's also something else," says Dr. Morris. Beta-carotene represents only one-fifth of the most common carotenoids found in orange and yellow fruits and vegetables. So it's entirely possible that whether you get your beta-carotene from a carrot or from a gelcap full of carrot oil, these other carotenoids may contribute to some of the effect that's being credited to beta-carotene.

"A second possibility is that there may be a kind of therapeutic window for beta-carotene," Dr. Morris continues. "In other words, some is good, but too much may cause problems. There's one theory, for example, that at higher levels, beta-carotene may interfere with the protective effects of something else." Just what that might be is pure speculation, he says.

Most of these reservations are not just the normal cautions that folks have come to expect from careful scientists. They are instead based on a mammoth study of 29,000 male Finnish smokers that was designed to tell whether beta-carotene and other synthetic supplements can prevent lung cancer and heart disease.

The problem is that most researchers expected to find that the supplements either reduced the chances of cancer and heart disease in the Finns or didn't do anything at all. Instead, the researchers found that male smokers who took 20 milligrams (about 33,000 international units) of synthetic beta-carotene a day actually increased their risk of both.

Some researchers have attributed this finding to the fact that heavy smokers are frequently heavy drinkers, and heavy drinking destroys beta-carotene in the body. Other researchers feel that taking a high dose of beta-carotene may inhibit the absorption or effect of other antioxidants.

Still others haven't a clue.

"Although most experts believe that the Finnish findings are unique, that doesn't warrant ignoring the data," says Dr. Hodis. "We have to wait until more data come in. And until it does, I think that people should stop smoking and eat a well-balanced diet that includes the Daily Values of all vitamins and minerals."

Vitamin C: The Antioxidant Attack Ship

Although the roles played by vitamin E and beta-carotene are becoming fairly well defined, vitamin C's role in preventing atherosclerosis is still emerging.

Some real-life studies indicate that after a decade of looking good in the laboratory, vitamin C may not do as much as scientists had hoped. But other studies indicate that it clearly contributes to preventing heart disease.

When researchers at the University of California, Los Angeles, checked the amounts of vitamin C taken by more than 11,000 men and women between the ages of 25 and 74, for example, they found that people who got more than 50 milligrams of vitamin C a day, in addition to a multivitamin/mineral supplement, reduced their risk of death from cardiovascular disease by 28 percent.

These findings seem to indicate that vitamin C is just as important as vitamin E and beta-carotene in preventing atherosclerosis, which makes sense when you look at what each of the nutrients does and how they complement one another's work.

To understand the value of these nutrients, "you have to distinguish between the two different classes of antioxidants," explains Dr. Frei. "One class is a group of water-soluble antioxidants that includes vitamin C. The other class is a group of fat-soluble antioxidants that includes vitamin E.

"The mechanisms by which they work are similar, but they work in different compartments of the body," says Dr. Frei. "The water-soluble antioxidants are present in blood and other water-containing solutions in the body, while the fat-soluble antioxidants are actually transported within the LDL particles themselves." The fat-soluble antioxidants get transported right into the body's fatty tissues and, on board the LDL, into the artery walls, Dr. Frei explains.

Vitamin C also seems to have one other role to play in defeating atherosclerosis, says Dr. Frei. When an LDL particle exhausts its vitamin E, vitamin C can regenerate the vitamin E, thus renewing its ability to prevent atherosclerosis. This observation has been made only in the laboratory, he adds, but there's no reason to think that it's not also happening in people.

The exact amount of vitamin C you need to achieve these results is still unknown, says Dr. Frei, but many cardiologists are recommending taking somewhere in the range of 250 to 500 milligrams a day.

Folic Acid Fights Heart Disease

Although antioxidants are clearly the major nutrients involved in defending your body against atherosclerosis, folate (the naturally occurring form of folic acid) may also have an important role to play.

That's because several years ago, researchers discovered that people who have elevated blood levels of homocysteine, an amino acid found in meats that can damage arterial walls and contribute to the development of atherosclerosis, frequently suffer from severe atherosclerosis and heart attacks in their twenties and thirties.

Some seem to have a genetic defect that makes their bodies unable to use homocysteine. But others seem to be suffering from deficiencies of vitamin B_6, vitamin B_{12} or folate.

Researchers are still not certain what causes excess levels of homocysteine in the blood, but they're beginning to figure out how to reduce them.

"Folate prevents the buildup of homocysteine," says Frank M. Sacks, M.D., associate professor of medicine and nutrition at Harvard School of Public Health.

In one study, researchers from Tufts University in Medford, Massachusetts, the Clinical Research Institute of Montreal and the Hospital Hotel-Dieu, also in Montreal, worked with 150 men and women between ages 28

Prescriptions for Healing

Although researchers now strongly suspect that low levels of vitamin E, beta-carotene and vitamin C may in fact put your body at increased risk for heart disease, most of these scientists are reluctant to recommend specific amounts of these nutrients that you should get from your diet or from supplements.

There are two reasons, researchers say. One is that there have not been enough large-scale studies in which huge numbers of people are given a specific amount of a nutrient and then tested for the effect. The second is that the amounts each person needs to eat or take to achieve therapeutic levels may be different, since each person absorbs each of these nutrients in his own individual way.

One researcher, however, has taken the bull by the horns.

In a study published in Britain, Dr. K. F. Gey of the Institute of Biochemistry and Molecular Biology at the University of Berne in Switzerland analyzed a number of nutrient studies from around the world. He postulates that when taken as a whole, these studies suggest that to protect against heart disease, individuals should aim for the levels listed below for the major antioxidants: beta-carotene, vitamin C and vitamin E. Dr. Gey states that these nutrients should be received together through a balanced diet rather than through individual supplementation.

Nutrient	Daily Amount
Beta-carotene	10,000–25,000 international units
Vitamin C	60–250 milligrams
Vitamin E	60–100 international units

and 59 with heart disease. They found that homocysteine levels can be reduced by taking either 50 milligrams of vitamin B_6 or 5,000 micrograms of folic acid every day.

Since these amounts are between 12 and 25 times the Daily Values of these vitamins, however, the researchers opted not to recommend such high doses until further studies reveal the long-term effects. (Vitamin B_6 is already known to cause nerve damage in high doses.) Lower doses may be as effec-

Several other nutrients also play roles in heart health. Because low levels of these nutrients seem to raise the risk of heart disease, most doctors recommend that people be sure to get the Daily Values of these nutrients through a well-balanced diet and, if necessary, a multivitamin/mineral supplement.

Nutrient	Daily Amount
Folic acid	400 micrograms
Iron	18 milligrams
Selenium	70–100 micrograms
Zinc	15 milligrams

MEDICAL ALERT: *If you have heart disease, you should discuss vitamin and mineral supplementation with your doctor.*

The recommendations for the antioxidants vitamin C and vitamin E exceed the Daily Values of these nutrients. A wide range is recommended for each vitamin because the exact amount consumed would vary from person to person.

If you are taking anticoagulant drugs, you should not take vitamin E supplements.

tive, but clinical trials are ongoing, says Jacques Genest, Jr., M.D., director of the cardiovascular genetics laboratory at the Clinical Research Institute of Montreal, who led the study.

In the meantime, advises Dr. Sacks, "eat some spinach or take a regular multivitamin/mineral supplement." That should help you meet the Daily Value of folic acid (400 micrograms) and help keep homocysteine levels low enough to prevent a big buildup to begin with.

Meet the Fighting Trio

Aside from helping you to meet your folate requirement, a well-balanced diet that emphasizes vegetables may help prevent heart disease for other reasons as well.

Researchers have found that low levels of at least three elements—selenium, zinc and iron, generally found in meats, seafood, cereals and vegetables—seem to increase your risk of heart disease.

In a study in Denmark of nearly 3,000 men between the ages of 53 and 74, researchers found that those with the lowest levels of selenium in their diets increased their risk of heart disease by 55 percent. What's more, the researchers suspected that close to 19 percent of the heart attacks among men in the study might in fact be caused by low levels of this nutrient.

The Daily Value for selenium is 70 micrograms. Most researchers agree, however, that you can take up to 100 micrograms daily without harm.

Zinc might also play a role in preventing atherosclerosis, researchers say. Laboratory studies at the University of Kentucky in Lexington indicate that zinc may be necessary to safeguard the heart's arterial walls from the damage triggered by high blood pressure, high cholesterol and tobacco smoke, which sets the whole atherosclerotic process into motion.

Zinc is involved in repairing and fortifying any breaches in the cells lining the heart's arteries. So it's possible that zinc can help prevent atherosclerosis by keeping arterial walls in such good shape that cholesterol and fatty acids do not enter the artery walls to form artery-clogging plaque.

The Daily Value for zinc is 15 milligrams a day.

A third mineral that may help your body fight heart disease is iron. A study of more than 4,000 men and women, conducted by the Hyattsville, Maryland, branch of the Centers for Disease Control and Prevention under the auspices of the National Institutes of Health in Bethesda, Maryland, revealed that people who had adequate levels of iron in the bloodstream were less likely to die from cardiovascular causes than people who had lower levels. The researchers noted that the data also indicated that adequate levels of iron may be protective against coronary heart disease.

Other researchers, however, believe that high levels of iron may be associated with increased risk of heart disease. So the benefit of high iron intake is an unresolved, controversial question.

The Daily Value for iron is 18 milligrams.

High Blood Pressure

Mineral Magic Can Bring It Down

You're not going to eat those potato chips. You refuse. You push them off your plate where the waiter has artfully piled them, dump them onto an extra plate and ask that they be removed from sight.

This isn't some little diet trick du jour, either. You're fighting in favor of your blood pressure. Your father's doctor said that salty foods such as potato chips, nuts and lunchmeats raised your father's blood pressure and helped set him up for his stroke. So not even one small salted chipette will find its evil little way into your mouth to cause the same problem. It's simply not going to happen to you.

Trying to lower high blood pressure so that you don't end up with a stroke, a heart attack or kidney disease—the three major health consequences of high blood pressure—is wonderful. But this particular antisalt strategy may backfire, because some researchers are now saying that by avoiding salt, you may be creating the very health threat that you're trying to avoid. Instead, high blood pressure is just as likely to be caused by low levels of potassium, magnesium and calcium in your body.

Taking a New Look at Salt

Until a few years ago, no one really had a firm handle on what makes blood pressure rise and fall. But that's beginning to change.

"A rise in blood pressure means you need to add minerals to your diet, not cut back on salt," says David McCarron, M.D., professor of medicine and head of the Division of Nephrology, Hypertension and Clinical Pharmacology at Oregon Health Sciences University in Portland. "Tragically, the idea that salt is bad for your blood pressure is one of the most generally accepted notions out there."

It's constantly repeated because an entire generation of doctors didn't have the research that now clarifies the connection between salt, which is about 40 percent sodium and 60 percent chloride, and other nutrients. Dr. McCarron explains that in addition to putting people on medication, many doctors consistently handed out just one piece of advice when confronted with a blood pressure reading that exceeded 140/90: Ditch the salt.

"It's tough to get a consensus in this area because the effects of sodium chloride on blood pressure are quite complex," says Dr. McCarron. "But our lab has found that people who experience rises in blood pressure when they take sodium chloride are probably responding to sodium only in the absence of potassium, calcium and magnesium.

"In other words, too much salt is not and never has been what jacks up your blood pressure," says Dr. McCarron. The problem is just as likely to be too little potassium, calcium and magnesium.

Salt: The Misunderstood Mineral

In retrospect, it's not hard to understand how doctors misread the effects of sodium chloride on blood pressure.

Nobody knew what causes most cases of high blood pressure. So in trying to figure what sends blood pressure through the roof, scientists conducted a series of studies in which they took blood pressure readings for a group of people, asked them about what they did or didn't eat, then ran the answers through a computer.

The results seemed to indicate that people who used a lot of salt frequently had slightly higher blood pressure readings. Actually, heavy salt users had nearly the same blood pressure readings as those who tended to restrict their salt intakes. In fact, so many heavy salt users—up to 67 percent in one study—remained unaffected when placed on a very low salt diet that researchers began to wonder if some people are salt-sensitive while others aren't.

Some people are, says Dr. McCarron. "But," he adds, "it's more likely the relative deficiency of other minerals in the diet—potassium, calcium and magnesium—that determines who is and who is not."

How is he so sure?

Part of the answer is that putting people on low-salt diets has not had the extensive impact on reducing the health consequences of high blood pressure that scientists had expected.

In a study at the Medical University-Polyclinic in Bonn, Germany, researchers put 147 men and women between the ages of 19 and 78 with normal blood pressure on a seven-day salt-restricted diet of 1,000 milligrams, or less than ½ teaspoon, a day. The researchers then compared the subjects' blood pressure readings with their readings after a seven-day high-salt diet of more than 15,000 milligrams, or about 7½ teaspoons, a day.

Food Factors

Although vitamins and minerals clearly play significant roles in preventing and perhaps treating high blood pressure, there are other dietary strategies that can also help keep your blood pressure where it belongs.

Cut calories. Obesity is one of the biggest risk factors for high blood pressure, reports the National Heart, Lung and Blood Institute in Bethesda, Maryland. It can make you two to six times more likely to develop the condition than if you were at a healthier weight. That's why the institute suggests that you lose weight by cutting 500 calories a day from your diet and that you find ways to burn off even more calories by becoming more physically active.

Eat fish. Fatty fish such as mackerel and salmon contain omega-3 fatty acids, a type of fat that, in large amounts, seems to reduce blood pressure. In at least one study, people with mild high blood pressure who took six grams of fish oil per day for 12 weeks found their blood pressure sank an average of two to four points. The National Heart, Lung and Blood Institute recommends that you chow down on fatty fish as often as possible. Provided the fish is not fried, the added fat isn't a harmful addition to your total fat budget, since it would likely replace unhealthy saturated fat.

Nix the drinks. The effect of alcohol on blood pressure is so significant that some researchers believe that it accounts for up to 5 percent of all cases of high blood pressure. Researchers at Harvard Medical School found that among 3,275 nurses who were 34 to 59 years old at the start of a four-year study, those who drank two to three alcoholic beverages daily increased their risk of high blood pressure by 40 percent. If you do drink, the National Heart, Lung and Blood Institute suggests that you limit your intake to two or less drinks a day.

Cut down on sugar. "Work from my laboratory shows that sugar—the kind in your sugar bowl and in foods—raises blood pressure," says Harry Preuss, M.D., professor of medicine at Georgetown University School of Medicine in Washington, D.C. Researchers don't yet know how much sugar it takes to cause a problem. "But it's always a good idea to limit sugar," Dr. Preuss advises.

The researchers found that the salt-restricted diet did in fact lower blood pressure in 17 percent of the people. But blood pressure readings remained largely unaffected in 67 percent, while blood pressure went up in 16 percent. What's more, levels of LDL cholesterol, the "bad" kind of cholesterol that sets the stage for heart disease and stroke, went up significantly.

The bottom line? A low-salt diet did not appear to lower blood pressure in approximately 80 percent of those in the German study. Instead, this research showed that such a diet may be just as likely to raise blood pressure as to lower it in people with normal blood pressure, and it may raise LDL cholesterol levels enough to increase the risk of heart disease.

In fact, that could be the reason that a study at Albert Einstein College of Medicine and Cornell University Medical College, both in New York City, showed that men with high blood pressure who ate the least salt (about 5,000 milligrams, or 2½ teaspoons) each day were four times more likely to have a heart attack—the very health consequence that a low-salt diet is supposed to prevent—than those who ate more than twice as much salt every day. While too few women were studied to draw a firm conclusion, the same pattern may be the case for them, too, the researchers observed.

It just doesn't make sense that sodium, a mineral that the body requires to survive, could be so harmful, says Dr. McCarron.

"There's a biological need for sodium chloride," he explains. "In my view, healthy people appear to seek between 3,500 and 4,200 milligrams in their diets. Without any salt at all, your blood pressure would be very low, and you could lose consciousness.

"You even have physiological mechanisms—whole systems of hormones—to conserve sodium chloride because it's so necessary," says Dr. McCarron. These systems wouldn't have evolved unless you needed the nutrient, he explains. Nor would the amount of salt that people eat remain relatively constant from person to person, even across international borders. Although some folks have tried to blame processed foods such as lunchmeats and fast-food megaburgers for the roughly 3,500 milligrams of salt that most of us eat every day, the truth is that people eat pretty much the same amount of salt, no matter what foods are commonly consumed. "Some reports show that the average American salt intake hasn't changed much since the 1870s, well before canned soups or fast-food restaurants," says Dr. McCarron.

"Every scientific survey, and not just in the United States but also in Mexico, Europe, Canada and Asia, shows that there is a very tight clustering of the population's sodium intake," says Dr. McCarron. "Every group of people takes in between 3,500 and 4,200 milligrams of sodium."

The fact is that "if you turn the human animal loose on this planet to forage for food, for whatever reason, that's the intake that he seeks," says Dr. McCarron.

The Power of Potassium

Although the body clearly needs a certain amount of sodium to maintain blood pressure, it also needs certain levels of other minerals, including potassium, to keep sodium levels in the body from getting too high, explains Dr. McCarron.

"Most researchers agree that we should get the Daily Value of 3,500 milligrams of potassium a day," says Dr. McCarron. But does that level lower blood pressure?

Yes. In a three-week study of 87 African-American men and women at the Johns Hopkins Medical Institutions in Baltimore, researchers took blood pressure measurements, divided the group in half, then gave potassium supplements of 3,120 milligrams a day to one group and placebos (fake pills) to the other.

The result? Systolic blood pressure, the top number in a blood pressure reading, went down an average of 6.9 points in the people who received the supplements. Diastolic pressure, the bottom number, went down an average of 2.5 points. There were no blood pressure changes in the people who took the placebos.

No one really knows exactly how potassium lowers blood pressure, reports Frederick L. Brancati, M.D., assistant professor of medicine and epidemiology at Johns Hopkins, who led the study. One theory suggests that potassium relaxes small blood vessels, while another holds that it helps the body eliminate water and salt.

Since most folks get only around 2,600 milligrams of the nutrient a day, however, Dr. McCarron suggests that most of us need to add at least three servings of potassium-rich fruits and vegetables, such as bananas and potatoes, as well as dairy products (a glass of milk has nearly as much potassium as a banana) to our diets every day.

People who have diabetes or kidney problems or who are taking anti-inflammatory drugs, potassium-sparing diuretics (water pills), ACE inhibitors or heart medicines such as heparin should not supplement potassium without medical supervision.

Magnesium's Magic

Along with potassium, magnesium seems to play an important role in keeping blood pressure down, particularly if you're magnesium-deficient to begin with.

In a study in Sweden of 71 people with mildly elevated blood pressure, researchers found that giving about 350 milligrams of magnesium to those who had deficiencies lowered their blood pressure readings several points.

How does it work in people with high blood pressure who may not have deficiencies?

Some studies indicate that it won't do much of anything, although at least one indicates that it might. That study, conducted by researchers in Belgium and the Netherlands, looked at the blood pressure readings of 47 women with high blood pressure. When the women were given 485 milligrams of magnesium every day for six months, their systolic readings dropped an average of 2.7 points, while their diastolic readings dropped 3.4 points. A few of the women had low levels of magnesium in their blood, but most did not.

That drop doesn't sound like a lot. But to someone with borderline-high blood pressure, it can mean the difference between taking medication and eating salmon, which is rich in magnesium.

Most people should get between 300 and 400 milligrams of magnesium daily to keep their blood pressure on an even keel, says Dr. McCarron. (The Daily Value for this mineral is 400 milligrams.) Only adult males in the United States get the full amount; women ages 30 to 60 get between 220 and 260 milligrams a day. Good food sources of magnesium are green, leafy vegetables, fish, whole grains, rice, legumes and nuts.

If you have heart or kidney problems, you should check with your doctor before taking supplemental magnesium.

Calcium for Kids and Moms

Although some studies have indicated that calcium might play a role in keeping blood pressure under control, a panel of experts at the National Institutes of Health in Bethesda, Maryland, has determined that most studies indicate the mineral's role is probably minor and that a recommendation to increase calcium intake for blood pressure control is unwarranted for most people at this time.

"The two exceptions may be pregnant women who suffer from high blood pressure during their pregnancies and children who are calcium-deficient," says Matthew W. Gillman, M.D., assistant professor of ambulatory care and prevention at Harvard Medical School, who has investigated the relationship between calcium and blood pressure.

In a study at the University of Florida Health Science Center/Jacksonville, for example, researchers found that 2,000 milligrams of calcium a day reduced the onset of high blood pressure in women during pregnancy by 54 percent.

Until scientists more clearly define whom calcium does and does not help, however, everyone should make sure to get the optimum daily intake, says Dr. McCarron.

The National Institutes of Health recommends the following optimum daily intakes:

- Men, ages 25 to 65: 1,000 milligrams
- Women, ages 25 to 50: 1,000 milligrams
- Pregnant and nursing women: 1,200 to 1,500 milligrams
- Women at menopause (ages 51 to 65) who are taking estrogen: 1,000 milligrams
- Women at menopause (ages 51 to 65) who are not taking estrogen: 1,500 milligrams
- Men and women over age 65: 1,500 milligrams

Unfortunately, federal surveys indicate that women ages 25 to 50 get only between 685 and 778 milligrams of calcium a day through diet. Women over age 50 get between 600 and 700 milligrams daily. Adult men get closer to the mark, generally getting between 700 and 1,000 milligrams daily.

A Role for Vitamin C

A number of studies indicate that vitamin C may also be involved in reducing blood pressure.

In analyzing the results of four separate studies conducted at Tufts University in Medford, Massachusetts, researchers found that the less vitamin C in the diet, the higher blood pressure is likely to be.

In one of these studies, researchers found that some individuals who consumed 240 milligrams or more of vitamin C a day were 50 percent less likely to have high blood pressure than those consuming less than 60 milligrams a day.

New studies to test whether adding vitamin C to the diet can actually lower blood pressure are under way. In the meantime, the level of vitamin C used in the Tufts study, in the neighborhood of 240 milligrams a day, is con-

Prescriptions for Healing

Several nutrients may play roles in keeping a lid on blood pressure. Here are the amounts that researchers recommend you get from dietary sources, if possible, or from vitamin and mineral supplements, if necessary.

Nutrient	Daily Amount
Calcium	1,000 milligrams for men ages 25 to 65, for women ages 25 to 50 and for women at menopause (ages 51 to 65) who are taking estrogen 1,200–1,500 milligrams for women who are pregnant or nursing 1,500 milligrams for women at menopause (ages 51 to 65) who are not taking estrogen and for men and women over age 65
Magnesium	300–400 milligrams
Potassium	3,500 milligrams
Vitamin C	240 milligrams

MEDICAL ALERT: *If you have been diagnosed with high blood pressure, you should be under a doctor's care.*

If you have heart or kidney problems, you should check with your doctor before taking supplemental magnesium.

People who have diabetes or kidney problems or who are taking anti-inflammatory drugs, potassium-sparing diuretics, ACE inhibitors or heart medicines such as heparin should not supplement potassium without medical supervision.

sidered safe, says Dr. McCarron. (Although the Daily Value is only 60 milligrams, consuming 240 milligrams every day is well within the safe limit for vitamin C.)

High Cholesterol

Protecting Yourself from the Bad Stuff

If you're like most Americans, you're struggling to reduce your cholesterol to a healthy level. You've probably sworn off eating eggs and liver and cut way back on your consumption of red meat. You're learning to carefully read labels to keep saturated fat and cholesterol from sneaking into your diet. And all of that vigilance is no doubt paying off. It's translating into a lower level of cholesterol in your blood, plus a reduced chance of heart disease and stroke.

So with your new healthy habits in place, you can now stop worrying and get on with living. Right?

That depends. The cholesterol level in your blood is usually divided into at least three numbers. One number reflects the total amount of cholesterol circulating in your blood. Another number reflects the part of that total that contains LDL cholesterol, the "bad" stuff that gets stuck in your arteries and helps initiate the disease process that can cause a heart attack or a stroke. And the third number reflects the amount of HDL cholesterol, the "good" kind that's known to put a half nelson on the bad stuff and escort it to the liver for disposal.

Some doctors recommend that you keep your total cholesterol below 200. But others, like William Castelli, M.D., former director of the Framingham Heart Study and now medical director of the Framingham Cardiovascular Institute in Massachusetts, suggest striving for an even lower number. "We have to remember that 35 percent of all heart attacks occur in people whose total cholesterol is under 200," says Dr. Castelli.

He looks for HDL numbers above 35 in both men and women and LDL under 160 if there are no other risk factors. If you have two or more risk factors—you have a family history of heart disease, you smoke or have diabetes, for example—your LDL should be below 130, he says. Dr. Castelli notes that for anyone with a total cholesterol reading of more than 150, it is the ratio of total cholesterol to HDL that's important. "If that ratio is four or above, your risk of heart disease is progressive and you should be following a diet and exercise program recommended by your doctor," he says. "If your total cholesterol is less than 150, you have nothing to worry about," says Dr. Castelli.

Food Factors

Several of the most important strategies for lowering artery-damaging LDL cholesterol and raising its artery-cleaning cousin HDL cholesterol involve tinkering with your diet. Here's how experts suggest it should be done.

Watch those numbers. Cut dietary cholesterol to less than 300 milligrams a day. Most experts agree that avoiding liver, limiting eggs, reducing consumption of red meat and adding up and monitoring the cholesterol amounts listed on packaged goods are good ways to keep your cholesterol down.

Lower fat. The key strategy behind any cholesterol-lowering effort is lowering the amount of saturated fat in your diet to less than 10 percent of calories, says Nancy Ernst, R.D., nutrition coordinator for the National Heart, Lung and Blood Institute in Bethesda, Maryland. That's because excess saturated fat overloads the body's cholesterol-clearing system and can lead to clogged arteries.

Start lowering saturated fat by choosing fish, poultry and very lean red meats, trimming all visible fat from meats, using low-fat dairy products and reading labels to determine exact fat content.

Redistribute your fat. Scientists suggest that you can lower your LDL cholesterol by changing the balance of fats in your diet. What's the best mix? For someone with high cholesterol, it's 7-10-13. Reduce saturated fat—the kind found in meats, for example—to less than 7 percent and polyunsaturated fat—the kind found in vegetable oils—to less than 10 percent of the calories in your diet. You should also increase monounsaturated fat—the stuff found in canola oil and olive oil—to 13 percent.

Keep in mind that for every 1 percent decrease in your diet's saturated fat, your cholesterol level goes down nearly two points. Just

Vitamin C Gives a Boost

Scientists have known for some time that keeping a close eye on your dietary fat intake and your cholesterol consumption is the key to lowering your LDL cholesterol level. The rule for cholesterol is simple: Eat less than 300 milligrams a day. The rule for fat is a little more complicated. By now we

don't lower your total dietary fat too much, because that can cause a drop in beneficial HDL, warns Margo Denke, M.D., an expert on women and cholesterol at the University of Texas Southwestern Medical Center at Dallas and a member of the panel of experts on HDL and heart disease of the National Institutes of Health in Bethesda, Maryland. Research shows that a diet that gets 30 percent of its calories from fat is best for cholesterol control.

Get hooked on fish. Studies measuring the effects of omega-3 fatty acids, found in fish such as tuna, mackerel, salmon and sardines, on HDL indicate that regularly adding fish to your diet anywhere from once a week to every day is a good way to reduce saturated fat intake.

What's more, an Australian study of more than 100 men between the ages of 30 and 60 found that eating fish once a day can counteract the drop in HDL that can be caused by eating a diet that's too low in fat.

Fill up on fiber. Adding fiber-rich foods such as whole-grain cereals and breads to your diet can also reduce your level of LDL cholesterol. But make sure that every bite is of the most fiber-dense sources you can find, since nutrition experts say that you need between 15 and 30 grams of fiber in your diet to affect cholesterol levels. You can get that much by adding one cup of blackberries or raspberries to your breakfast, a half-cup of baby lima beans to your lunch, one cup of whole-wheat spaghetti to your dinner and five dried peach halves as a snack.

Look for soy. Soy products, such as tofu and the texturized vegetable protein often added to ground meat, contain natural plant chemicals called isoflavones. Studies indicate that these chemicals may help flush artery-damaging cholesterol out of your body.

have all heard that a diet in which you get less than 25 percent of your calories from fat is best. But for someone with high cholesterol, that's not the case. Research has shown that a diet too low in fat will lower not only your level of damaging LDL but also your level of beneficial HDL. A diet that gets 30 percent of its calories from fat is better for someone with high cholesterol, because it lowers LDL levels without lowering HDL.

While being careful not to lower your HDL is important, you should also take action to pump up your level of this good cholesterol. Researchers are just beginning to learn how you can do that.

Some studies indicate that a little alcohol (one or two drinks a day), heart-pumping exercise several times a week and avoiding tobacco are three strategies that will raise HDL. And several studies from researchers at Tufts University in Medford, Massachusetts, indicate that the higher the level of vitamin C in your blood, the higher your HDL level.

Blood levels of vitamin C and HDL were tested in 1,372 men and women at Tufts. Those who had the highest levels of vitamin C in their blood had 10 percent more HDL than those with the lowest vitamin C levels.

In a study at the Jean Mayer USDA Human Nutrition Research Center on Aging at Tufts University in Boston, 138 men and women ages 20 to 65 took 1,000 milligrams of vitamin C a day for eight months. "We saw significant increases in HDL cholesterol—an average of 7 percent—among those volunteers who started with low levels of vitamin C in their blood," says Paul Jacques, Sc.D., an epidemiologist at the center and one of the authors of the study. More than half of the adults in the United States who don't take supplements containing vitamin C have low levels of this vitamin in their blood, according to vitamin C expert Robert A. Jacob, Ph.D., a research chemist in micronutrients at the U.S. Department of Agriculture Western Human Nutrition Research Center in San Francisco. Dr. Jacob suggests increasing these levels with "three to four servings a day of the top vitamin C sources, such as citrus fruits, potatoes, broccoli, cauliflower, strawberries, papayas and dark green, leafy vegetables."

Researchers who are following up on these studies for the Baltimore Longitudinal Study on Aging, of the National Institute on Aging in Bethesda, Maryland, agree. The Baltimore researchers measured blood levels of vitamin C in 316 women and 511 men between the ages of 19 and 95, then asked them about the amount of vitamin C they consumed through either foods or supplements.

The result? The researchers found that the more vitamin C people got, the higher their HDL—but only up to a point. The study indicated that women who took 215 milligrams a day and men who took 346 milligrams a day increased their bodies' HDL to maximum levels.

Doctors who recommend vitamin C for high cholesterol suggest taking 250 milligrams a day, an amount that's more than four times the Daily Value of 60 milligrams but that's generally considered to be quite safe.

Niacin: Nutrient or Drug?

Doctors are beginning to suspect that niacin is not the risk-free "natural" alternative to high-tech cholesterol-lowering drugs that they had thought.

It does lower cholesterol. Studies show that daily doses of 2,000 to 3,000 milligrams reduce total cholesterol and LDL cholesterol, the bad stuff that clogs your arteries, by an average of 20 to 30 percent.

That's not bad. But what is bad are the side effects. "When niacin is taken in high doses to lower cholesterol, 100 times higher than what you need for nutritional adequacy, it really has to be looked at as a drug, because it has adverse effects," says Frank M. Sacks, M.D., associate professor of medicine and nutrition at Harvard School of Public Health.

"At high doses, there are common, bothersome side effects that aren't serious. Flushing, like the hot flashes that women have during menopause, is one. Skin rashes are another. But there are a few serious things that niacin can do as well, such as make gout or an ulcer worse."

Twenty-five percent of those who begin to take large doses of niacin abandon the vitamin because of these side effects. A slow-release form of the vitamin, however, has proven to be less of a problem in terms of these particular side effects.

What researchers have found is that slow-release niacin creates problems of its own. When scientists at the Virginia Commonwealth University Medical College of Virginia in Richmond teamed up with researchers at Pennsylvania State University College of Medicine in Hershey to compare the slow-release and immediate-release versions of niacin, they found that liver enzymes were three times higher than normal in half of the people taking slow-release niacin. Twenty-five percent of them actually showed symptoms of liver malfunction, including fatigue, nausea and loss of appetite.

Fortunately, once everyone was off the niacin, their livers returned to normal within four weeks.

Nevertheless, concluded the researchers, no one should take slow-release niacin, and no one should take the immediate-release form without being under a doctor's watchful eye.

Prescriptions for Healing

Lowering cholesterol is a key strategy in the fight against heart disease. And although scientists have not yet figured out all of the different ways that nutrients can help, studies indicate that these two vitamins can be of assistance.

Nutrient	Daily Amount
Vitamin C	250 milligrams
Vitamin E	100–400 international units

MEDICAL ALERT: *If you have been diagnosed with high cholesterol, you should be under a doctor's care.*

If you are taking anticoagulant drugs, you should not take vitamin E supplements.

Vitamin E: The Neutralizer

Vitamin C is a water-soluble vitamin and is found in blood and other water-containing solutions in the body. But vitamin E is a fat-soluble vitamin, which means it actually becomes part of an LDL particle in the bloodstream. Vitamin E helps prevent the LDL from oxidizing or going rancid and thus clogging arteries, explains Balz Frei, Ph.D., associate professor of medicine and biochemistry at Boston University School of Medicine. With plenty of vitamin E around, the LDL particle harmlessly passes into the artery wall instead of forming plaque. Vitamin C acts as a helper by regenerating vitamin E when stores are low.

The Daily Value for vitamin E is 30 international units. Doctors who recommend vitamin E supplements to prevent heart disease, however, generally call for at least 100 international units a day. Up to 600 international units daily is a safe dose, according to medical experts, although people taking anticoagulants should not take vitamin E supplements.

HIV

Aggressive Nutrition Prolongs Life

A nutrition specialist based in Chicago is on the phone trying to set up an appointment with someone who needs her expertise.

"Well, Wednesday I'm in Chicago, Thursday I'm in Charlotte, and Friday, I think, I'm in your area. Monday I'm in Indianapolis . . ."

Meet Cade Fields-Gardner, R.D., the woman whom every person infected with the human immunodeficiency virus (HIV) wants to see. She is the director of services for Cutting Edge Consultants, a group of dietitians who use their expertise to set up and monitor HIV nutritional programs for hospitals, industries and individuals across the country. And she is someone who is trying to make a difference in the lives of those who are infected with HIV, the virus that destroys the immune system and causes AIDS.

Fields-Gardner is hot. Physicians speak of her with respect. People who test positive for HIV speak of her with reverence. She can read lab reports the same way a Wall Street broker reads the Dow-Jones. She has the information that may help people stay alive.

Studies show that the majority of those who are HIV-positive are likely to have major deficiencies of a slew of vitamins and minerals at different stages of the disease. But figuring out exactly what that means and how to correct it has turned Fields-Gardner and her colleagues in HIV care into nothing less than medical detectives. "Almost all of us in HIV care are often flying by the seat of our pants," says Fields-Gardner.

A study at the University of Miami of 112 men who were HIV-positive, for example, found that 67 percent had at least one nutrient deficiency, while 36 percent had more than one. Thirty percent were deficient in vitamin B_6, 30 percent in zinc, 20 percent in vitamin E, 16 percent in vitamin A and 11 percent in vitamin B_{12}.

None of these men had any symptoms of nutritional deficiency—fatigue or memory loss, for example—and the majority of them were eating balanced diets that provided all of the Recommended Dietary Allowances. Many were also taking supplements. Yet when vitamin B_{12} was measured, for example, only those men taking 25 times the Recommended Dietary Allowance demonstrated even adequate B_{12} levels.

A Body That Can't Fight Back

Why would a well-nourished body experience almost a half-dozen nutrient deficiencies?

"Nutrition in HIV is complex," says Fields-Gardner. In some cases, the virus may indirectly injure the intestinal wall, which can make it difficult for the body to absorb nutrients. Doctors know that opportunistic infections, such as intestinal viruses and bacteria from undercooked foods, are common in people with HIV and can also affect the body's ability to absorb nutrients. Medication-induced diarrhea and malabsorption as well as metabolic changes resulting from additional liver or pancreatic disease, often seen in people with HIV, also contribute to lower blood levels of nutrients. Compounding the situation is the fact that the body seems to increase the rate at which it uses nutrients. And it may actually use them differently.

All of these factors add up to malnutrition, which has three major effects on those who are HIV-positive, experts agree. It contributes to the weight loss that frequently leads to a wasting syndrome in which more than 10 percent of total body weight, mostly lean muscle, is lost. It can decrease the effectiveness of drugs designed to prolong life, or it can increase the toxicity of other drugs. And it can sabotage already compromised immune system cells, which are charged with fighting off HIV as well as any opportunistic infections and even the cancers that frequently try to gain a foothold during HIV infection.

"Any type of malnutrition can contribute to immune dysfunction," says Fields-Gardner.

A vitamin B_6 deficiency, for example, can reduce the number of natural killer cells that the immune system has available to target marauding viruses. And it directly reduces the number of what are known as CD4 cells, the immune system's first line of defense against HIV. In fact, since HIV attacks CD4 cells first, doctors can count the number of CD4 cells in a blood sample as a means of tracking how well—or how poorly—a person's immune system is fighting the HIV invasion.

The Beta-Carotene Lesson

Although malnutrition is common in those with HIV, there's a wide spectrum of opinion about why it exists and what should be done about it.

"Although it may seem obvious that any deficiency should be corrected, we don't know if there's a purpose for the deficiency, so we have to proceed cautiously," says Fields-Gardner. "We have to play detective, do trial and error, then monitor the results closely with appropriate blood tests and other tests."

Studies at Oregon Health Sciences University in Portland, for example, revealed that levels of carotenoids—lutein, alpha-carotene, beta-cryptoxanthin and the more well known beta-carotene—are reduced early in an HIV infection and that the more advanced the disease, the lower the levels of these nutrients.

Since carotenoids are known to boost levels of body chemicals that may help fight off the destructive effects of HIV, logic seems to dictate that you do everything you can to raise levels of these chemicals as high as you can, such as taking beta-carotene supplements.

But such may not be the case. Researchers in Oregon did exactly that and found that there may be one group of HIV-positive people for whom beta-carotene is beneficial and a subgroup for whom beta-carotene is actually harmful. The problem is, no one can tell who falls into which group.

The bodies of people with a particular disease may not use nutrients in the same way that the bodies of healthy people do, explains Fields-Gardner. Healthy people, for example, will turn orange if they get more beta-carotene than their bodies can use. "But we've had reports of people who've had signs of toxicity, including high levels of triglycerides, without even turning orange first. This is worrisome in people who may have problems with the pancreas." (Triglycerides are fat molecules in the blood that are markers for heart disease.)

Aggressive Nutrition

Keeping in mind that supplementing various nutrients in those who are HIV-positive can have unexpected problems, HIV experts are increasingly viewing aggressive nutrition as the defining battle in the war against AIDS. Nutrition may not be the primary therapy directed against the virus; an alphabet soup of drugs designed to slow the virus bears that standard. But many experts feel that winning the nutrition battle can at least raise the quality of life on the battlefield or even prolong the war.

A six-year study at Johns Hopkins School of Hygiene and Public Health in Baltimore of 281 HIV-positive men, for example, found that the highest levels of thiamin, niacin and vitamin C from both foods and supplements were associated with slower progression to AIDS. Between 9,000 and 20,000 international units of vitamin A a day, two to four times the Daily Value, was associated with a 43 percent decrease in the risk of progression to AIDS, although amounts of vitamin A over that amount were associated with an increased risk. (The Daily Value for vitamin A is 5,000 international units.)

Consumption of vitamins B_{12}, D and E, plus calcium, folic acid, iron and copper, was not associated with AIDS in one way or another. But increasing consumption of zinc was actually associated with an increased risk of AIDS. Men with higher zinc intakes were more likely to develop AIDS.

"There's a growing body of evidence suggesting that micronutrient intake may be significant in helping the body to keep its immune system at the best level to help control the virus," says Neil M. H. Graham, M.D., associate professor of epidemiology at Johns Hopkins School of Hygiene and Public Health and the study's senior investigator.

"On the other hand, it's worth pointing out that nutritional supplements are certainly not a cure. There seems to be progression to AIDS despite supplementation, but at a slower pace," he says.

Nutrients against AIDS

But if proper nutrition can slow the progression of HIV to AIDS, won't it also slow the progression of AIDS to death? In short, won't it buy people with AIDS more time?

Alice M. Tang, a doctoral candidate working with Dr. Graham and lead author of the study at Johns Hopkins, had the same question. She followed the survivors of the initial study for another two years and launched the first study in the nation to examine the relationship between nutrients and survival in people with AIDS.

The result? "There was a 40 to 50 percent increase in survival during the study among those who consumed the highest levels of certain vitamins," says Tang.

The highest consumption of thiamin, riboflavin, vitamin B_6 and niacin was associated with more than one year of increased survival time. Much of the protective effect appears to be from supplements rather than foods. The intake of B_6 supplements at a level more than twice the Recommended Dietary Allowance was associated with a 37 percent decrease in mortality. Similar effects were seen with thiamin and riboflavin at levels more than five times the Recommended Dietary Allowances.

"We don't know if the supplements are bringing the nutrients up to normal levels in the patients' bodies or if they're giving nutrient levels an extra boost," says Tang.

A Nutritional Surprise

Although increased levels of B vitamins seem to prolong life, more is not always better when it comes to nutrients.

"We also looked at beta-carotene and vitamin A," says Tang. Between 7,622 and 11,179 international units of beta-carotene a day was associated with a 42 percent increase in survival. But in one of those odd nutritional quirks found so often in HIV, more or less beta-carotene did not result in any improvement.

The same thing occurred with vitamin A, which is chemically related to beta-carotene. Between 9,098 and 20,762 international units a day was associated with protection.

Those therapeutic windows were not the only nutritional surprises found by Tang and her colleagues. "The intake of zinc in the population we studied appeared to be harmful," she says. "Scientists have done studies in which very high levels of zinc were toxic to the immune system. But never has anybody found that ranges around the Recommended Dietary Allowance, about 15 milligrams a day, could be harmful. Yet when we looked at zinc supplements separately from food, people who were taking any zinc supplement had a 50 percent increase in their risk of mortality."

She suspects that taking zinc supplements may be like feeding HIV a spoonful of fertilizer.

"Studies show that the virus has something called zinc fingers," says Tang. The fingers may actually grab zinc as the virus replicates itself.

If that's true, she adds, giving the body even a milligram more zinc than it needs to carry out basic functions might be counterproductive.

"There may be a fine balance between boosting your immune system and not giving the virus too much to work with," she concludes. It should be noted that these findings have yet to be confirmed by other studies, so the issue remains controversial.

The Nuances of Nutrition

Given the surprises that frequently emerge in HIV nutrition, many experts are reluctant to recommend even the Daily Value of a particular vitamin or mineral.

Others say that since people with HIV are running out of time, they're willing to suggest whopping doses that may in fact prove toxic just on the chance that they might help.

"Everyone may be well-meaning, but the issue is very emotional," says Fields-Gardner. "If you suggest small amounts of vitamins and minerals, people say you're allowing your patients to die. If you suggest large amounts, people say you're killing them."

But there is a middle ground, one that's based solidly on the available research.

"There are very preliminary data and no clinical trials, so you have to be careful," says Dr. Graham. "But anything you can do to tip the immune system in your favor seems to be a good idea."

His recommendation? Load up on B vitamins, keep zinc at or below the Daily Value of 15 milligrams and do not exceed twice the Daily Values of fat-soluble nutrients such as vitamins A, D and E. Vitamin D in doses exceeding 600 international units daily should be taken only under medical supervision. And research has found that taking 10,000 international units of vitamin A daily in early pregnancy can cause birth defects. For this reason, women of childbearing age should consult their doctors before supplementing this much vitamin A. Women who are pregnant should not use this therapy.

"If you're going to take B vitamins, take all of them in reasonably solid doses," says Dr. Graham. Take thiamin, riboflavin, vitamin B_6, vitamin B_{12}, folic acid and niacin in the range of two to four times their Daily Values. You should check with your doctor before supplementing B_{12} if you have any kind of infection. And folic acid in doses exceeding 400 micrograms daily should be taken only under your doctor's supervision, as this vitamin can mask signs of a B_{12} deficiency.

"It's also suggested that if you're going to take supplements, you should start very early, because the virus is replicating right from the word go," says Dr. Graham.

The Promise of Selenium

Scientists originally thought that HIV invaded the immune system and then laid low until some unknown trigger finally catapulted it into rabid replication.

Scientists now realize, however, that there is a "titanic struggle" going on between the immune system and the virus all of the time, says Dr. Graham.

In fact, the body's immune system seems to be able to mount a vigorous response and keep the virus in check for years. Eventually, however, HIV destroys more immune cells than the body can replace, and the virus spreads

Food Factors

Although vitamins and minerals may play important roles in holding off the development of AIDS in those infected with the human immunodeficiency virus (HIV), medical experts say that these nutrients cannot do their jobs without three other dietary constituents. Here's what they recommend.

Stay liquid. "For those who are HIV-positive, fluids are the number one priority, because they are the medium in which everything occurs," says HIV nutrition specialist Cade Fields-Gardner, R.D., director of services for the Chicago-based Cutting Edge Consultants, a group of dietitians who use their expertise to set up and monitor HIV nutritional programs for hospitals, industries and individuals across the country. All of the micronutrients in the world won't do you any good unless you have enough fluid in your body to process and transport them, she says. Try to get at least eight to ten glasses of fluids a day, preferably those that contain calories (juices and nectars are good sources). Coffee and alcoholic beverages don't count, since they may cause dehydration.

Increase calories. "Calories are the number two priority," says Fields-Gardner. They give people the sheer raw energy with which to live and to be able to use vitamins and minerals.

The nutrient-dense calories found in the basic food groups (grains, vegetables, fruits, dairy and meats) are preferable to the calories in foods that are high in fat and sugar. To increase calories, choose higher-calorie foods such as nonfat ice cream or frozen yogurt, dried fruits and low-fat condiments.

Level out your protein intake. Protein is the third priority for those who are HIV-positive, because most of the body is made up of protein, says Fields-Gardner. And protein is a key player in keeping the immune system on its toes.

To increase the amount of protein in your diet, try fortifying milk, soups, shakes and other foods with nonfat dry milk. Add eggs to soups and other items that will be cooked thoroughly. You should check with your dietitian to be sure you need additional protein before adding too much, however, since excess protein may cause dehydration.

Prescriptions for Healing

The body's ability to absorb and use nutrients can be affected by the human immunodeficiency virus (HIV) in unexpected ways, according to experts. That's why they maintain that each individual who is HIV-positive needs a battery of blood tests to define his exact nutritional state as well as regular consultation with an HIV nutrition specialist, who can work with the individual's doctor to custom-tailor a nutritional plan. Based on evolving research, here are some recommendations for daily nutrient consumption that experts suggest you and your HIV health practitioners consider.

Nutrient	Daily Amount
Folic acid	800–1,600 micrograms
Niacin	40–80 milligrams
Riboflavin	3.4–6.8 milligrams
Selenium	200–400 micrograms
Thiamin	3–6 milligrams
Vitamin A	5,000–10,000 international units
Vitamin B_6	4–8 milligrams
Vitamin B_{12}	12–24 micrograms
Vitamin D	400–800 international units
Vitamin E	30–60 international units

throughout the body, usually precipitating a drop in the immune system's CD4 cells (the fighters) and the onset of full-blown AIDS. CD4 cells are a type of white blood cell called a T-helper lymphocyte. These cells are often referred to as the conductors of the immune system, because they coordinate the response of all other immune cells by using chemical messengers called cytokines. They also help other cells increase their antiviral effects.

MEDICAL ALERT: If you are HIV-positive, you should be under a doctor's care.

Folic acid in doses exceeding 400 micrograms daily should be taken only under your doctor's supervision, as this vitamin can mask signs of a vitamin B_{12} deficiency.

Doses of selenium in excess of 100 micrograms a day should be taken only under medical supervision.

Vitamin A has been linked to birth defects when taken during early pregnancy in doses of 10,000 international units daily. Women of child-bearing age should consult their doctors before taking this much vitamin A. Women who are pregnant should not use this therapy.

You should check with your doctor before supplementing vitamin B_{12} if you have any kind of infection.

Vitamin D in doses exceeding 600 international units daily should be taken only under medical supervision.

If you are taking anticoagulant drugs, you should not take vitamin E supplements.

A study at Johns Hopkins School of Hygiene and Public Health in Baltimore has found an association between zinc and the progression of HIV infection to AIDS. Do not take zinc supplements without first consulting your doctor.

What causes HIV to suddenly overwhelm the immune system is a matter of intense speculation in the scientific community. But one theory suggested by Gerhard N. Schrauzer, Ph.D., a researcher at the University of California, San Diego, is that HIV breaks out of its immune system hosts only after it has exhausted their available supplies of selenium.

In other words, the virus is hungry. For selenium.

What makes Dr. Schrauzer think this might be the case? For one thing, studies indicate that the less selenium in the body, the more advanced an HIV infection is likely to be. For another, a group of French scientists has found that adding selenium to HIV in cell cultures blocks the virus's replication. And third, an ongoing investigation by Dr. Schrauzer and a colleague in Germany seems to indicate that supplementing the diet with somewhere between 100 and 300 micrograms of selenium a day reduces symptoms and prevents life-threatening weight loss in those with AIDS.

But the proof of Dr. Schrauzer's theory may actually come from research conducted by Will Taylor, Ph.D., an AIDS researcher at the University of Georgia in Athens. Dr. Taylor has found theoretical genetic evidence supporting the idea that there are actually selenium-containing proteins on the genes that may regulate HIV replication.

"This means that HIV may be regulated by selenium levels," says Dr. Taylor. "And there may actually be a molecular switch controlling the virus that is sensitive to selenium levels and that would be turned on when selenium levels get too low."

Dr. Schrauzer emphasizes that a person infected with HIV should seek a medical doctor open to all approaches of treatment and healing. "Selenium is important," he says, "but any single agent or treatment has its limitations. The best results have been obtained with comprehensive treatments."

The bottom line? "Selenium should be a key complementary therapy in any AIDS program," says Dr. Schrauzer. "I recommend 200 to 400 micrograms a day." Doses of selenium in excess of 100 micrograms a day should be taken only under medical supervision.

Immunity

Fortifying the Troops

If you wanted to learn how to wage war, you could examine the battlefield strategies of history's great generals.

Or you could study your immune system, a mind-boggling array of internal defenses designed to protect your body from the assault of disease-causing troublemakers.

Your immune system carries on a never-ending battle against a relentless horde: airborne microscopic spike-covered cold and flu viruses trying to attach themselves to your nose and throat. Cancer-causing particles sucked into your lungs. Fungus clinging to your feet after a shower at the gym. Even bacteria breeding on your unrefrigerated roast beef sandwich.

Your own standing army of immune system defenders fights a continuing battle. Is there anything you can do to help the troops fight the good fight? Yes, a great deal!

Soldiers Need Their Rations

Medical researchers have long recognized the connection between good nutrition and the strength of your immune system. They know, for example, that in impoverished countries, millions of children die each year from measles, pneumonia and diarrhea because they don't get enough vitamin A to keep their immune systems up to par.

While they're usually less extreme, nutritional deficiencies present an immune system problem in America as well. Some experts believe that subtle vitamin and mineral deficiencies as well as enhanced nutrient requirements at different stages of life can cause your immune system to falter in its important work.

"We know that in many older folks, for example, immune response is compromised," says Adria Sherman, Ph.D., professor and chair of the Department of Nutritional Sciences at Rutgers University in New Brunswick, New Jersey. "It's not clear whether this is an inevitable characteristic of aging, a physiological process, years of nutritional depletion, poor eating habits or increased needs. But in my opinion, it's probably some combination of all of these." Dr. Sherman is certainly not alone in this opinion.

"Several surveys show that almost one-third of apparently healthy elderly people have reductions in the intake of several nutrients," according to Ranjit Kumar Chandra, M.D., research professor at Memorial University of Newfoundland and director of the World Health Organization's Center for Nutritional Immunology, also in Newfoundland. "The most common deficiencies are those of iron, zinc and vitamin C. Correction of these deficiencies by following nutritional advice or by taking dietary or medicinal supplements results in a significant improvement in immunity."

While the whole story isn't yet in, researchers are slowly identifying the roles that specific nutrients play in helping your immune system keep you free of disease and infection.

Food Factors

Eating right can help keep your immune system running strong. Besides a diet based mainly on whole grains, fruits and vegetables, here's what the experts recommend.

Juice up your iron. Drinking a glass of vitamin C–rich orange juice while eating meat or a whole-grain food helps your body better absorb the iron in the food. But oranges need not be your only source of vitamin C. Eating broccoli, spinach, cantaloupe or strawberries with your steak works just as well, says Adria Sherman, Ph.D., professor and chair of the Department of Nutritional Sciences at Rutgers University in New Brunswick, New Jersey.

Avoid the sweet stuff. Medical studies have found that antibody production drops after people have as little as 18 grams of sugar, about as much as you'd find in half of a can of regular soda.

Vitamin A: An Immune Enhancer

Vitamin A seems to top the A-list of nutrients that are vital for a strong immune system.

While studying the effects of vitamin A in children, Dr. Chandra observed that even a moderate deficiency can weaken the immune defenses of a child's respiratory tract. Vitamin A deficiency causes damage to the naturally protective mucous membrane barrier of the respiratory tract, and it's thought that bacteria and viruses take advantage of that damage.

How might that affect a child's health? After a flu virus attacks, for example, the lining of a normal throat will repair itself. Not so in those who are vitamin A–deficient. "Instead, you might get that once-healthy cell replaced by an abnormal cell," says Charles B. Stephensen, Ph.D., associate professor in the Department of International Health at the University of Alabama in Birmingham. "That may predispose you to having a more severe episode of an infection or having another infection on top of a viral infection."

"The link between vitamin A deficiency and the severity of respiratory disease is very well established," agrees Susan Cunningham-Rundles, Ph.D., associate professor of immunology at Cornell University Medical Center in New York City and editor of *Nutrient Modulation of the Immune Response*.

Such deficiencies are common in poorer countries, where foods high in vitamin A, such as green, leafy vegetables and fortified milk, are not readily available or are not utilized. And as a result, health officials in those countries routinely prescribe vitamin A supplements to prevent measles and other infections, particularly diarrhea, from becoming life-threatening. This strategy has cut deficiency-related deaths by 30 percent in some countries.

Many experts believe that immune-compromising vitamin A deficiencies are also widespread among children in the United States. Some 28 percent of children in the United States may be vitamin A–deficient, according to Martha Rumore, Pharm.D., associate professor at the Arnold and Marie Schwartz College of Pharmacy and Health Sciences in Brooklyn. In a published review of vitamin A research, Dr. Rumore found that vitamin A deficiency has been correlated with decreased resistance to pneumonia, tuberculosis, whooping cough and infectious diarrhea.

Another study, this one of 20 U.S. children with measles, showed that half were vitamin A–deficient.

How could children in a land so well-supplied with milk shakes and salad bars be vitamin A–deficient? For one thing, measles actually depletes vitamin A. And for another, many people, especially kids, just don't eat foods that contain vitamin A.

"There's no doubt about it. All of the continuing food consumption survey studies have shown that vitamin A intakes are low among children, especially in poverty areas," says Adrianne Bendich, Ph.D., a clinical research scientist in the human nutrition research department at Hoffmann–La Roche in Nutley, New Jersey.

How much vitamin A is enough? The Daily Value for vitamin A is 5,000 international units.

Beta-Carotene: Immune Booster

Beta-carotene is the pigment that helps turn carrots, cantaloupe and other fruits and vegetables orange or yellow. But researchers are discovering that this nutrient does a lot more than add color to your favorite produce.

In fact, studies have shown that beta-carotene does quite a bit of immune-boosting work of its own.

Researchers in one study found that the number of T-helper cells in male volunteers jumped 30 percent after the men took 180 milligrams (almost 299,000 international units) of beta-carotene a day for two weeks. (T-helper cells are important components of the immune system.)

In another study, this time at the University of Arizona in Tucson, groups of men and women were given daily doses of 15 milligrams (about 25,000 international units), 30 milligrams (about 50,000 international units), 45 milligrams (about 75,000 international units) or 60 milligrams (almost 100,000 international units) of beta-carotene for two months, according to Ronald R. Watson, Ph.D., research professor at the University of Arizona College of Medicine. An enhanced immune response was noticeable at 30 milligrams and above, with increased numbers of both natural killer cells and activated lymphocytes, which are also important immune system components.

In studies of AIDS patients and in studies of older patients with precancerous oral lesions, a similar immunological effect was seen with 30 milligrams of beta-carotene a day during a three-month period. The effect declined after the three months, however.

Levels being tested in clinical trials are between 50,000 and 100,000 international units a day. These dosages are considered safe as well as potentially effective in preventing both cancer and heart disease.

No toxic level of beta-carotene has been shown in research so far. A potential side effect is discoloration of the skin, which fades as the dosage is decreased.

Most research has found that smokers benefit the most from beta-carotene supplementation, as lung cancer usually shows the strongest association with low levels of beta-carotene. And lung cancer risk is reduced the most in smokers who consume high levels of beta-carotene-containing foods or supplements. Most doctors and researchers, however, still recommend eating more fruits and vegetables and eliminating smoking.

There is no Daily Value for beta-carotene, but nutrition experts generally recommend getting 8,300 to 10,000 international units a day. Most people get 1,600 to 3,300 international units a day from foods.

B_6: You May Need More

Researchers at Tufts University School of Nutrition in Medford, Massachusetts, discovered that when healthy elderly people had vitamin B_6 almost completely taken out of their diets, immune response went down. Even more telling: The amount of B_6 needed to restore strength to the immune system was higher than the Daily Value of 2 milligrams. When the study participants were provided with 50 milligrams of B_6 daily, immunity was boosted to a level that was even better than before the study began.

"These data tell us two things," says Dr. Bendich. "One is that the Daily

Value of vitamin B_6 is not high enough for optimum function in the elderly. The other is that taking a B_6 supplement enhances immunity."

Several other studies, in fact, have shown that older folks in general don't seem to eat enough vitamin B_6. One study of older residents of New Mexico showed that they eat barely one-fourth of the B_6 that they need each day.

Whether you're young or old, you can boost your vitamin B_6 intake by eating chick-peas, prune juice, turkey, potatoes and bananas. A banana provides 33 percent of your Daily Value of B_6, while an eight-ounce glass of prune juice provides 28 percent.

Vitamin C Gets Votes

There is general agreement in the medical community that vitamin C is vital to the production of white blood cells, the foot soldiers of your immune system.

"The best experimentation that I've seen suggests that vitamin C is in some way or another stimulating the white blood cells to function better," explains Elliot Dick, Ph.D., professor of preventive medicine and chief of the respiratory virus research laboratory at the University of Wisconsin–Madison and one of the country's leading cold researchers. "White blood cells attack the infected cell, gather around it, destroy it and then clean up."

By the same token, at least one study has shown that levels of vitamin C don't have to be very low, even in otherwise healthy men between ages 25 and 43, to cause a decline in immune function. During a three-month study, researchers at the U.S. Department of Agriculture Western Human Nutrition Research Center in San Francisco found that getting 20 milligrams or less of vitamin C a day caused a delayed reaction to a skin test designed to provoke an immune response, such as swelling or a rash. What's more, "the researchers could not bring the levels of vitamin C back up to where they were before the deficient diet until the volunteers were given 250 milligrams of vitamin C a day for three weeks," says study investigator Robert A. Jacob, Ph.D., research chemist in micronutrients at the Western Human Nutrition Research Center.

While the Daily Value for vitamin C (60 milligrams) is lower than the amounts used in many of these studies, many people don't get even that much.

"You'll find a significant number of people who do not get even 75 percent of the Daily Value of vitamin C, a vitamin that is very abundant, to say the least," says Vishwa Singh, Ph.D., director of the Human Nutrition Re-

Prescriptions for Healing

Good nutrition is an important key to having a healthy immune system. Experts recommend taking a multivitamin/mineral supplement that contains the Daily Values of all of the vitamins and most minerals. If the multivitamin/mineral supplement does not contain the nutrients listed below at the levels recommended, additional supplements may be needed, according to Adrianne Bendich, Ph.D., a clinical research scientist in the human nutrition research department at Hoffmann–La Roche in Nutley, New Jersey.

Nutrient	Daily Amount
Beta-carotene	8,300–10,000 international units
Iron	18 milligrams
Vitamin A	5,000 international units
Vitamin B_6	2–50 milligrams
Vitamin C	500 milligrams
Vitamin D	400 international units
Vitamin E	400 international units
Zinc	15 milligrams

MEDICAL ALERT: *If you are taking anticoagulant drugs, you should not take vitamin E supplements.*

search Department at Hoffmann–La Roche. No one should be deficient in vitamin C, he maintains, not when so many fruits and vegetables have such high amounts. An eight-ounce glass of orange juice has 200 percent of the Daily Value, for example. And a half-cup of chopped raw red bell peppers provides 158 percent.

But is the Daily Value enough to keep your immune system functioning in tip-top form? That's the question. And researchers simply don't know the answer yet. Many nutrition experts, however, recommend that you get at least 500 milligrams a day.

Delivering Potential Benefits with Vitamin D

Vitamin D is also developing a reputation as a key player in a healthy immune system. When researchers at the University of Wisconsin–Madison tested vitamin D–deficient laboratory animals, they found that the thymus gland was not doing its job of generating a sufficient number of immune system cells. And it took eight weeks of a diet with normal vitamin D levels to restore proper immunity.

The Daily Value for vitamin D is 400 international units. The nutrient is found in eggs and fortified milk. You even create your own supply as a natural reaction when sunlight touches your skin.

So who wouldn't get enough? Experts say people who avoid milk to bypass stomach problems or who stay out of the sun for fear of getting wrinkles could be putting themselves at risk for a shortage. "It could be more of a problem in the elderly than in the young," says Dr. Bendich. "What we're finding is that elderly people aren't able to make vitamin D in their skin as well as younger people. They don't go out in the sun as much. They use more skin protectors—sunscreens that block the formation of vitamin D. And they don't drink a lot of milk." The elderly need to get their Daily Value of vitamin D from a multivitamin/mineral supplement, according to Dr. Bendich.

Vitamin D is in most multivitamin/mineral supplements as well as most calcium supplements and is safe at the levels in these supplements, according to Dr. Bendich.

Vitamin E: A Well-Known Aid

The story on vitamin E and immunity is long and positive. For years, researchers have been finding dramatic immune-enhancing effects using vitamin E supplements, including increased levels of interferon and interleukin. Both of these biochemicals are produced by the immune system to fight infection.

In one study, Tufts University researchers divided older volunteers into two groups: 18 who took daily 800-milligram vitamin E supplements and 14 who took placebos (inactive look-alike pills). At the end of 30 days, the researchers found that the vitamin E takers had a 69 percent increase in levels of interleukin-2 and a decrease in levels of a substance called prostaglandin, which can reduce the number of white blood cell soldiers patrolling your body.

"The work at Tufts has very clearly shown that giving the elderly doses of vitamin E can improve immune response," says Dr. Singh.

Vitamin E also helps prevent oxidative damage in the body. This is a kind of damage that has been linked to lowered immune response. It seems that when immune system killer cells such as macrophages do their jobs of attacking and absorbing viruses, bacteria and other foreign invaders, dreaded free radicals are created as a by-product. Free radicals are unstable molecules that steal electrons from healthy molecules to balance themselves, weakening or damaging cells in the process. Vitamin E tames these free radicals by offering them its own electrons, helping to shield healthy cells from abuse.

How much vitamin E is enough to create this immune-boosting effect? Experts generally recommend getting 400 international units a day.

Iron: Tops for Immunity

Not only is iron an important mineral for healthy immune system functioning, but iron deficiency is fairly common, says Dr. Sherman. The deficiency can be caused by not eating enough iron-containing foods such as red meat and green, leafy vegetables. Menstruating women often have low iron stores because of the monthly loss of iron-rich blood. Stomach problems such as ulcers also cause the loss of blood, as do parasitic infections and, of course, serious injuries, she says.

Stored in the liver, spleen and bone marrow, iron is used first and foremost to produce hemoglobin in the blood. You're not considered iron-deficient until your blood hemoglobin level begins to fall, according to Dr. Sherman.

The Daily Value for iron is 18 milligrams, which is considered enough to keep the immune system up to par. Many researchers urge caution in taking more. Getting too much can cause abdominal pain, diarrhea and constipation.

Think Zinc

Like iron, zinc is crucial for making sure that the first wave of immune fighters, lymphocytes, has enough troops.

"When the body is exposed to a pathogen, one of the things that happens is that immune cells begin to proliferate. That is the beginning of all of the steps in killing the offender," says Dr. Sherman. "And both zinc and iron are involved in that process." Less zinc means that lymphocytes will respond more slowly to the foreign invader and that fewer will even make it to the battlefield.

Fortunately, serious zinc deficiencies are rare. Far more common, however, are moderate zinc deficiencies. Strict vegetarians are often at the greatest risk for zinc deficiency because they shun meats and seafood, the best sources of zinc.

Getting the Daily Value of zinc (15 milligrams) should be enough to keep the immune system functioning properly. And getting that amount shouldn't be a problem. Just three ounces of any lean red meat delivers about 32 percent of that amount, while six steamed oysters provide five times the amount of zinc that you need.

Taking Some Multivitamin Insurance

There's also a good deal of research that supports the idea of taking a multivitamin/mineral supplement every day. In a yearlong study of 100 elderly Canadians, for example, Dr. Chandra gave half of the group daily multivitamin/mineral supplements with extra vitamin E and beta-carotene. The other half simply received placebos each day. At the end of the study, Dr. Chandra found that the group taking supplements had half as many colds, flus and other infection-related illnesses as the group taking placebos. And when they did get sick, those taking supplements recovered in half the time, on average.

Since then, another multivitamin/mineral study has produced similar results. Researchers used skin tests to measure immune responses to proteins from bacteria and fungi that cause tuberculosis, diphtheria, tetanus and other ailments. After one year, the supplement takers in the study had significantly more virile immune systems than did the people who took placebos for the same amount of time, according to research leader John Bogden, Ph.D., professor in the Department of Preventive Medicine and Community Health at the University of Medicine and Dentistry of New Jersey/New Jersey Medical School in Newark.

Why would a simple multivitamin/mineral tablet make such a difference in the performance of your immune system? Dr. Bogden thinks he has the answer, at least for the elderly. "We think it may be either that older people have increased requirements or that the Recommended Dietary Allowances, or levels near the Recommended Dietary Allowances, are not adequate to support optimum immunity," he says.

Infertility

Improving Your Chances

For all of the aggravation and expense that most of us go through to prevent it, you'd think that getting pregnant would be a breeze. And for most people, it is. More than 900,000 babies are conceived each day worldwide, the overwhelming majority by low-tech means.

But about one in six couples has trouble conceiving. They've tried for a year or more, without luck, to produce a baby.

Often the problem proves to be "mechanical." A blocked fallopian tube may prevent an egg from hooking up with eager sperm. Or a varicocele, a varicose vein in a testicle, may interfere with sperm production by making blood pool in the testes, causing an increase in temperature or other changes that may decrease sperm production. Both these of conditions are usually fixed with surgery.

Sometimes, however, the problem is not so obvious and may be related to hormonal or metabolic imbalances. And here, experts say, is where it pays to do some detective work to see if your eating habits and lifestyle are jeopardizing your chances for procreation.

In both men and women, stress, smoking and alcohol are well-known roadblocks when it comes to making babies. Exposure to toxic chemicals and drugs can also play a role, as can nutritional deficiencies or excesses.

"Even in my practice of well-educated, well-off people, there is evidence that some people don't eat well," says G. David Adamson, M.D., director of Fertility Physicians of Northern California in Palo Alto. Usually, a few well-focused questions about eating habits ferret out the fast-food feeders, he says. And even some people who eat pretty well—vegetarians, for instance—may have certain dietary shortcomings that affect fertility.

Here's what research shows.

Vitamin C Keeps Sperm Moving

Imagine trying to move through a crowd if everyone was stuck together: No one would go anywhere very fast. That's what seems to happen to sperm when a man's body isn't getting enough vitamin C.

A lack of vitamin C makes sperm clump together, a problem called agglutination that can easily be diagnosed when sperm are examined under a microscope, says Earl Dawson, M.D., Ph.D., associate professor of obstetrics and gynecology at the University of Texas Medical School at Galveston.

Dr. Dawson and his colleagues found that in men who took 500 milligrams of supplemental vitamin C twice a day, the percentage of sperm that stuck together dropped from above 20 percent to below 11 percent.

"We've also found that supplemental vitamin C improves sperm count, motility and viability in male smokers and reduces the number of abnormally formed sperm," he adds.

Toxic chemicals from cigarette smoke eventually get into semen, the fluid that sperm swim in, Dr. Dawson explains. Vitamin C, which is highly concentrated in semen, neutralizes these chemicals, helping to keep them from doing a nasty number on sperm.

Dr. Dawson found that only amounts above 200 milligrams a day were helpful and that the greatest improvement was noted in the men taking 1,000 milligrams of vitamin C daily for at least one month. To get that high amount from foods, you'd have to eat about 25 cups of chopped rutabaga or kohlrabi, not exactly the kind of meal to get you in the mood. So doctors feel that supplements are in order. But don't forget vitamin C–rich foods, too. Try citrus fruits and juices, sweet peppers and (ahem!) passion fruit.

Check Up on Zinc

Think of it as a manly mineral.

Although zinc is essential for both men and women, it plays a particularly important role in the production of testosterone, the main male hormone. "A low zinc level leads to a reduction in the production of testosterone, which can lead to impaired fertility," explains Ananda Prasad, M.D., Ph.D., professor of medicine at Wayne State University School of Medicine in Detroit and a leading zinc researcher.

In one study, Dr. Prasad and his colleagues found that men on a diet deliberately low in zinc had significant drops in testosterone levels and in sperm count. When the men's zinc intakes were restored to levels on a par with the Daily Value of 15 milligrams, both testosterone levels and sperm count slowly rose back to normal in 6 to 12 months.

Zinc also influences sperm motility, or their ability to wriggle and thrash through the female reproductive tract en route to an egg, says Fouad Habib, Ph.D., a cell biologist at the University of Edinburgh Medical School in

Food Factors

Dietary changes are about as low-tech as it gets when it comes to treating infertility. "But doctors don't make money offering this sort of advice, so they don't always mention it," one doctor confides. Here's what to watch for.

Find your most fertile weight. Body fat plays an important role in hormone levels, especially for women but also, apparently, for men.

"Thin women may have too little estrogen, and overweight women too much, to become pregnant," says G. William Bates, M.D., vice-president for medical education and research of the Greenville Hospital System in South Carolina.

Thin men, such as marathon runners, may have low sperm counts, while obese men have low testosterone levels and high estrogen levels, which impede sperm production, Dr. Bates says.

He has both men and women aim for an ideal body weight based on height, using the 1985 Metropolitan Life height-to-weight table as a guide. "We use a medium weight for a medium frame," he says.

Thin women need to gain enough weight to normalize their menstrual cycles, he says. While overweight women don't need to become svelte, they do need to lose enough weight to allow their periods to normalize.

Scotland. "Low levels of zinc reduce sperm motility, while optimum amounts restore it," he explains.

Some experts think that low sperm counts or slow sperm can be caused by anything from too-tight shorts to lead-laden drinking water. "In my opinion, not many men in the United States are so deficient in zinc as to be infertile," says Rebecca Sokol, M.D., a specialist in male infertility at the University of Southern California in Los Angeles. This is why measuring blood levels of zinc is not routinely done in infertile men, she says.

If you find that your dietary zinc intake is low, then it might be useful to take zinc supplements under medical supervision, Dr. Habib suggests, and to have your blood level of zinc monitored.

Most experts say that you can safely get the Daily Value (15 milligrams) by eating zinc-rich foods and taking supplements as necessary. But it's best to

After a man reaches his ideal weight, Dr. Bates says, he needs to allow three to four months—the time it takes for a new batch of sperm to be produced—to see results.

"We have about a 90 percent success rate with women and about a 50 percent success rate with men," he says. "This is something every doctor should address before beginning hormone treatment."

Your best bet for help: a doctor who specializes in reproductive endocrinology.

Lay off the hard stuff. Experts agree that alcohol is a reproductive tract toxin for both men and women. And the more you drink, and the longer you drink, the greater the impairment of fertility may be.

How much is too much? A study by Harvard University researchers found that women who had more than seven drinks a week were 60 percent more likely to be infertile because of ovulation problems than women who did not drink. And even moderate drinkers (those having four to seven drinks a week) had a 30 percent increased risk of infertility.

One drink equals a 12-ounce beer, 4 ounces of table wine or a shot of straight spirits.

work with a doctor, Dr. Habib says, because too much zinc can be counterproductive and toxic, since it might interfere with copper absorption. "The amount needed varies from person to person, and frankly, we are not sure of optimum amounts," he says. If you're very low in zinc, you may need to start at a high amount, then cut back as your blood level reaches normal.

Studies show that men generally get between 10 and 15 milligrams of zinc a day, mostly from meats and seafood. Most likely to be coming up short: vegetarians, dieters and older people, who may be getting less than two-thirds, and in some cases less than one-half, the Daily Value.

The absolute best source of zinc is eastern oysters. Six of these succulent mollusks offer 76 milligrams of zinc (but make sure they're cooked!). Beef, veal, lamb and crab and other seafood are also good sources, as are wheat germ, miso and whole grains.

Save Your Heart, Save Your Love Life

You can be packing millions of ready-to-go sperm. But not one of those eager swimmers is ever going to fertilize an egg if your penis can't deliver the goods. We're talking here about potency, or the ability to maintain an erection for intercourse.

Although impotence can occur for a multitude of reasons, in men ages 40 and older it's often associated with circulation problems related to atherosclerosis, says Kenneth Goldberg, M.D., founder and director of the Male Health Center in Dallas. The same fatty deposits that clog up the arteries to your heart can build up in the tiny arteries to your penis. The result: too little blood to pump up the spongy cylinders that cause an erection.

Drugs used to treat high blood pressure and nerve damage caused by diabetes can also cause impotence.

So to stay frisky into your fifties and sixties and even longer, stick to the same lean diet that saves your heart.

The Salt-and-Pepper Approach

Lots of other nutrients are recommended for fertility problems in both men and women. Magnesium, vitamins B_6, B_{12} and E and other nutrients are all touted now and then as being helpful, even though there is little research to support their use.

"Many times doctors just don't know what to do. So they'll add a little 'salt and pepper,' trying a bit of this and that without knowing for sure what's helpful and what's not," Dr. Sokol says. But when it comes to hard scientific evidence, there's no one recipe for making babies.

So use common sense, experts advise. "It may sound boring, but your best bet really is to eat a healthy balanced diet that offers at least five servings of fruits and vegetables, along with whole grains and some good-quality protein such as meats, fish, eggs or milk," Dr. Adamson says. And take a multivitamin/mineral supplement (or, if you're a woman, a prenatal supplement) to cover your bases, he suggests. If you're a vegetarian, he adds, make sure that you're not shortchanging yourself on zinc, vitamin B_{12}, iron and other essential nutrients.

Prescriptions for Healing

Doctors agree that eating a healthy, balanced diet is the first step toward successful conception. But in some cases where conception is difficult, nutritional supplements may prove helpful. Here's what is recommended.

Nutrient	Daily Amount
For Men	
Vitamin C	200–1,000 milligrams
Vitamin E	400–800 international units
Zinc	15 milligrams
Plus a multivitamin/mineral supplement containing the Daily Values of all essential vitamins and minerals	
For Women	
Vitamin E	400–800 international units
Plus a prenatal multivitamin/mineral supplement containing the Daily Values of all essential vitamins and minerals	

MEDICAL ALERT: *More is not necessarily better. Experts say that a too-high amount of any nutrient can impair fertility.*

Some doctors recommend that women start taking prenatal supplements a few months before they stop using birth control.

Consult your doctor before taking more than 600 international units of vitamin E daily. If you are taking anticoagulant drugs, you should not take vitamin E supplements.

And if you want to take protective amounts of vitamin E, stick to 400 to 800 international units, Dr. Adamson says. It's a good idea to check with your doctor before taking vitamin E in doses exceeding 600 international units a day.

Insomnia

Resetting the Sleep Clock

The late-night talk show hosts look more familiar than most of your relatives. You and the night cashier at the 7-Eleven are on a first-name basis. You can't remember the last time you paid full price for a long-distance call; in fact, you could use more friends in faraway time zones who would still be up when you are.

If you sometimes have trouble sleeping, you're far from alone. About 30 percent of adults have an occasional bad night that keeps them from functioning at their best the following day. That, by the way, is how the experts decide whether your insomnia is a problem.

"It is not how many hours you sleep but how you feel during the next day that's important," says Peter Hauri, Ph.D., director of the insomnia program at the Mayo Clinic Sleep Disorders Center in Rochester, Minnesota. "Some people routinely sleep only four hours a night but feel fine during the day. They don't have insomnia."

But while an occasional bad night won't ruin your life, a whole string of them can pose some serious problems. Some of the worst industrial accidents of the century have been linked to errors made by sleep-deprived workers, according to Dr. Hauri. If you're among the 9 percent of Americans who suffer from chronic insomnia, you know that sleepless nights make a big difference in the way you feel, the way you work and the way you relate to other people.

Sleuthing beneath the Surface

"Insomnia is not a disease. It's just an indicator that something is wrong," says Dr. Hauri. In about half of all cases, the underlying problem is psychological. Depression, job stress and marital problems can all lead to insomnia.

Sometimes the cause is physical, such as an allergy or chronic pain, says Dr. Hauri. If that's the case, finding an effective treatment for those symptoms should end insomnia as well.

Sleepless nights can also be caused by environmental factors (noise), bad sleep habits (sleeping late on weekends) and circadian rhythm problems (feeling sleepy at the wrong times).

Finally, a growing body of research shows that sleep can be affected, positively or negatively, by what you put in your mouth. "There are so many other factors—illness, stress, depression, lifestyle—that are likely to have much stronger effects on your sleep than nutrition would," says James G. Penland, Ph.D., head researcher with the U.S. Department of Agriculture Grand Forks Human Nutrition Research Center in North Dakota. "But once those factors have been ruled out, our research suggests that getting more or less of certain nutrients can improve the quality of sleep."

Copper Gets a Medal

A study by the U.S. Department of Agriculture found that low intake of copper was associated with poor sleep quality in premenopausal women. Women on a low-copper diet of less than one milligram daily took longer to fall asleep and felt less rested in the morning than women who consumed the same diet but also got a two-milligram copper supplement daily, says Dr. Penland, who directed the study.

The Daily Value for copper is two milligrams—a tiny amount, but more than the average American is getting. Most of us get about one milligram of copper a day. That is not enough of a deficiency to cause obvious symptoms, but it may be enough to affect the way we sleep. The best food sources of copper are lobster and cooked oysters. Seeds, nuts, mushrooms and dried beans also contain copper, but you'd have to eat several servings a day to meet the Daily Value, says Dr. Penland.

Iron Makes a Difference

Another mineral that seems to have an effect on sleep quality is iron. One study by the U.S. Department of Agriculture found that women who got only one-third of the Recommended Dietary Allowance for iron experienced more awakenings during the night and poorer sleep quality than those who got the full Recommended Dietary Allowance. And while both low-iron and low-copper diets cause total sleep time to increase, that's not necessarily a good thing, says Dr. Penland. "When people are sick, they sleep more," he says. "Greater total sleep time often indicates that the body is trying to cope with some kind of challenge, which may be the case if you're not consuming enough copper or iron."

Food Factors

When it comes to insomnia, what you're eating may be just as important as what you're not eating. Here's how to make sure your diet isn't sabotaging sleep.

Eliminate the usual suspects. That means coffee, tea, cola and anything else containing caffeine. Everyone knows that too much caffeine can interfere with sleep. What we may not know is just how much is too much. "Some people with insomnia are very sensitive to caffeine, and even one or two cups of coffee is too much," says Peter Hauri, Ph.D., director of the insomnia program at the Mayo Clinic Sleep Disorders Center in Rochester, Minnesota.

Bag the nightcap. The late-night cocktail is one of the oldest sleep remedies in the book. But while a nightcap may help you drop off faster, it's also likely to wake you up during the night, says Dr. Hauri.

Keep it light. Eating a heavy meal before bed can kick your digestive system into overdrive and keep you awake. Have a light but satisfying dinner, suggests Dr. Hauri, and skip any foods that tend to trigger heartburn for you.

Stop raiding the refrigerator. Try to break the habit of getting up in the night for a snack, counsels Dr. Hauri. If you often wake up hungry, have a high-protein snack before bedtime, such as yogurt or a bowl of cereal with milk. This often prevents nocturnal hunger pangs.

If you suspect that low copper or iron intake is affecting your sleep, a multivitamin/mineral supplement is a safe, easy way to correct the problem, says Dr. Penland. Just be sure that the supplement contains 2 milligrams of copper and the Recommended Dietary Allowance of iron, which is 15 milligrams for menstruating women and 10 milligrams for men and nonmenstruating women.

Aluminum Can Foil Sleep

Another mineral that seems to have an effect on sleep quality is aluminum. Dr. Penland and his colleagues compared the sleep quality of women

Tripping to Dreamland

Until a few years ago, the top nutritional remedy for insomnia was the amino acid tryptophan. Sold in health food stores, tryptophan was used successfully by thousands of people to get a better night's sleep. That changed around 1990, when several people came down with a rare blood and muscle disorder that was linked to contaminated tryptophan supplements from a Japanese manufacturer.

"If I could be sure it was pure tryptophan, I would still recommend it to people," says Peter Hauri, Ph.D, director of the insomnia program at the Mayo Clinic Sleep Disorders Center in Rochester, Minnesota. But while tryptophan supplements are no longer sold in the United States, some people find that eating foods rich in tryptophan just before bedtime seems to help them sleep, says Dr. Hauri. "It doesn't work for everyone, but it's certainly worth trying for a couple of weeks to see if it helps." Good sources of tryptophan include turkey, spinach and milk, which may have something to do with why a cup of hot milk before bedtime became such a popular folk remedy.

who consumed over 1,000 milligrams of aluminum a day with the sleep quality of women who consumed only 300 milligrams of aluminum a day. The women who consumed more aluminum reported poorer sleep quality.

We all absorb small amounts of aluminum from air and water as well as from aluminum cooking utensils and some antiperspirants, but it probably isn't enough to cause a problem, says Dr. Penland. But if you regularly take an antacid, especially a liquid, you should be aware that many brands contain as much as 200 to 250 milligrams of aluminum per teaspoon. If you take an antacid and find yourself waking up during the night, try giving it up for a few weeks to see if your sleep improves, suggests Dr. Penland. You can also try switching to tablets, which are usually aluminum-free. Check the active ingredients on the label to be sure.

Keep an Eye on Magnesium

Some research suggests that a low magnesium level can also lead to shallower sleep and more nighttime awakenings. "Low magnesium status means

Prescriptions for Healing

Some doctors recommend these nutrients to send you nightly to the Land of Nod.

Nutrient	Daily Amount
Copper	2 milligrams
Iron	10 milligrams for men and nonmenstruating women 15 milligrams for menstruating women
Magnesium	400 milligrams

MEDICAL ALERT: *People with heart or kidney problems should consult their doctors before taking magnesium supplements.*

that your magnesium intake is very low on a daily basis, probably less than 200 milligrams a day," says Dr. Penland. "It isn't uncommon, especially among people with reduced caloric intakes, such as the elderly and people on weight-loss diets."

Even if your magnesium intake is normal, certain medications can keep your body from absorbing the mineral efficiently. The most common are probably diuretics (water pills) prescribed for high blood pressure. If you're taking them, your doctor should keep an eye on your magnesium level. Just make sure your physician knows about any medications that you're taking, especially if you're being treated by more than one doctor.

The Daily Value for magnesium is 400 milligrams. If you opt for a supplement, this amount should be enough to prevent sleep problems, says Dr. Penland. If you have heart or kidney problems, be sure to consult your doctor before taking magnesium supplements.

Intermittent Claudication

Improving Circulation

The fight to save H. Stanley Andrews's left leg from intermittent claudication may not sound like a major medical battle—until you learn what happened to his right leg. Seeing little alternative, doctors removed it.

Andrews's wife, Gertrude, knew that there had to be a better way to fight the circulatory disease caused by impeded blood flow in the legs. Suffering from heart problems herself, she explored ways to keep both herself and her husband healthy and away from the surgeon's knife.

Today, pounds lighter and free of pain, these Valrico, Florida, residents practice a wellness strategy that includes low-fat eating and vitamins. And there's no doubt in their minds, or in the mind of their new doctor, Donald J. Carrow, M.D., a physician in private practice in Tampa, Florida, with a particular interest in nutritional therapy, that supplements of vitamin E and fish oil have helped both of them turn the corner on the road to better health.

"His leg was going cold," Gertrude Andrews says. "He doesn't have pain, but he did. At 82, he's out raking the yard right now."

Clogging Up the Works

It's rare that intermittent claudication costs someone his leg. More commonly, the condition creates mild to severe pain during exertion.

The same things that contribute to heart disease, such as smoking and too much dietary fat, also contribute to intermittent claudication. Fatty deposits build up along artery walls, impeding circulation and reducing the amount of blood reaching the legs.

If you have this condition, at first you might find that you are able to walk long distances and suffer only minor pain. But eventually, as blood flow continues to slow, even a short walk can cause difficulty. Skin becomes weak and susceptible to wounds from lack of proper amounts of blood, oxygen and nutrients. Pain can develop in the hips, thighs, calves and feet. People with advanced cases can develop sores on their toes and heels.

The Nutrient Catch of the Day

Think fish. What do fish have to do with improving your ability to walk farther and faster?

Some doctors recommend getting more omega-3 fatty acids, which are found in fish oil, because of their ability to help reduce both blood fat levels and the "stickiness" of blood platelet cells. Both of these benefits will help improve your ability to walk.

"We know that fish oil has the ability to reverse the effects of plaqueing material," says Donald J. Carrow, M.D., a physician in private practice in Tampa, Florida, with a particular interest in nutritional therapy.

Depending on the severity of intermittent claudication, Dr. Carrow recommends taking 2.1 grams of eicosapentaenoic acid fish oil daily, divided into three doses. That's a total of seven 300-milligram (0.3-gram) capsules. You can take the capsules at lunch and dinner and before going to bed.

You can also get more of these beneficial fatty acids by eating more of the right kinds of fish. A three-ounce portion of dry-cooked Atlantic herring provides 1.82 grams of omega-3's. A similar amount of canned pink salmon provides 1.45 grams, and dry-cooked swordfish, 0.9 gram. Just avoid deep-fried fish. Deep-frying fish destroys the omega-3 fatty acids. (And if you have intermittent claudication, you should be avoiding high-fat foods.)

Vitamin E Helps Open Arteries

To help get the blood flowing again, more doctors are turning to a vitamin that first showed promise decades ago and that has captured the attention of modern researchers as well: vitamin E.

The rage for helping to prevent and treat heart disease, vitamin E also has quite a history of use for intermittent claudication. Back in 1958, Canadian researchers divided 40 men with intermittent claudication into two groups: one that received 954 international units of vitamin E a day and one that received placebos (blank pills). The study lasted 40 weeks.

Although only 17 men from each group completed the study, 13 of the vitamin E takers were able to walk farther without experiencing pain than the placebo takers. The researchers who conducted the study noted one finding that they considered important: "We also found that there is a considerable delay before any response can be noted, and we conclude that therapy should be continued for at least three months before being abandoned."

A long-term study in Sweden, published in 1974, gave the Canadian theory a boost. For two to five years, the Swedish researchers tracked 47 men with intermittent claudication. Half of the group took 300 international units of vitamin E a day; the other half took drugs designed to increase blood flow to their legs.

After 4 to 6 months, 54 percent of the vitamin E takers were able to walk nearly a mile without stopping, while just 23 percent of those who took drugs were able to cover the same distance without stopping. Arterial blood flow also improved in the vitamin E group 12 to 18 months into the study, and by 20 to 25 months, they had a 34 percent increase in the amount of blood flowing through their legs.

Laboratory study seems to confirm the claims of those who advocate vitamin E for intermittent claudication, says Mohsen Meydani, Ph.D., associate professor of nutrition at the Jean Mayer USDA Human Nutrition Research Center on Aging at Tufts University in Boston. Researchers at Tufts have found that when the linings of arteries are bathed in vitamin E, plaque-forming cells are less likely to stick to them than to arteries without the vitamin E treatment, he says. "It's just my clinical observation, mind you, but it makes sense that vitamin E would be useful," says Dr. Meydani.

Food Factors

The same dietary factors that help treat heart disease also help intermittent claudication. That's because both conditions are caused by narrowing of the arteries. Here's what doctors recommend.

Go low-fat. While high-fat foods are known to contribute to heart disease and other circulation woes, switching to an eating plan that gets about 10 percent of its calories from fat has been shown to actually reverse heart disease. (The average American diet gets approximately 40 percent of its calories from fat.) You can do this by eating very little red meat and more fruits and vegetables.

Kicking Intermittent Claudication

The well-muscled legs of the Italian professional soccer team and the painful legs of people with intermittent claudication may not seem to have much in common. But it appears that both can benefit from L-carnitine, an amino acid–like compound found in red meat and dairy products.

In fact, since Italy's 1984 World Cup soccer victory, European researchers have been exploring the benefits of L-carnitine for intermittent claudication, in large measure because of the soccer team's success.

"L-carnitine started getting used for a lot of things that relate to muscle weakness: cramps, stamina, endurance, over-the-counter remedies for increasing your strength and those kinds of things," says Loran Bieber, Ph.D., professor of biochemistry and associate dean of research at Michigan State University in East Lansing.

In one study, Italian researchers gave 20 people who had intermittent claudication either placebos (blank pills) or two grams of L-carnitine for three weeks and then measured the distance that they were able to walk on a treadmill. For the next three weeks, the groups switched pills and then took the walking test again. The results showed that 12 people had a 60 percent increase in walking distance and 4 people had 25 to 59 percent improvement when taking L-carnitine. Only 4 of the study participants showed no improvement.

Researchers say that L-carnitine has some mechanism other than increasing blood flow that is responsible for its ability to increase walking time and reduce pain. In someone with intermittent claudication, the body's ability to deliver fuel and oxygen to the tissues is compromised, explains Dr. Bieber. "My guess is that if L-carnitine can help you use the fuel a little more efficiently or get more oxygen to the muscles, that might be what's at work here."

L-carnitine can be found in meats, especially red meat. Vegetarians can get enough L-carnitine if they follow a diet that supplies a reasonable amount of protein, says Dr. Bieber. If you choose to supplement your diet, L-carnitine supplements can be found in most health food stores.

Prescriptions for Healing

Some doctors recommend one nutrient, vitamin E, to prevent and treat intermittent claudication.

Nutrient	Daily Amount
Vitamin E	1,600–4,000 international units, taken as 3 divided doses, or 400 international units for each 40 pounds of body weight

MEDICAL ALERT: *If you have intermittent claudication, you should be under a doctor's care.*

It's best to check with your doctor before taking vitamin E in doses that exceed 600 international units daily. If you are taking anticoagulant drugs, you should not take vitamin E supplements.

There are at least two more reasons that vitamin E seems to help improve intermittent claudication, experts say. Even though reduced blood flow prevents adequate oxygen from getting to muscles in the legs, vitamin E helps the muscles use what little oxygen they get more efficiently. It also helps muscles get by on less oxygen.

More important, vitamin E seems to reduce the ability of blood cells to stick together and form clots. Actually, it's a good thing that blood can form clots. "If I cut my finger and hold it in front of me, blood will stop pumping out of it before I die from loss of blood," says Dr. Carrow. "It's an inherent, built-in safety mechanism."

This same safety mechanism causes problems, however, after fatty deposits called plaque have built up along the walls of your leg's arteries. Sensing injury at the scene of the plaque, blood cells pile on like cars at a traffic accident, clotting and further decreasing the flow of blood.

By making your blood cells less sticky, vitamin E helps prevent any further decrease in blood flow and might even reverse some of the damage, says Dr. Carrow. "Most people with intermittent claudication learn that they can walk to the point of discomfort and then walk through it," he explains. "Now this is not true in the later stages, but when you use vitamin E and fish oil, it is almost always true."

Dr. Carrow generally advises taking between 1,600 and 4,000 international units of vitamin E a day, in three divided doses throughout the day, for a limited period of time.

Vitamin E is also recommended by Paul J. Dunn, M.D., a physician in private practice in Oak Park, Illinois, as part of a multifaceted treatment program for intermittent claudication. His prescription: about 400 international units of vitamin E daily for each 40 pounds of body weight.

For both doctors, a recommendation for vitamin E supplementation comes only after a diagnosis based on the results of a comprehensive medical history, thorough examination and testing. "Based on all of that information, I design an integrated, multifaceted treatment program that includes lifestyle changes, diet, exercise and supplements. If you come in with pain in the calves when you walk three blocks, I wouldn't just say, 'Here is some vitamin E,' " says Dr. Dunn. "Vitamin E is a helpful adjunct to treatment, but it's not the sole treatment."

It's best to check with your doctor before taking vitamin E in doses that exceed 600 international units daily.

Kidney Stones

Dissolving a Painful Problem

Take a look at a kidney stone under a microscope, and you'll understand why the pain of passing a stone is unforgettable. Most stones are spiked with razor-sharp crystals. No wonder those who've gone through the experience say the agony is equivalent to a knife in the back.

Kidney stones develop when urine concentrations of minerals and other dissolved substances get so high that the minerals can no longer remain dissolved. Stones can also form if the pH (acid-alkaline balance) of urine is too high or too low. In all cases, the minerals form insoluble crystals and precipitate, or drop out, of the urine, exactly the same way too much sugar drops to the bottom of a glass of iced tea. The crystals collect in the kidney ducts, slowly solidifying into stones.

Most doctors these days rely on both dietary measures and drugs, often diuretics (which decrease urinary calcium and increase urine flow), to keep kidney stones from coming back.

Know Your Stone

While some dietary changes seem to help prevent all kinds of kidney stones, a few work for only certain types of stones. So it's important to know the kind of stone you have formed, doctors say. The only way to do that is with laboratory analysis of a captured stone. The most common type of kidney stone, made of calcium oxalate, is found in more than 80 percent of cases.

"It's also important to know why you're forming stones. The only way to do that is with urine and blood tests and measures of levels of some hormones, such as parathyroid hormone, which regulates body levels of calcium," explains Freda Levy, M.D., clinical associate professor at Methodist Medical Center in Dallas. "People form stones for lots of different reasons, including metabolic abnormalities and infections."

Check with your doctor to make sure you're selecting the best dietary changes for your specific condition before you try any of these measures, she adds.

Magnesium May Counterbalance Calcium

The chemistry behind kidney stone formation is complex. Some doctors believe that the ratio of calcium to magnesium, another essential mineral, in the diet is important. They recommend that people who've had one or more bouts of calcium oxalate stones make sure that they get at least the Daily Value of magnesium, 400 milligrams, through diet and supplements, if necessary.

Most kidney specialists believe that there's only a minor role, if any, for magnesium in the treatment of kidney stones. They might recommend supplemental magnesium to someone whose urine is low in magnesium and high in calcium, which is a rare condition, says Fred Coe, M.D., professor of medicine and physiology and chief of nephrology at the University of Chicago Pritzker School of Medicine.

But some researchers and some doctors with an interest in nutrition believe that magnesium's potential for preventing stones has not been fully appreciated. They maintain that getting an optimum amount can help prevent stones in many people.

"Doctors think it doesn't work because they don't try it," says Stanley

Food Factors

Many doctors consider the following dietary adjustments proven and effective kidney stone stoppers. Here's what they recommend.

Stay well-watered. The more water that you take in, the less chance that minerals in your urine will form crystals that lead to stones. "Aim for at least a half-gallon of water a day or an eight-ounce glass every other waking hour," says Fred Coe, M.D., professor of medicine and physiology and chief of nephrology at the University of Chicago Pritzker School of Medicine. If you care to measure, you should be producing about two liters of urine a day. (Large plastic soda bottles contain almost two liters, or roughly a half-gallon.) Drinking enough water helps prevent all types of stones, and it's especially important for people who live in hot, dry climates.

Shake the salt habit. Too much salt raises urine calcium levels, which ups your risk of kidney stones. Some doctors aim for a maximum daily salt intake of about 2,400 milligrams, about half of the usual intake. To go that low, avoid most processed foods, especially lunchmeats, soups and frozen dinners, and toss out your saltshaker.

Don't be so sweet. "Sweet treats raise urine calcium levels at the same time they decrease urine volume, causing a very high concentration of calcium in the urine," Dr. Coe explains. If you must eat dessert, make it a small one. And avoid sweet snacks.

Don't have a cow (or a pig or a chicken). For people eating the typical American diet, high meat consumption is associated with calcium oxalate stones, studies show. Animal protein increases the concentration of both calcium and uric acid in the urine, Dr. Coe says. "Many men with kidney stones are big meat-eaters," he adds.

Gershoff, Ph.D., professor of nutrition and dean emeritus at Tufts University School of Nutrition in Medford, Massachusetts.

In a study that Dr. Gershoff did years ago, 149 people who had had at least two stones annually for five years saw their stone formation drop dramatically when they started taking 300 milligrams of magnesium a day. (They also took 10 milligrams of vitamin B_6 a day, which is discussed below.) The people were followed for 4½ to 6 years. Over 90 percent had no stones

"We try to get them under ten ounces a day, and the less, the better."

Don't cut back on calcium. Cutting back on dairy products and other calcium-rich foods used to be standard advice for people with kidney stones. Turns out, though, that people who get more calcium in their diets are less likely to develop kidney stones than people who get less calcium. If you're taking calcium supplements, though, don't go above 1,000 milligrams a day without your doctor's okay, Dr. Coe says.

Go easy on C. The Daily Value for vitamin C is a mere 60 milligrams, but many people ingest more to take advantage of vitamin C's many healing benefits. It's especially important for people who've had kidney stones to not jump on the vitamin C bandwagon with too much enthusiasm. Some doctors recommend that if you are taking vitamin C supplements, you stay below 500 milligrams. That's because one by-product of vitamin C metabolism may be oxalate, which is half of the most common kidney stone, says Dr. Coe.

Scratch oxalates off your grocery list. Beans, cocoa, instant coffee, parsley, rhubarb, spinach and black tea are all loaded with stone-causing oxalates. And ask your doctor about others. "We give our patients a list of the oxalate contents of about 200 foods," Dr. Coe says.

Don't worry about coffee—or beer. Although both of these beverages up calcium excretion, they also increase urine volume, so there's no increase in calcium concentration in the urine. In fact, some people rely on beer's strong diuretic effects to flush out kidney stones, Dr. Coe says.

during that period, Dr. Gershoff says. Only 12 people continued to make stones, but with much less frequency, he adds. "I think magnesium is definitely worth a try," he says.

Studies also show that magnesium-deficient animals are more likely than normal to develop calcium oxalate crystals in their kidneys, making stones more likely.

In Dr. Gershoff's studies, urine from people taking supplemental magnesium was capable of holding more than twice as much calcium oxalate in solution compared with urine from people not taking magnesium. This finding held even when the pH and the amount of calcium in the urine were adjusted so that they were exactly the same for both groups.

"Magnesium helps prevent calcium oxalate from crystallizing, although exactly how it does that isn't known," Dr. Gershoff says. One theory, that magnesium competes with calcium to bind with oxalate and forms a soluble compound that can be excreted from the body, is intriguing but not proven, Dr. Gershoff says.

He recommends that anyone who has passed a calcium oxalate stone take 300 milligrams of supplemental magnesium a day. "That amount worked just fine in our study," he says. Some other doctors recommend taking 400 to 500 milligrams daily.

Studies show that most men get about 329 milligrams a day and most women get about 207 milligrams a day through foods.

Stick to the lowest dose that works for you and get medical supervision, especially if your kidneys have been damaged or if you have a heart problem, Dr. Gershoff says.

Good food sources of magnesium are green vegetables, nuts, beans and whole grains.

Vitamin B_6 Provides Anti-oxalate Protection

Along with magnesium, some doctors recommend vitamin B_6 to people who get kidney stones.

"A vitamin B_6 deficiency throws up a roadblock in the body's metabolism, so more oxalic acid is made, which means that high amounts get into the urine," Dr. Coe explains. Oxalic acid then combines with calcium to form insoluble calcium oxalate, the stuff from which stones form.

In one study, conducted in India, researchers found that people with a history of kidney stones who took 40 milligrams of vitamin B_6 a day were much less likely to form stones than they were prior to beginning the vitamin. (A few people required up to 160 milligrams a day before they stopped forming stones.)

Most kidney stone specialists, however, discount the idea that people in the United States could be so shortchanged when it comes to vitamin B_6 that they develop kidney stones as a result. "It might be given to someone whose urine is very high in oxalic acid, but in my opinion, most stone-formers aren't B_6-deficient," Dr. Coe says. People with stones are seldom tested for B_6

Prescriptions for Healing

Some doctors recommend these nutrients, in a range of amounts, as part of a program to prevent a recurrence of kidney stones. Check with your doctor first to determine whether these supplements might help you.

Nutrient	Daily Amount
Magnesium	300–500 milligrams
Potassium	3,500–4,500 milligrams
Vitamin B_6	Up to 50 milligrams (including the amount in a multivitamin/mineral supplement containing the B-complex vitamins)

MEDICAL ALERT: No supplement program dissolves kidney stones that have already formed.

If you have kidney or heart problems, check with your doctor before taking supplemental magnesium.

People taking potassium-sparing diuretics or who have kidney disease or diabetes should not use potassium supplements without first consulting their doctors.

Some doctors recommend taking no more than 50 milligrams of vitamin B_6 without medical supervision. Large doses have been associated with nerve damage. Stop taking B_6 if you develop numbness in your hands or feet or unsteadiness in walking.

deficiency or asked about their intakes of B_6-rich foods such as fish, bananas and nuts. (Studies show that in the United States, both men and women get less than the Daily Value of 2 milligrams of B_6. Men average 1.87 milligrams a day; women, 1.16 milligrams a day.)

If you're supplementing vitamin B_6, stick to no more than 50 milligrams a day without medical supervision, says Dr. Coe. In large doses, B_6 has been associated with nerve damage. Stop taking B_6 if you develop numbness in your hands or feet or unsteadiness in walking. Medical experts suggest that if you're taking B_6 supplements, make sure you're also taking a well-balanced multivitamin/mineral formula that includes the array of B-complex vitamins. (B vitamins work in harmony with each other.) But again, be sure that the two supplements combined give you no more than 50 milligrams of B_6 a day.

Protection with Potassium Power

Medical experts agree that eating grains, vegetables and fruits helps avert kidney stones, and one reason for this may be that vegetarian fare offers lots of potassium. Low levels of this mineral can increase the risk of stone formation.

"People with low potassium levels, and especially those on potassium-draining diuretics such as thiazides, are likely to be prescribed potassium supplements and to be told to get more potassium in their diets," explains Lisa Ruml, M.D., assistant professor of medicine and a researcher in the Department of Mineral Metabolism at the University of Texas Southwestern Medical Center at Dallas. "Low potassium can lead to low urine citrate, which is the direct reason for increased stone risk."

Doctors who recommend potassium as a preventive for kidney stones generally suggest aiming for 3,500 to 4,500 milligrams daily. You can get this amount by eating at least five servings of fruits and vegetables, including plenty of citrus fruits and juices, every day.

One form of this mineral, potassium citrate, which is available by prescription, may be helpful not only for people with low blood levels of potassium but also for many who form calcium oxalate stones, Dr. Ruml adds.

In a study done by researchers at the University of Texas Southwestern Medical Center at Dallas, people cut their chances of forming new stones to close to zero during three to four years of daily potassium citrate therapy.

"Potassium citrate changes the pH of urine, making it able to hold more calcium oxalate without forming crystals because citrate is increased," Dr. Ruml explains. "Instead of forming stones, the calcium oxalate is excreted in the urine. We use potassium citrate now in most of our patients who get calcium stones."

Potassium citrate supplements should be taken only under medical supervision, Dr. Ruml says. People taking potassium-sparing diuretics or who have kidney disease or diabetes should not use potassium supplements of any kind without first consulting their doctors.

Leg Cramps

◆

Stopping the Squeeze

Troubled by a series of health problems that included an excruciating, wake-you-up-out-of-a-sound-sleep case of leg cramps, Geraldine Young got some interesting advice from, of all people, her surgeon: "Take 400 international units of vitamin E a day, and let's see what happens."

You can probably guess the rest. As her nightly cramps loosened their grip, the Lebanon, Ohio, resident fell in love with vitamin E. "It's fabulous," she says. "My mother takes it now, and she doesn't have leg cramps anymore, either."

Though a hit with many, vitamin E is by no means the only treatment for leg cramps, mainly because there are all kinds of causes of this not-so-serious yet painful condition.

The Cause of the Cramp

Defining a cramp is simple enough: It's nothing more than the short, involuntary contraction of a muscle. One of your muscles literally decides to flex, and to briefly stay that way, without your permission.

Exactly what provokes this display of belligerence is a little more difficult to get a handle on. For one thing, researchers can't seem to get muscles to cramp on cue. "To have a cramp actually happen in a laboratory situation, when you're in a position to study it, can only be described as fortuitous," says Lorraine Brilla, Ph.D., associate professor of exercise physiology at Western Washington University in Bellingham.

Doctors do know that those who are more muscular seem to have more leg cramps. They also know that pointing your toes a certain way while swimming can cause cramps. Getting your feet trapped in tight bedsheets can elicit a similar response. But bodybuilding, swimming and playing footsie with your bedspread are among the least innocuous causes of leg cramps.

Low levels of certain minerals known as electrolytes—magnesium, potassium, calcium and sodium—have long been linked to leg cramps. (Marathon runners sweating out the miles are particularly prone to this variety.) Certain drugs, such as diuretics (water pills) for the heart and for high blood pressure,

Food Factors

These dietary tips can help you keep magnesium and vitamin E, the nutrients that help ward off leg cramps, where you need them: in your body.

Cut the cocktails. Even a single drink containing alcohol may decrease the supply of magnesium in your body, says Lorraine Brilla, Ph.D., associate professor of exercise physiology at Western Washington University in Bellingham.

Trim the fat. Dietary fat makes magnesium harder to absorb, increasing the chances that it will be wasted, Dr. Brilla says.

Cap your sweet tooth. Eating sugary foods forces your body to use magnesium just to metabolize the sweet stuff, adds Dr. Brilla.

Can the cola. Soft drinks contain phosphates, which experts say also deplete your body of magnesium and calcium.

have also been cited as a cause of leg cramps. Dialysis patients, who have their blood filtered by a machine because their kidneys don't work properly, often complain of leg cramps. And pregnancy, it seems, is also a factor.

What do these last four causes have in common? Studies have found that each sometimes responds to vitamin and mineral therapy.

Victory with Vitamin E

Fred Whittier, M.D., professor of internal medicine at Northeastern Ohio Universities College of Medicine in Canton, owes his foray into the world of vitamin E to a rash. As part of his regular medical practice, he prescribed quinine for one woman's leg cramps. Quinine normally is an effective treatment for leg cramps, but this particular woman experienced an unpleasant side effect: It made her skin break out.

While researching other possible treatments, Dr. Whittier and his staff spotted a letter in a medical journal that reported good results using vitamin E for leg cramps. He decided to give it a try. Sure enough, a short time after the woman began taking vitamin E, her cramps disappeared.

Encouraged by his success in that case, Dr. Whittier and his associate began studying the effects of vitamin E on leg cramps. In one study, they gave 40 people who were on dialysis and who regularly suffered from leg cramps either 400 international units of vitamin E or quinine at bedtime.

A month after starting treatment, both groups went from an average of 10 leg cramps a month to 3.5 a month. If anything, the vitamin E group performed a little better.

Although he's still not sure why vitamin E seemed to help these people, Dr. Whittier does have a theory. Dialysis treatment may clean the blood, but it doesn't work as well as your own kidneys. As a result, toxins, including renegade molecules known as free radicals, which damage healthy molecules by stealing electrons to balance themselves, are left behind to irritate the muscles. Just as vitamin E soaks up free radicals linked to heart disease and cancer, it may also attack those causing leg cramps, Dr. Whittier suggests. "We know vitamin E is a scavenger. It may be picking up those irritable agents," he says. These same irritating agents may also be roaming the muscles of some people who are not undergoing dialysis, he adds.

While Dr. Whittier's research looked just at people undergoing dialysis, several older studies showed the benefits of vitamin E for people without kidney problems.

In one of the largest studies, 103 of 125 people who had been experiencing leg and foot cramps at night reported relief after taking vitamin E. A daily dose of 300 international units was effective for half of the participants, while the others required 400 international units or more for relief.

While not all studies have demonstrated that vitamin E is effective treatment for leg cramps, Dr. Whittier stands behind this remedy. "I don't think it's unusual in medicine to have two studies reporting opposite results," he says. "Vitamin E is just as good a remedy as quinine and probably safer, too."

When using vitamin E as a therapy, doctors frequently prescribe many times the Daily Value of 30 international units. Good food sources of vitamin E include wheat germ (one-quarter cup provides 39 percent of the Daily Value), safflower oil, corn oil, oatmeal and pastas. But even these fine sources provide relatively small amounts of the vitamin.

Studies have shown that some people can tolerate up to 1,600 international units of vitamin E a day without experiencing side effects, but some experts caution against taking more than 600 international units a day.

Making a Case for Magnesium

You've seen those sports drink ads on television, the ones featuring weary, sweat-soaked weekend warriors gulping bottles of fluid filled with electrolytes. Electrolytes—magnesium, potassium, calcium and sodium—are

Prescriptions for Healing

Doctors recommend these nutrients to help end leg cramps.

Nutrient	Daily Amount
Calcium	800–1,200 milligrams
Magnesium	800–1,200 milligrams, taken as 2 or 3 divided doses
Vitamin E	400 international units

MEDICAL ALERT: Pregnant women should not take any supplement without first discussing it with their doctors.

If you have kidney or heart problems, don't take magnesium supplements without medical supervision. Excess magnesium can also cause diarrhea in some people.

If you are taking anticoagulant drugs, you should not take vitamin E supplements.

some of the most important and most well known nutrients in the fight against cramping. What most folks don't know, however, is that you're likely to run out of magnesium before any other electrolyte.

"The truth is, most people in this country just don't eat enough foods containing magnesium," says Robert McLean, M.D., clinical assistant professor of medicine at Yale University School of Medicine and an internist in New Haven, Connecticut. And even if you do eat plenty of green, leafy vegetables and other foods rich in magnesium (such as nuts, figs and pumpkin seeds), there are many things that rob your body of this important nutrient. Certain medications used to treat heart disease and high blood pressure, for example, flush magnesium from the body.

So what's the connection between magnesium and muscle cramps? Think of a key and a lock. Normally stored in muscle and bone, magnesium acts like a key that unlocks muscle cells, allowing potassium and calcium to move in and out when needed as a muscle does its job.

Without adequate levels of any of these three nutrients, the muscle becomes irritable, says Dr. McLean. "It's a crude analogy, but to keep the muscle cell adequately healthy and alive, you need to get potassium into the cell, and you need to have magnesium to open up the door to let the potassium in," he explains.

Make no mistake: Both potassium and calcium are also vital to this process. It's just that the body generally has adequate amounts of these two electrolytes on hand, says Dr. Brilla. If the body is going to get low on any electrolyte, it is most likely to be magnesium, she says.

Doctors have long marveled at magnesium's powerful relaxant effect on muscles. In massive intravenous doses, this mineral is the preferred treatment for stopping premature labor contractions and a dangerous condition called preeclampsia, which causes extreme swelling and high blood pressure in pregnant women. (*Note:* Pregnant women should not take any supplement without first discussing it with their doctors.)

Before recommending magnesium supplements to ease muscle cramps, Dr. McLean does a blood test to determine an individual's blood magnesium level, to make sure that it is not unexpectedly high. If the blood level is low or even normal, then body magnesium stores may be low. Unfortunately, a normal blood level does not ensure that body magnesium stores are adequate.

Based on the results of the tests as well as the person's muscle cramp symptoms, Dr. McLean usually recommends taking one 400-milligram magnesium capsule two or three times a day. "I wouldn't go higher than that, because too much magnesium can cause you to develop diarrhea," he says. (Magnesium salt is the ingredient that makes Phillips' Milk of Magnesia, a popular bowel cleanser, do its job.)

But be careful: If you have kidney problems, taking magnesium supplements may make you accumulate the mineral too quickly, which could be toxic, says Dr. McLean. If you have kidney or heart problems, you should check with your doctor before taking magnesium supplements.

Some people taking magnesium may get relief from leg cramps right away, but a long-standing deficiency can take weeks to overcome with supplements, says Dr. Brilla. "We like to recommend supplementing for four weeks," she says. "That's how long we feel it takes before we have some kind of measurable outcome."

Calcium Can Help

By now nearly everyone on the planet knows that calcium can help ward off osteoporosis. But here's another reason to make sure you have at least one cup of skim milk or low-fat yogurt every day: Calcium can help your body absorb the magnesium you're taking to fight your leg cramps, says Dr. Brilla.

"Calcium by itself may not have much benefit for leg cramps, but calcium helps magnesium absorption. You're going to absorb more if they are both taken together," says Dr. Brilla.

Getting enough calcium may be as simple as taking your magnesium supplement with skim milk. A single glass of skim milk provides 350 milligrams of calcium, which is 35 percent of the Daily Value, says Dr. Brilla. (The Daily Value for calcium is 1,000 milligrams.) If you'd rather take a calcium supplement, shoot for one that contains between 800 and 1,200 milligrams. You might also consider a supplement that combines calcium and magnesium in one tablet, she says.

Lou Gehrig's Disease

A Potentially Radical Solution

Theoretical astrophysicist Stephen Hawking is in his third decade of a disease that kills most people in five years.

He can't tell you exactly how he made it this far, but he can tell you that in the space of all of those "extra" years, he has developed the concepts of black holes, space-time and how the universe got started. And in his spare time, Hawking—who can move only a few facial muscles and a single finger on his left hand—wrote the 5.5 million–copy best-seller *A Brief History of Time*.

Hawking's disease is amyotrophic lateral sclerosis (ALS), the progressively degenerative condition that most of us know as Lou Gehrig's disease. It's a disease in which nerve cells of the spine and the lower part of the brain are killed off little by little. The result is a progressive muscle weakness that affects the limbs, trunk, breathing muscles, throat and tongue. Sense of touch remains normal, as do the bladder, the bowel and sexual function. Intellect is not affected. There are apparently two forms: one that seems to occur at random and one that may have a genetic base. Currently, there is no treatment. But there is one therapy being studied that holds out some hope for the future. And that therapy involves vitamin E and other nutrients.

"We have no idea what causes most ALS," says Gabriel Tatarian, D.O., medical director of the ALS Clinic at Hahnemann University Hospital in Philadelphia.

Food Factors

The major nutritional difficulty for those with amyotrophic lateral sclerosis (ALS), or Lou Gehrig's disease, is getting enough calories to keep their weight up, says Fran Grabowski, R.D., a dietitian who develops eating strategies for people attending the ALS Clinic at Hahnemann University Hospital in Philadelphia. "Calorie needs may be increased in some people, others may have loss of appetite, and still others may have difficulty swallowing," she says.

In any case, here's what she suggests.

Eat cheesecake. "Of course, we want a person to eat fruits, vegetables, meats and dairy, plus whole grains," says Grabowski. "But sometimes people need to eat simple carbohydrates. I usually suggest to people with ALS that they blend two tablespoons of nonfat powdered milk into cheesecake. The cheesecake becomes an easy disguise for some added protein, thus making it more nutritious."

Is this a license to eat cheesecake? "Yes," says Grabowski. "I try to widen the choices people have to meet their caloric needs."

Don't restrict cholesterol or sugar. "People need to look at what they eat and how they eat in a whole new way," says Grabowski. "Cholesterol restriction is not good, and sugar should not be of concern."

Eat soft foods. "Let's get back to cheesecake. It is very easy to eat because of its texture. By paying attention to the texture of foods, we are able to get around some swallowing problems. Foods that are sticky, crumbly, flaky or stringy make it much more difficult to chew and swallow," says Grabowski.

Customize your eating. Check with the ALS Association for a list of clinical care facilities near you that can provide the customized nutritional advice necessary to handle this condition. The association's address is 21021 Ventura Boulevard, Suite 321, Woodland Hills, CA 91364.

"The most information we have is on the hereditary form of the disease, which affects something like one in ten of those with ALS. In probably 20 percent of those cases, we've identified an abnormal gene, the copper- and zinc-dependent superoxide dismutase gene, as a problem."

The gene to which Dr. Tatarian refers is one that controls the body's abil-

Prescriptions for Healing

Although no one knows for sure, some researchers suspect that certain nutrients may help prevent the death of nerve cells in people with Lou Gehrig's disease. Researchers are now testing several nutrients—beta-carotene, selenium, vitamin C and vitamin E—in doses that are several times higher than the Daily Values. They are also testing coenzyme Q_{10} and N-acetylcysteine, both of which function like vitamin E in the body.

The study results are not yet in, and researchers are not yet able to say for certain that any of these nutrients will be helpful. They are also not yet able to make recommendations about specific amounts. So if you'd like to try nutritional therapy using high doses of these vitamins and minerals, you should discuss with your doctor whether this approach is appropriate for you. If it's okay for you to try this therapy, your doctor will have to suggest the specific dosages for you.

Here are some things to be aware of when using these nutrients.

Vitamin C in doses exceeding 1,200 milligrams daily can cause diarrhea in some people.

If you are taking anticoagulant drugs, you should not take vitamin E supplements.

If you have Lou Gehrig's disease, you are undoubtedly already under the care of a doctor. It's really important not to engage in nutritional experimentation on your own, because your physical response to large doses of vitamins and minerals should be monitored closely.

ity to make a natural antioxidant called superoxide dismutase, or SOD.

Antioxidants are substances that mop up the maverick molecules, sometimes called free radicals, that are set loose in the body like a bull in a china shop by normal, everyday body processes. These free radicals steal electrons from your body's healthy molecules to balance themselves. Antioxidants rein in free radicals by offering their own electrons, protecting healthy molecules from harm.

Several nutrients are antioxidants; so is SOD. "Within the body, there are several different types of SOD," says Carol Troy, M.D., Ph.D., a neurologist at Columbia University College of Physicians and Surgeons in New York

City. "Their presumed function—and not everything is clear on this—is as a first line of defense against free radicals."

Laboratory studies indicate that excessive levels of these free radicals kill nerve cells and that when cells have chronically low levels of the antioxidant SOD, it is impossible to protect them from free radical damage.

"It's controversial as to what is going on," says Dr. Troy. "Certainly, we know that the cells have SOD for a reason. And when there are alterations in the cells, we know that there are problems, such as ALS."

To see if they could get a better handle on what happens, Dr. Troy and her colleagues set up small dishes of nerve cells in the laboratory and lowered the amount of SOD, just as it seems to occur in ALS.

And just as they did in people, the cells died.

Dr. Troy took new dishes of cells, lowered the SOD, then added a nerve growth factor to see if it would protect the cells. Again, the cells died.

She took a third batch of cells, lowered the SOD, then added the antioxidant vitamin E.

The cells lived.

Vitamin E Sparks New Hope

Whether or not vitamin E or any other antioxidant nutrient can prevent nerve cell death in humans with ALS is unknown. Nevertheless, that's exactly what scientists are hoping.

A few studies using low levels of vitamin E and other antioxidants have been tried in the past with poor results. But now researchers at Massachusetts General Hospital in Boston have developed an antioxidant cocktail that they hope will be powerful enough to do the job.

The recipe?

"We combine coenzyme Q_{10}, N-acetylcysteine, vitamin E, vitamin C, beta-carotene and selenium into four pills that people take every day," says Merit Cudkowicz, M.D., a researcher in neurodegenerative disease at Massachusetts General. (Coenzyme Q_{10} and N-acetylcysteine are antioxidant boosters that also naturally occur within the body.)

The pills are being given to half of the participants in a controlled study that is designed to test the effects of antioxidants on ALS. The other half of the study's participants are being given placebos (dummy pills).

"There's no proof yet that these will work," says Dr. Cudkowicz. "But we do not think that they will be harmful. People with ALS don't have a lot of time to wait."

Dr. Tatarian agrees. "People with ALS are very quick to jump on treatments that aren't orthodox. They'll do anything and take anything they can to feel better. But as long as it doesn't hurt and there are some theoretical indications for it, it would be reasonable to use."

Even scientists are not standing around waiting for the results of clinical trials. Dr. Troy, for example, is still testing nerve cells in her laboratory. And should vitamin E be as effective in people as it is in her laboratory, she's already prepared to mix up a batch.

It turns out that vitamin E plus nerve growth factor prevents cell death even better than vitamin E alone. A medication combining the two is not yet available. In the meantime, you might want to talk to your physician about taking the antioxidants used in Dr. Cudkowicz's study.

Lupus

Fighting Off an Immune System Attack

Most of the time your immune system is your best friend, fighting off invading microbes and keeping you healthy. But in certain cases—in someone with lupus, for example—the immune system gets confused about who the enemy is.

A painful and potentially life-threatening illness, lupus occurs when the immune system turns renegade and attacks the body's own tissues, causing inflammation and damage. Skin, kidneys, blood vessels, eyes, lungs, nerves, joints—just about any part of the body can be involved.

At the same time, in severe cases the immune system sometimes shirks its normal protective duties, making infections of all sorts more likely. "No one knows what sets off the immune system in the first place, but a genetic tendency and exposure to some sort of outside trigger, perhaps a virus, may be involved," explains Sheldon Paul Blau, M.D., clinical professor of medicine at the State University of New York at Stony Brook and co-author of *Living with Lupus*.

Lupus affects about 1 in 2,000 people, mostly women between puberty and menopause (ages 13 to 48) and, more frequently, African-American women. Some get the more common form of the disease, systemic lupus ery-

Food Factors

Revamping your eating habits can go a long way toward controlling the symptoms of lupus and warding off heart problems and kidney damage, its worst side effects, says Sheldon Paul Blau, M.D., clinical professor of medicine at the State University of New York at Stony Brook and co-author of *Living with Lupus*.

Don't chew the fat. Saturated fat, that is. "Evidence that this fat contributes to inflammation and promotes heart disease is a good reason to keep the fat out of your diet as much as possible," Dr. Blau says. One way to do that: Stick to small servings of lean meats and reduced-fat salad dressings and cheeses and load up on whole grains, fruits and vegetables.

Avoid alfalfa. According to Dr. Blau, alfalfa sprouts, tablets and tea all contain an immune system–stimulating compound called canavanine. In large amounts, this compound can trigger immune problems, says Dr. Blau.

Only two cases have been reported of people whose symptoms flared in response to alfalfa. One took 15 tablets a day for nine months; the other, 8 tablets a day for more than two years. Since alfalfa could be a problem for people with lupus, Dr. Blau recommends that his patients avoid it.

Stay away from cured meats and hot dogs. Both contain compounds that in large amounts can aggravate symptoms in people with lupus, says Joseph McCune, M.D., associate professor of rheumatology at the University of Michigan Hospitals in Ann Arbor.

Take it easy on mushrooms and beans. They add flavor to any dish, but both contain hydrazines and amines, compounds that in large amounts can aggravate lupus symptoms, says Dr. Blau.

Load up on garlic. Numerous studies show that garlic has a remarkable ability to reduce blood cholesterol levels and help prevent clotting in the arteries.

thematosus, which affects the entire body. Another form of the disease, discoid lupus erythematosus, can cause disfiguring skin problems. Both conditions can flare up, then subside.

Lupus may be treated with corticosteroid drugs, such as prednisone

Should Fish Be Your Dish?

If you have lupus, you may have heard about the potential beneficial effects of fish oil for this condition. Doctors sometimes suggest fatty fish for several autoimmune diseases, including lupus, rheumatoid arthritis, Raynaud's disease, psoriasis and scleroderma. (Autoimmune diseases are the result of the immune system turning on the body.) These conditions involve inflammation, or pain and swelling, of the joints, skin and vital organs. But since they don't involve infection, drugs such as antibiotics usually don't help.

"Fish oil apparently reduces inflammation by substituting for other fats when your body makes inflammation-generating biochemicals," explains William Clark, M.D., professor of medicine at the University of Western Ontario in London, Ontario, and a leading researcher of lupus and fish oil.

Your body normally makes two groups of potentially inflammatory biochemicals, prostaglandins and leukotrienes, using whatever fats are available. If you eat meats and eggs, your body uses a component of the fats found in these foods, arachidonic acid, to make very potent forms of these biochemicals. (To a much lesser extent, your body can also use corn oil, safflower oil and sunflower oil to make these biochemicals.) If fish oil is abundant, however, your body uses it to produce forms of prostaglandins and leukotrienes that are less likely to cause inflammation.

Does fish oil really help control the symptoms of lupus? "Studies of mice with lupus that were fed large amounts of fish oil instead of other dietary fats show that these diets do help reduce inflammation and improve kidney function and immunity," says Richard Sperling, M.D., assistant professor of medicine at Harvard Medical School and a

(Deltasone), which reduce inflammation and suppress the immune response. "But most people newly diagnosed with lupus don't need steroids," Dr. Blau says. "They may do well on nonsteroidal anti-inflammatory drugs such as aspirin or with some dietary changes."

It's still important to see a doctor, preferably a rheumatologist (one who specializes in arthritis and autoimmune diseases), for assessment and long-term follow-up, Dr. Blau says. One good reason: People with lupus can de-

rheumatologist at Brigham and Women's Hospital in Boston. "In the few studies done so far with humans, however, results have been disappointing, with no clear benefits."

That doesn't mean that fish oil is a bust, however. It's possible that the people in these studies got too little fish oil and too much of other fats, says Dr. Sperling. It's also possible that they started the diet too late in the course of their disease or were followed for too little time to see benefits, he speculates.

If you have lupus and you decide that you want to try fish oil, your best bet may be to substitute fatty fish (broiled or poached—not fried!) for meats and eggs, experts say. Amounts as small as 6 grams a day may help reduce inflammation, but up to 15 to 18 grams a day may be necessary for cardiovascular protection, Dr. Clark says. One fish oil capsule contains only 300 milligrams (0.3 gram) of fish oil, so you'd still have to take about 60 capsules a day (ugh!) to reach the 18-gram level.

One seven-ounce serving of mackerel, Pacific salmon or fresh albacore tuna offers 5 grams of omega-3's, about as much as you would get in 16 capsules. (Omega-3 fatty acids are the beneficial part of the oil found in fish.) The same amount of Atlantic herring has 4.24 grams of omega-3's; canned anchovies, 4.1 grams; canned pink salmon, 3.38 grams; and bluefin tuna, about 3 grams.

Some doctors worry that combining fish oil with anti-inflammatory medicines such as aspirin may prolong the amount of time it takes for blood to clot. But in one study of people with rheumatoid arthritis who had been taking anti-inflammatory drugs such as aspirin, there was no increase in bleeding time, Dr. Sperling says.

velop inflammation in their kidneys, blood vessels and other organs but have no obvious symptoms until damage is severe. Your doctor can periodically check your kidneys with blood and urine tests.

Nutritional therapy for lupus involves correcting drug-induced deficiencies and eating a balanced diet to help prevent heart disease. Women with lupus are much more likely than normal to develop heart disease. People with kidney disease also need to follow special protein restriction guidelines.

In addition, some doctors recommend so-called antioxidant nutrients that may help reduce inflammation and protect against heart disease. "There's good evidence that vitamins C and E can help prevent heart disease, and since that's such a big risk, even in these young women, I feel these vitamins are essential," Dr. Blau says.

Some doctors also recommend fish oil, which helps fight inflammation. Here are the nutrients that may help the symptoms of this disease.

Antioxidants May Offer Protection

Inflammation produces unstable molecules called free radicals, which damage cells by grabbing electrons from healthy molecules in a cell's outer membrane. Antioxidants help stop a free radical free-for-all by generously offering up their own electrons.

There's no doubt that inflammation produces free radicals. And lupus creates inflammation, sometimes all over the body. Doctors who recommend vitamins C and E, the mineral selenium and beta-carotene (the yellow pigment found in carrots, cantaloupe and other orange and yellow fruits and vegetables) to people with lupus are hoping that over time, these nutrients will help reduce the inflammation by mopping up some of the free radicals.

"Studies of animals with lupus do show that these nutrients can help stop the damage from inflammation," Dr. Blau says. "I give these nutrients to all of my patients, from day one."

He recommends a daily intake of 1,000 milligrams of vitamin C, 1,000 international units of vitamin E, 25,000 international units of beta-carotene and a supplement that includes 50 micrograms of selenium and 15 milligrams of zinc, which is used by the body to produce a free radical–dousing enzyme. Dr. Blau urges all people with lupus to discuss any vitamin or mineral treatment with their doctors.

In two studies, people with discoid lupus, a form of lupus typically characterized by red, inflamed skin in a butterfly pattern on the nose and cheeks, who took more than 300 international units of vitamin E daily (most took 900 to 1,600 international units daily) saw clearing of their inflamed skin. And a British doctor reported that large doses of beta-carotene (50 milligrams, or 83,000 international units, three times daily) completely cleared up sun-induced skin rashes in three of his patients with discoid lupus.

Vitamins C and E and beta-carotene are considered safe, even in fairly large amounts. Both selenium and zinc have much smaller ranges of safety. It's best not to take more than 100 micrograms of selenium or 15 milligrams of zinc a day without medical supervision, experts say.

Prescriptions for Healing

Drugs, not supplements, are standard treatment for lupus. But some experts believe that these nutrients may help ease symptoms.

Nutrient	Daily Amount
Beta-carotene	25,000 international units
Calcium	1,000 milligrams
Selenium	50 micrograms
Vitamin C	1,000 milligrams
Vitamin D	400 international units
Vitamin E	1,000 international units
Zinc	15 milligrams

MEDICAL ALERT: Anyone with lupus should be taking vitamin and mineral supplementation only after discussing it with a physician.

Vitamin D can be toxic in large amounts, so supplements should be taken only under medical supervision.

It's a good idea to consult your doctor before taking vitamin E in doses exceeding 600 international units daily. If you are taking anticoagulant drugs, you should not take vitamin E supplements.

Bone Up with Calcium and Vitamin D

Frequently, people with severe lupus need to take corticosteroid drugs such as prednisone. These drugs get inflammation under control, but at a price. One side effect is bone loss.

"If these drugs are being given to women in their twenties and thirties, a time when they should be maintaining optimum bone mass, chances are that they will begin to develop osteoporosis fairly early in life, by their forties or fifties," says Joseph McCune, M.D., associate professor of rheumatology at the University of Michigan Hospitals in Ann Arbor. Osteoporosis, which literally means porous bones, can lead to painful, crippling fractures.

That's why doctors who treat lupus recommend that anyone taking corticosteroid drugs for the condition get at least 1,000 milligrams of calcium a day through foods and supplements, if necessary. They also keep an eye on vitamin D, aiming for the Daily Value of 400 international units, to help calcium absorption. Some doctors recommend supplements; others reserve vitamin D supplements for those who are already showing signs of osteoporosis on special x-rays that measure bone density. Vitamin D can be toxic in large doses, so supplements should be taken only when approved by your doctor.

A glass of 1 percent low-fat milk, a top source of calcium, offers 300 milligrams, so you'll need to drink slightly more than three glasses a day to reach 1,000 milligrams. That same amount of milk provides almost 400 international units of vitamin D. Egg yolks and fatty fish such as salmon are also excellent sources of vitamin D.

Macular Degeneration

Protecting Vision into the Later Years

If you think of your eye as a camera, then the retina is the film. It's a sheet of light-sensitive cells lining the back of the eyeball. The retina captures images focused on it by the lens, converts the images to nerve impulses and sends the impulses straight to your brain, which then has the task of figuring out whether you've set your gaze on a sock, a parking ticket or a double-dip ice cream cone.

Smack in the middle of the retina is an area called the macula. Dense with cells that provide the brain with finely detailed, color-saturated images, the macula is the biological equivalent of Kodachrome. It doesn't get any sharper or more brilliant than this.

The macula gets the most focused light of any part of the eye. But as vital as light is to vision, it has a mean side. Focused year after year on the retina, light interacts with oxygen and may damage the retina's cells, causing the accumulation of waste material and sometimes the abnormal growth of tiny blood vessels under the retina. These blood vessels sometimes leak, swell and cause scars that can permanently blur your sight. This whole vision-damaging process is called macular degeneration. After cataracts, it's the leading cause of blindness in people ages 50 and older.

Fighting for Vision

Symptoms usually develop slowly. "People find it difficult or impossible to see clearly at long distances, to do close work, to see faces or objects clearly or to distinguish different colors," says Ronald Klein, M.D., professor of ophthalmology at the University of Wisconsin Medical School in Madison. You might mistake that double-dip cone of Bing cherry vanilla for rocky road, for instance.

Treatment for macular degeneration sometimes includes sealing off leaking blood vessels with a laser, a process that at least temporarily stops the spread of damage but that also destroys some retinal cells, Dr. Klein says. So preventing macular degeneration is definitely the way to go.

There's some evidence that retinal damage involves oxidative chemical reactions, the same reactions that make iron rust and oil turn rancid. In fact, macular degeneration is sometimes called rusting of the retina.

Oxidative reactions occur when oxygen interacts with other substances, setting off a game of molecular musical chairs as unstable molecules lose electrons and then grab electrons from other molecules to balance themselves. Oxidative reactions damage cell membranes and genetic material.

There's also some evidence that certain dietary components known as antioxidants can help prevent macular degeneration. Vitamins C and E and beta-carotene, a vitamin A precursor, seem most helpful. These nutrients can inhibit oxidative reactions. Some minerals, such as zinc, copper and selenium, may also be involved. These minerals are needed in small amounts for the body to make antioxidant enzymes that help protect the eye.

Multivitamins Get Some Votes

Several over-the-counter multivitamin/mineral products, including Icaps and Ocuvite (available in health food stores), are marketed to people with either macular degeneration or cataracts. And at least two small studies suggest that multivitamin/mineral supplements may help people with macular degeneration.

In one study, one-third of the people with macular degeneration scored better on vision tests after taking supplements for six months, while only 10 percent of the people not taking supplements scored better. In addition, about 40 percent of the people in the nonsupplement group continued to have deteriorating eyesight compared with only 22 percent of the people in the supplement group.

"There's certainly good reason to look further at possible nutritional protection for macular degeneration," Dr. Klein says. He and some other researchers, however, feel the case is far from solid, at least right now. They're waiting for the results of the Age-Related Eye Disease Study, a ten-year nationwide study now in progress that is looking to see whether a mix of vitamins and minerals, including vitamin C, vitamin E, beta-carotene and zinc, can cut people's risk of developing macular degeneration.

"If my patients ask about nutrients for macular degeneration, I tell them the facts: that there's some suggestion of benefit but nothing conclusive," Dr. Klein says. "I don't encourage them one way or the other."

Other ophthalmologists do recommend nutrients. "I'm not saying the evidence is in, either. But the facts so far seem promising enough for me to tell my patients that certain nutrients may help," says Randall Olson, M.D., professor and chairman of the Department of Ophthalmology at the University of Utah School of Medicine and director of the John A. Moran Eye Center, both in Salt Lake City.

Here's what research shows may help slow down macular degeneration.

Beta-Carotene Gets an A for Eyes

There's no doubt that vitamin A plays an important role in vision. In the retina, a form of vitamin A helps convert light to nerve impulses. Two signs of vitamin A deficiency are night blindness and trouble recovering vision after being temporarily blinded by bright light, such as the headlights of an oncoming car.

When it comes to macular degeneration, however, it seems to be beta-carotene and perhaps other related compounds that provide the protection. These nutrients act as antioxidants, stopping chain reactions of free radicals, those unstable molecules that cause so much damage, by offering their own electrons.

So far, evidence is limited to several dietary studies that suggest that people who eat plenty of beta-carotene-rich fruits and vegetables are less likely than normal to develop macular degeneration. A study at Harvard Medical School, for instance, found that people who got at least 8,700 international units of beta-carotene a day had 50 percent less risk of developing macular degeneration than those getting less than that amount.

In another study, people who ate beta-carotene-packed carrots, broccoli, spinach and apricots on a daily basis had only about half of the risk of macular generation of people who ate hardly any of those foods.

Food Factors

Antioxidant nutrients seem to get all of the attention when it comes to eye protection, but researchers are interested in other, less widely studied food components as well. Here's what shows promise.

Go after glutathione. In test tube experiments, this micronutrient helped stop oxygen-induced damage to retinal tissue. (It helps form an important antioxidant enzyme called glutathione peroxidase.) Look to fresh green, yellow and red vegetables for your supply of this nutrient. Canned and frozen vegetables lose all of their glutathione in processing.

Doctors who recommend over-the-counter beta-carotene supplements to prevent macular degeneration or slow its progression prescribe 25,000 international units daily, Dr. Olson says.

Even though beta-carotene supplements are being used in ongoing studies, these supplements have not yet been proven to help prevent macular degeneration. That fact, along with the possibility that other nutrients in fruits and vegetables besides beta-carotene may be offering protection, leads many researchers to recommend food sources of beta-carotene rather than supplements. You'll be well into the high-intake range found protective in studies if you get five servings of orange, yellow or dark green, leafy vegetables every day.

Orange Aid for Eyes

Need another good reason to stock up in the produce section the next time you're shopping for groceries? It turns out that vitamin C, an antioxidant that's highly concentrated in the eye, may help shield retinal cells from oxygen-generated damage.

Studies suggest that people who get plenty of vitamin C in their diets are less likely to develop macular degeneration than those whose vitamin C intakes are low. Harvard University researchers, for instance, found that about 80 milligrams of vitamin C a day reduced the risk of macular degeneration by about 30 percent.

Doctors who recommend vitamin C to prevent or slow the progress of macular degeneration suggest 500 milligrams or more daily. That's many

Prescriptions for Healing

Some doctors recommend these nutrients to help prevent or slow the progress of macular degeneration.

Nutrient	Daily Amount
Beta-carotene	25,000 international units
Copper	1.5–9 milligrams (1 milligram for every 10 milligrams of zinc)
Selenium	50–200 micrograms
Vitamin C	500 milligrams
Vitamin E	400–800 international units
Zinc	15–90 milligrams

Plus a multivitamin/mineral supplement containing the Daily Values of all essential vitamins and minerals

MEDICAL ALERT: *If you have macular degeneration, check with your doctor before taking supplements.*

Selenium supplements in excess of 100 micrograms daily should be taken only under medical supervision.

It's a good idea to check with your doctor before beginning vitamin E supplementation that exceeds 600 international units daily. People who are taking anticoagulants should not take vitamin E supplements.

Don't take more than 15 milligrams of zinc daily without medical supervision.

times the Daily Value of 60 milligrams. One researcher, Ben C. Lane, O.D., director of the Nutritional Optometry Institute in Lake Hiawatha, New Jersey, believes that there is good reason to limit your vitamin C intake to less than 3,000 milligrams daily. He has found that this much vitamin C is associated with retinal macular puckering and increased risk of retinal detachment, which involves the retina pulling away from the back of the eyeball. (If you are very nearsighted, Dr. Lane adds, you should take no more than

1,000 milligrams daily. Nearsighted people are at higher than normal risk for retinal detachment.)

Vitamin E Eye Guard

Along with vitamin C and beta-carotene, vitamin E is a well-known antioxidant. Incorporated into the fatty membranes that enclose cells, vitamin E shields cells from free radical damage. In the retina, vitamin E may help dampen the reactions between light and oxygen that may eventually cause retinal cells to malfunction.

A few studies suggest that vitamin E can be helpful in preventing macular degeneration. Researchers at Johns Hopkins University School of Medicine in Baltimore, for instance, found that people with high blood levels of vitamin E had only half of the risk of developing macular degeneration compared with people with low blood levels.

"I feel that we don't yet know enough about how nutrients such as vitamin E work in the retina to make recommendations regarding supplement use," says Sheila West, Ph.D., associate professor of ophthalmology at Johns Hopkins University School of Medicine and the study's main author.

Doctors who do recommend vitamin E generally stay in the range of 400 to 800 international units, Dr. Olson says. Even diets that include lots of vitamin E–rich foods such as wheat germ and almonds can't provide these high amounts, so supplementation may be in order. The Daily Value for vitamin E is 30 international units. (It's a good idea to talk to your doctor if you're considering taking more than 600 international units of vitamin E daily.)

Zinc May Slow Down Damage

It's well-known that the retina contains high concentrations of zinc, an essential mineral. "Zinc appears to play an important role in the metabolism of the retina," Dr. Lane says. Zinc-deficient animals show signs of retinal breakdown, and people who are shortchanged when it comes to zinc seem to be at higher than normal risk for macular degeneration. But the zinc needs to be in balance with other minerals and not excessive, says Dr. Lane.

One study, from the Louisiana State University Eye Center in New Orleans, seems to show that zinc can help keep sight sharp as we age. That study included 151 older, healthy people with early signs of macular degeneration. Half took daily doses of 100 to 200 milligrams of zinc sulfate for 18 to

24 months. The other half took placebos (harmless blank pills).

The eyes and vision of the people in both groups were checked before and after the study. Those taking supplemental zinc were found to have significantly less loss of vision compared with those taking the placebos.

Doctors who recommend zinc to prevent or slow macular degeneration suggest amounts ranging from the Daily Value of 15 milligrams up to 80 or 90 milligrams a day. Dr. Olson recommends 50 milligrams, while Dr. Lane bases his initial dosage on each person's zinc status. "It may be necessary to start a person at a fairly high amount, then cut back as his status returns to normal," he says. Over-the-counter supplements such as zinc amino acid chelate, zinc gluconate and zinc aspartate are good sources of zinc, Dr. Lane adds.

One thing is for sure with zinc: More is not necessarily better, and doses that exceed the Daily Value deserve medical supervision. Why? For one thing, zinc competes with copper in the body, which means that too much zinc can make you deficient in copper. "That's bad, because copper also apparently plays a role in macular degeneration," Dr. Lane says. (Copper, along with zinc, is needed for the body to produce a potent antioxidant enzyme called superoxide dismutase.)

You should be getting one milligram of copper for every ten milligrams of zinc. And as with zinc, don't overdo copper. It is possible to accumulate too much copper, even when it's taken in fairly small amounts. This can be bad for your health.

Selenium Adds Antioxidant Power

Doctors sometimes fill out their antioxidant prescriptions with selenium, a mineral that is involved in the body's production of glutathione peroxidase, yet another protective enzyme found in the eye and in other parts of the body.

"In theory, selenium should be helpful in preventing macular degeneration, but in reality, there is no good proof yet that it is," Dr. Lane explains. He recommends supplements only to people found to be deficient. Dr. Olson does not recommend individual selenium supplements, but he does recommend multivitamin/mineral products such as Icaps and Ocuvite, which contain selenium.

Doctors who recommend supplements suggest 50 to 200 micrograms a day. Doses of more than 100 micrograms daily should be taken only under medical supervision; even in small amounts, selenium can be toxic. For foods rich in selenium, try garlic, onions, mushrooms, cabbage, grains and fish.

Memory Loss

Helping Your Brain to Work Better

You've heard of the tree of knowledge? Think of your brain. Inside that four-pound organ sitting inside your skull is a root and branch system of truly biblical proportions.

Hundreds of billions of brain cells called neurons stretch toward each other with rootlike growths called axons and dendrites.

Close as they might get, the tiny nerve endings of one axon never touch those of the dendrites branching toward it. Instead, memories and other thoughts have to hurdle what are called synaptic gaps.

Without chemicals called neurotransmitters (such as dopamine, norepinephrine, serotonin and acetylcholine) bridging them, these tiny gaps may as well be as wide as the Grand Canyon. Information just can't get from one neuron to the other. And that means memories, though stored throughout your brain, are just out of reach.

"You know that if you have a phone, I can call you," says Michael Ebadi, Ph.D., professor of pharmacology and neurology at the University of Nebraska College of Medicine in Omaha. "But if you don't have a phone, there's nothing I can do. That's the way it is with neurotransmitters. In order for things to occur, you know you need transmitters. In the absence of transmitters, biological function is halted."

Turning Memories into Mush

If neurotransmitters are the stuff that helps transmit memories, then what makes neurotransmitters? Although the brain's primary fuel is glucose, experts believe that key vitamins and minerals supply the raw material for many of these neurotransmitters.

And that may be what's at the heart of many memory loss problems. Although Americans eat a lot of food, they don't always choose the right kinds. As a result, many of us just don't get enough brain-boosting nutrients. And even if you are among the few who are getting the Daily Values of these essential nutrients, you may not be home free as far as memory is concerned.

Food Factors

These dietary tips can help you keep the memories flowing.

Control your cocktails. Excessive drinking can deplete your body's stores of B vitamins, says Michael Ebadi, Ph.D., professor of pharmacology and neurology at the University of Nebraska College of Medicine in Omaha. "There is a whole syndrome of B vitamin and zinc deficiencies that occurs in alcoholics, causing memory loss and even seizures," he says.

Not only that, but drinking often takes the place of healthy eating, thus lowering the amounts of essential nutrients that you eat. Alcohol can also make it difficult for the body to digest and absorb nutrients. When should you say when? If you're going to drink at all, make sure that you don't have more than two drinks a day, says Dr. Ebadi.

Eat low-fat. Details from the famous Framingham Heart Study show that the higher the blood pressure, the lower the scores on a series of mental tests, including memory tests. Researchers theorize that higher blood pressure may cause changes in blood flow to the brain. One proven strategy to bring down high blood pressure is to eat a diet that gets no more than 25 percent of its calories from fat.

Some doctors wonder whether the Daily Values are set high enough to meet all of the body's needs. Not only that, but it's possible to consume all of the nutrients in all of the right amounts and still be shortchanged if your body isn't doing a good job of absorbing the nutrients. This is a situation most likely to develop among older people, precisely the population that is most likely to be beset by memory problems.

Malabsorption of vitamin B_{12}, which means that your body can't get sufficient B_{12} from foods no matter how much you eat, is thought to affect at least one in five older adults, says Sally Stabler, M.D., associate professor of medicine at the University of Colorado Health Sciences Center School of Medicine in Denver.

Mix already poor nutrition with improper or impaired nutrient absorption, and you have a recipe for memory loss.

Benefits of B_6

It's one thing to occasionally misplace your car keys. It's another to forget where you parked your car—especially when it's in the garage, where you usually keep it. Yet that's what some research shows could happen if you don't get proper amounts of vitamin B_6, also called pyridoxine.

One study showed that over 80 percent of the healthy, independent-living, middle-income elderly surveyed in Albuquerque, New Mexico, had vitamin B_6 intakes below three-fourths of the Daily Value. (The Daily Value for B_6 is two milligrams.)

A group of researchers in the Netherlands decided to see what would happen if they added vitamin B_6 to the diets of healthy older men. First the men were given a mental test that included things such as being able to remember different objects flashed on a screen and the names and occupations of people in a list. Then one group took 20 milligrams of B_6 a day, while the others took placebos (blank pills).

At the end of three months, the men were tested again. The memories of those in the vitamin B_6 group showed "modest but significant" gains, especially in long-term memory. The bottom line: The researchers felt that their study made a strong case for taking B_6 supplements.

There's a good reason that vitamin B_6 helps memory. Remember those all-important neurotransmitters with the long names? Vitamin B_6 apparently helps create dopamine, serotonin and norepinephrine, says Dr. Ebadi.

The Daily Value of two milligrams should be sufficient to help keep your memory in good working order. You can easily get this amount as part of a B-complex supplement that supplies the Daily Values of all B vitamins. You should never take B_6 by itself without medical supervision, as amounts above 100 milligrams can be toxic.

Boosting the Brain with B_{12}

In one study, when 39 people were treated for neurological symptoms related to vitamin B_{12} deficiency—things such as memory loss, disorientation and fatigue—all of them improved, sometimes dramatically. "B_{12} deficiency causes problems in the nervous system, including burning points in the feet and mental problems such as difficulty with recent memory and the ability to calculate, that sort of thing," says Dr. Stabler. A B_{12} deficiency has even been known to change brain wave activity, she says.

Nearly one-third of people over age 60 can't extract the vitamin B_{12} they need from what they eat. That's because their stomachs no longer secrete enough gastric acid, the stuff that breaks down food and helps turn it into fuel for your brain and body.

And taking supplements won't help, because they are also broken down in the stomach. So doctors who suspect vitamin B_{12} deficiencies in people with memory problems give them B_{12} shots, thus bypassing the faltering digestive system.

Vitamin B_{12} deficiency caused by diet is rare when the digestive system is in good working order. That's because eating just small portions of dairy products or animal protein gives you enough of this vital nutrient. About the only eating plan that seems to put you at risk are diets that completely eliminate meats and dairy products. But even then you have to adhere to such a diet for at least several years before a deficiency develops, says Dr. Stabler.

Virtually all animal products, such as milk, cheeses, yogurt and lean beef, contain vitamin B_{12}. The Daily Value for B_{12} is six micrograms.

Fortification at Its Finest

Both thiamin and riboflavin, other important B vitamins, are routinely added to most flours, cereals and grain products.

Even mild deficiencies of these vitamins can have an impact on your thinking and memory. While checking brain function and nutrition status of 28 healthy folks over age 60, a U.S. Department of Agriculture study showed that those with low thiamin registered brain activity impairment. On the other hand, the folks with adequate thiamin had better memories.

Thiamin deficiencies have also been found to cause mood changes, vague feelings of uneasiness, fear, disorderly thinking and other signs of mental depression—symptoms that researchers say often affect memory.

Fortunately, it doesn't take much thiamin to make a difference. One study showed that women who were restricted to 0.33 milligram of thiamin a day became irritable, fatigued and unsociable. These symptoms improved with just 1.4 milligrams of thiamin a day.

The Daily Value for thiamin is 1.5 milligrams, while the Daily Value for riboflavin is 1.7 milligrams.

The Lecithin-Choline Connection

As a doctoral candidate overwhelmed by the vast amounts of information she had to study, Florence Safford took lecithin supplements to help keep her memory sharp—and she told her friends about the benefits.

Her friends don't have to just take her word for it any longer. Twenty years later, Dr. Safford, now professor of social work and gerontology at Florida International University in Miami, has conducted two studies that help shed light on how lecithin and choline, a B vitamin, can actually boost memory.

Lecithin is a common food additive; it's used in ice cream, margarine, mayonnaise and chocolate bars to help wed the fat in these foods with water. It has healthful qualities as well, such as mildly increasing the amount of choline in your brain. And more choline means more acetylcholine, an important neurotransmitter that you need for your memory to function.

In one study, 61 volunteers between ages 50 and 80 were divided into two groups: 41 took two tablespoons of lecithin a day, while 20 were given placebos. At the end of five weeks, the volunteers who took lecithin had "significant improvement" in memory test scores and fewer memory lapses than those who took the placebos, says Dr. Safford.

In another study, 117 volunteers were divided into three groups according to their ages: 35 to 50, 50 to 65 and 65 to 80. These groups were then subdivided, with half taking 3.5 grams of a form of lecithin a day and the other half taking placebos. At the end of three weeks, those who took the lecithin recorded almost half as many memory lapses on average, says Dr. Safford.

"The fascinating thing about lecithin is that when it helps, it's right away," says Dr. Safford. "It's one of the few substances like alcohol, which crosses the blood-brain barrier and produces an immediate reaction." (In a bid to prevent harmful substances from reaching your brain, you're equipped with what is called the blood-brain barrier. Like an armed guard at a checkpoint, your blood-brain barrier allows only certain chemicals in your blood to pass into your brain.)

Dr. Safford recommends two tablespoons of lecithin granules a day. Just mix it in with foods such as yogurt, applesauce and cereals.

Iron and Zinc to Help You Think

While researchers have established the importance of iron and zinc in the mental development of infants, you have to dig into the scientific literature before you'll find studies showing that these minerals help make for better memories in adults as well.

In one small preliminary study, researchers measured the effects of mild zinc or iron deficiency on short-term memory in 34 women between ages 18 and 40, a group at risk for low levels of both minerals.

Prescriptions for Healing

Some doctors recommend these nutrients to help avoid memory loss.

Nutrient	Daily Amount
B-complex supplement containing . . .	
Riboflavin	1.7 milligrams
Thiamin	1.5 milligrams
Vitamin B_6	2 milligrams
Vitamin B_{12}	6 micrograms
Iron	18 milligrams
Zinc	15 milligrams

For eight weeks, researchers gave the women either 30 milligrams of zinc, 30 milligrams of iron or both or supplements containing other micronutrients. A mental test found that the short-term memories of those taking zinc or iron improved by 15 to 20 percent, says Harold Sandstead, M.D., professor in the Department of Prevention Medicine and Community Health at the University of Texas Medical Branch at Galveston.

Those who took iron supplements had better short-term verbal memory, while visual memory, or the ability to remember pictures, was improved by both zinc and iron.

Although the women received supplements during the study, Dr. Sandstead says that foods are much better sources of these nutrients. Steamed clams and oysters, Cream of Wheat cereal, soybeans and pumpkin seeds are all good sources of iron, while whole grains, wheat bran, wheat germ, seafood and meats are top sources of zinc.

Women who menstruate need between 2 and 2.5 milligrams of iron a day to offset loss of the mineral, explains Dr. Sandstead. (The Daily Value for iron is much higher—18 milligrams—because your body doesn't absorb all of the mineral that you take in.) "If they have heavy menstrual loss, the level goes up even more," he adds. Men need about 1 milligram of iron a day.

And how does iron help memory? Experts believe that pumping up your iron intake helps build those all-important brain neurotransmitters, among other things.

For a closer look at zinc's role in helping you to think, researchers at the U.S. Department of Agriculture Grand Forks Human Nutrition Research Center in North Dakota fed ten men living at the center meals containing one, two, three, four or ten milligrams of zinc every day for five weeks each.

At the end of the 25-week study, researchers noted that the week the men ate ten milligrams of zinc a day, they were better able to remember shapes and responded faster to simple motor tasks, says James G. Penland, Ph.D., head researcher at the center and author of the study. "There was a very clear improvement at ten milligrams versus the other amounts, with the others being more or less the same," he says.

And how does zinc help memory? Apparently, vitamin B_6 can't do its job without zinc pitching in, says Dr. Ebadi. "In the absence of zinc, active B_6 is not formed properly in the brain, and as a result, neither are key neurotransmitters," he says. Not only that, but large amounts of zinc have been found in the brain's memory center, the hippocampus.

Some experts say that some elderly people may get less than half of the zinc that they need. (The Daily Value for zinc is 15 milligrams.)

Ménière's Disease

Stopping the Spinning

If you've ever been so drunk that you feel like the room is spinning, you know exactly what someone experiencing an acute attack of Ménière's disease is going through. This disorder affects the part of the inner ear that controls balance: a tiny set of membranes and nerve endings that respond to motion. When this part of the ear is damaged, it sets off a reaction that results in stop-the-world-I-want-to-get-off vertigo that only time resolves.

"I've gotten so dizzy and nauseated that I had to hold on to things to keep my balance," says Linda Dowell of Gardiner, Maine, who has had Ménière's disease since 1986. Her first bout woke her up in the middle of the night and was so frightening that it necessitated an ambulance ride to the emergency room. Less serious attacks leave people feeling nauseated, weak and disoriented.

Food Factors

Virginia Fitzgerald of Phoenix is a grandmother. And as the facilitator of one of the country's largest Ménière's disease and tinnitus support groups, she offers the same grandmotherly advice to anyone who cares to listen.

"I'm always telling people to make sure they eat right," she says. "I feel like that really is the best advice I can give them."

Ear doctors and their patients agree that healthy eating can go a long way toward alleviating ear problems, for plenty of reasons. Here are the details.

Nibble away at fat. A damaged inner ear is particularly sensitive to high blood levels of cholesterol. Some researchers believe that fat in the blood actually makes the blood more viscous, or thick, and impairs blood delivery through the tiny artery that leads to the inner ear.

So cut fat, especially saturated fat, from your diet. This means filling up on fresh vegetables and fruits, whole grains, beans, low-fat dairy products, fish and lean cuts of meat. Eat only the low-fat versions of lunchmeats, mayonnaise, cheeses, frozen desserts and baked goods.

Battle your sweet tooth. Loading up on sugar does several things. It prompts your body to pump up insulin production. (Insulin is a hormone that your body uses to get energy from sugar.) Too much sugar in your diet can also send your blood sugar level to extremes of high and

Normally, the fluid in your inner ear is contained in two balloonlike chambers. The purpose of the fluid is to help you sense where your head is in reference to the rest of the world. This is done by a series of receptors in the inner ear that are sensitive to motion.

In Ménière's disease, something, perhaps a virus, interferes with the proper balance of fluid in the inner ear. Fluid pressure builds, eventually rupturing a tiny membrane in the inner ear. The rupture is often preceded by a feeling of fullness or ear pressure, followed by a loud, roaring noise and hearing loss that can be temporary or permanent. Other symptoms may include nausea and vomiting as well as tinnitus, in which there's persistent noise such as hissing or buzzing in the ear.

While the vertigo typically lasts for 10 to 60 minutes, the entire attack often encompasses hours. "I could be wiped out for days, and rest was the

low, says Charles P. Kimmelman, M.D., professor of otolaryngology at New York Medical College in Valhalla and a physician at Manhattan Eye, Ear and Throat Hospital. Your ears don't like that, he says.

It's easy enough to avoid the usual sugar-laden snacks: cookies, candy and soda. But the sweet stuff also lurks in some unsuspected foods. Low-fat cookies and other snacks, fruit-flavored yogurt, flavored teas and breakfast cereals can all pack a sugar wallop. If you're really looking to curb your sweet tooth, enjoy these foods only in moderation.

Know your salt sources. To cut salt, nutrition experts recommend reading labels carefully and avoiding foods with more than 150 milligrams of sodium per serving. Either eliminate potato chips, corn chips, pickles, olives, ham, hot dogs, canned foods (soups, beans and vegetables), hard cheeses, cottage cheese, tomato juice, tuna, lunchmeats, biscuits, pancakes, breads and pizza, or use low-sodium or no-sodium versions of these foods.

You can reduce the salt in some canned foods up to 80 percent by rinsing and draining the food for one minute.

Try using onion powder or garlic powder as seasoning rather than salt. In fact, there's a whole world of tastes worth exploring. Try sage or savory on chicken and rosemary or marjoram on meats, and add dried mushrooms and tomatoes to casseroles.

only thing that really helped," Dowell says. Ménière's disease can be helped by certain allergy drugs that are also ideal for relieving the symptoms of dizziness. If nausea and vomiting are major components of an extended attack, then antinausea suppositories may be used. For temporary relief, doctors frequently prescribe diuretics (water pills) to reduce fluid buildup in the ear. Some doctors also make several dietary recommendations.

Shake the Salt Habit

For most doctors, tops on the list of dietary advice for people with Ménière's disease is to cut way back on sodium, an essential nutrient that's too abundant in most diets. "Some people with Ménière's seem to be extremely sensitive to salt, almost as though their ears pick up any extra salt they can," explains Michael Seidman, M.D., director of the Tinnitus Center at Henry Ford Hospital in Detroit.

Once salt is concentrated in the fluid within the inner ear, it draws in additional fluid, increasing the pressure in the inner ear until the membrane ruptures, setting off a dizzying attack. Eventually, the membrane heals and the ear settles down.

Some doctors ask their patients to make sure that they get no more than 1,000 to 2,000 milligrams of sodium per day. The higher amount is for active people living in hot climates. One study of soldiers estimated that they got about 11,000 milligrams a day! (There are 2,000 milligrams of sodium in one teaspoon of salt.)

So it's obvious that people with Ménière's disease should cut back on salt. But they should also be looking at other mineral needs as well.

Other Minerals Balance Salt

Magnesium, calcium and potassium are other minerals that are critical to the normal functioning of the inner ear, explains Charles P. Kimmelman, M.D., professor of otolaryngology at New York Medical College in Valhalla and a physician at Manhattan Eye, Ear and Throat Hospital.

Because these minerals are so important to healthy ears, some doctors tell their patients with Ménière's disease to make sure that they get at least the Daily Values of these nutrients.

For magnesium, that's 400 milligrams a day. Studies show that most people come up short, with men usually getting about 329 milligrams a day and women getting about 207 milligrams a day. Whole grains, nuts and beans are your best magnesium sources. Green vegetables are good sources, but bananas are the only fruit that provides much magnesium.

For calcium, doctors recommend aiming for the Daily Value of 1,000 milligrams. One cup of 1 percent low-fat milk offers about 300 milligrams of calcium; one ounce of hard cheese (part-skim mozzarella), about 181 milligrams; and eight ounces of low-fat yogurt, about 415 milligrams.

To get a healthy amount of potassium—3,500 milligrams or more a day—load up on fresh fruits and vegetables and their juices. A cup of tomato juice, for instance, has about 537 milligrams of potassium; orange juice, 496 milligrams; and prune juice, 707 milligrams. Potatoes, yams, avocados, Swiss chard and bananas are also good sources. Since potassium is leached out by boiling water, you'll want to stick to fresh, baked or lightly steamed fruits and vegetables.

Note: Diuretics, pills that increase your flow of urine, are frequently prescribed for people with Ménière's disease, says Dr. Kimmelman. Some types of diuretics can deplete the body of potassium and sometimes of magnesium. If you're taking this kind of diuretic, he says, check with your doctor to make sure that you get enough supplemental potassium and magnesium to make up for the loss. Don't take potassium and magnesium supplements on your own in this situation, however. Too much of either mineral can be harmful, especially if you have heart or kidney problems or diabetes.

Other Vitamins May Deter Dizziness

Do any other vitamins or minerals help Ménière's disease? A number of ear doctors and other hearing specialists recommend a multivitamin/mineral supplement to their patients with Ménière's disease, but they're hard-pressed

Prescriptions for Healing

Doctors recommend cutting back on salt and adding these nutrients to a healthy diet to reduce the dizziness of Ménière's disease.

Nutrient	Daily Amount
Calcium	1,000 milligrams
Magnesium	400 milligrams
Potassium	3,500 milligrams
Plus a multivitamin/mineral supplement containing the Daily Values of all essential vitamins and minerals	

MEDICAL ALERT: Some diuretics, which are often prescribed for people with Ménière's disease, can deplete the body of potassium and magnesium. Before taking supplements of either nutrient, however, talk to your doctor. Too much of either mineral can be harmful.

If you have heart or kidney problems, be sure to consult your doctor before supplementing magnesium.

Talk to your doctor before taking potassium supplements if you have kidney problems or diabetes.

to come up with the kind of scientific proof that most doctors insist on before recommending something as effective.

"We found out by accident that women taking a multivitamin/mineral formula for premenstrual problems had a reduction, or sometimes a complete abatement, of their Ménière's or tinnitus symptoms," says Susan J. Seidel, an otologist (hearing specialist) at the Greater Baltimore Medical Center. The women were taking Optivite, an over-the-counter multivitamin/mineral supplement that offers, among other nutrients, 300 milligrams of vitamin B_6 and 250 milligrams of magnesium.

"We now recommend this supplement to people who have a sense of fullness or pressure in the ear or dizziness," says Seidel. "We don't know what in the vitamin is helping, but some people with these symptoms do say that it helps."

Another doctor, George E. Shambaugh, Jr., M.D., professor emeritus of otolaryngology and head and neck surgery at Northwestern University Medical School in Chicago, prescribes a hefty multivitamin/mineral supplement called Basic Preventive, from Advanced Medical Nutrition in Hayward, California. This supplement contains a long list of ingredients, including 500 milligrams of calcium, 500 milligrams of magnesium, 100 international units of vitamin D, 20 milligrams of zinc and an array of other vitamins and minerals. He prescribes it, he says, because his patients report that it works. "Their ears often improve, along with other health problems that they may have," Dr. Shambaugh says.

Even if you decide to take a multivitamin/mineral supplement, make sure that you follow the dietary measures recommended in "Food Factors" on page 382 as well. While nutrients can make up for some dietary indiscretions, says Dr. Shambaugh, it's unrealistic to expect them to overcome constant bad eating habits.

Menopausal Problems

Reinventing the Change of Life

Some women have a miserable time at menopause. Others barely notice that it's happening.

Either way, as the century turns, more women all over the world will go through "the change" than at any other time in history.

Menopause is not really a single event but rather a process that can last a decade or longer. The average woman has her last period between the ages of 48 and 52, but menopausal changes actually begin much earlier. Women often notice changes in their cycles when they're in their early forties or even before then. Periods may be shorter or longer, lighter or heavier; they may come closer together or farther apart.

The Estrogen Connection

It's during this time, known as perimenopause, that the ovaries gradually slow their production of the female hormone estrogen and that a woman begins to notice the effects this has on her body. So why do some women experience such discomfort at menopause, while others never have so much as a single hot flash?

It may be because some women experience more drastic drops in their estrogen levels than others do, says Margo Woods, D.Sc., associate professor of community health at Tufts University School of Medicine in Boston. Dr. Woods is doing research on the effects of soy on menopausal symptoms. Asian women, who have lower estrogen levels before menopause than Western women, experience less drastic drops in estrogen, which may be one reason that they report fewer menopausal symptoms, says Dr. Woods. Many researchers feel that diet may influence menopausal symptoms.

And some lucky women, about 25 to 30 percent, don't entirely stop producing estrogen, says Susan M. Lark, M.D., director of the PMS and Menopause Self-Help Center in Los Altos, California, author of *Menopause: Self-Help Book* and a physician specializing in women's health. Even after their ovaries stop producing estrogen, their adrenal glands and one small area of each ovary called the stroma continue to produce small amounts of this hormone. These glands don't produce enough estrogen to promote menstruation, but they do produce enough to keep the most bothersome symptoms of menopause at bay, explains Dr. Lark.

"Some women are just good estrogen producers," she says. "We don't know why."

The amount of estrogen that the body continues to produce is out of a woman's hands, adds Dr. Lark. But there are plenty of other factors that a woman can control that can reduce menopausal discomfort. "Women who avoid stress, who don't overdo caffeine and who get regular exercise have a much easier time of it than women who don't do those things," she says.

"There isn't much hard evidence to prove it, but it has been my experi-

Fighting Back with Phytoestrogens

If you're fed up with menopause, move to Japan. In the Land of the Rising Sun, hot flashes and night sweats are virtually unheard of. "Oriental women and American women report such dramatically different experiences of menopause that it's easy to wonder if we're talking about the same thing," says Margo Woods, D.Sc., associate professor of community health at Tufts University School of Medicine in Boston. Dr. Woods is researching the effects of soy on menopausal symptoms.

Of course, Japanese women don't have an easier time with menopause just because of where they live. Researchers believe that it has more to do with their traditional diet. Besides providing more vegetable protein and less animal protein than a Western diet, it's also low in fat and high in soy products such as tofu. These foods are rich in plant compounds known as phytoestrogens, which seem to mimic some of the biological activities of female hormones.

"Japanese women of all ages have lower estrogen levels than their American counterparts," says Dr. Woods. "At first we thought it was just because of their lower-fat, higher-fiber diet. Now it looks as if phytoestrogens might also play a role."

While the phytoestrogen content of soy foods varies considerably from brand to brand, one or two servings of tofu, soybeans or soy milk a day is equivalent to the usual intake of the Asian population. It also contains approximately 35 milligrams of phytoestrogens, a reasonable goal to shoot for, says Dr. Woods.

Japanese women eat from 2½ to 3½ ounces of tofu per day, says Dr. Woods.

"If you are having hot flashes and night sweats and don't want to take hormones, I certainly think it would be worthwhile to try it. It can't hurt," says Dr. Woods. "Legumes, vegetables and soy foods are safe, nutritious and good for you, whether you're having hot flashes or not."

ence that women who have a history of premenstrual syndrome and bad menstrual cramps also have more hot flashes and other symptoms of menopause," says Dr. Lark. And here again, lifestyle factors come into play. "These women tend to have very stressful lives, poor diets and poor coping skills," she maintains.

Finally, nutrition apparently plays an important role in determining whether your menopause will be an endurance contest or a walk in the park. Here's what experts say you can do to make the transition as comfortable as possible.

Vitamin E Snuffs Out Hot Flashes

A hot flash—that sudden, intensely hot feeling in your face and neck that makes you wish for a walk-in refrigerator—can happen anytime, anywhere: at home, at work, while you're driving in traffic or even while you're sleeping.

Caused by hormonal surges, hot flashes usually last for three to five minutes, but they can feel like an eternity. Some women get flushed, sweat profusely and even have heart palpitations. Other women have flashes so mild that they barely notice them. About 80 percent of all women going through menopause have hot flashes at one point or another.

Studies show that thin women are more prone to hot flashes than heavier women. This is because even after the ovaries slow their hormone production, fat cells continue to produce small amounts of estrogen. So women with a lot of fat cells go through less drastic estrogen withdrawal than their leaner sisters.

While hot flashes can be relieved by hormone replacement therapy, there may be another, less drastic option: a daily vitamin E supplement.

Vitamin E can act as an estrogen substitute, explains Dr. Lark. Studies have shown that it can relieve hot flashes, night sweats, mood swings and even vaginal dryness. "Vitamin E is really an essential part of a supplement program for women during the menopause years," she says.

If vitamin E is so effective, why hasn't your doctor recommended it? Chances are she has never heard of it, or if she has, she's waiting to see some hard scientific proof that it works. And sad to say, there isn't any. While a number of studies were done in the 1940s on vitamin E and menopause, the connection hasn't been investigated recently. A number of doctors who use nutritional therapies as part of their medical practices recommend it, however, and find that it often works.

If you get hot flashes and would like to try vitamin E, Dr. Lark recommends a fairly high dose: about 800 international units a day. And while vitamin E is nontoxic at this level, she says, women should get their doctors' okay before taking this high amount, especially if they have diabetes or high blood pressure.

Food Factors

Menopause is an excellent time to take stock of your eating habits and make healthy adjustments, says Susan Lark, M.D., director of the PMS and Menopause Self-Help Center in Los Altos, California, author of *Menopause: Self-Help Book* and a physician specializing in women's health. The following simple changes, she says, can make a big difference in your health during menopause and in the years to come.

Shake the salt habit. Eating too much salt can contribute to water retention, a common problem among women going through menopause, says Dr. Lark. "It's not enough to stop adding salt to your foods," she cautions. "I tell women to eliminate fast foods, salty snacks and other highly processed foods and to use garlic and herbs instead of salt in cooking."

Switch to decaf. "A number of studies show that women who use caffeine have more hot flashes than those who don't," says Dr. Lark. Caffeine used in excess also increases anxiety, irritability and mood swings. It depletes the body's stores of the B-complex vitamins, explains Dr. Lark, which can be a real problem for some women during menopause.

With all of these negative side effects, Dr. Lark recommends either dramatically cutting down on caffeine or eliminating it entirely. Because cutting out caffeine can cause withdrawal symptoms such as irritability and headaches, she suggests eliminating caffeine gradually. And don't forget that tea, chocolate and cola drinks also contain caffeine, she adds.

Be a teetotaler. Alcohol depletes the body's B-complex vitamins, disrupts the liver's ability to metabolize hormones and can worsen hot flashes, says Dr. Lark. "Excessive drinking is also a risk factor for osteoporosis, which all menopausal women should be concerned about," she adds. If you can't cut out cocktails altogether, she suggests limiting yourself to one or two drinks a week.

Eat more fruits and vegetables. Fresh produce is full of important vitamins and minerals, says Dr. Lark. And because they're low in fat and high in fiber, eating more fruits and vegetables can help prevent weight gain, a common problem for women of menopausal age, according to Dr. Lark.

Reduce Bleeding with Nutrients

Many women approach menopause expecting menstrual flow to taper off and finally stop. But for a good percentage, periods during perimenopause are heavier than ever.

Besides the inconvenience—perimenopausal bleeding is often so irregular that women have to be prepared anytime, anywhere—frequent heavy bleeding can seriously endanger a woman's iron stores, says Dr. Lark.

Heavy bleeding can be treated effectively with nutrients, says Dr. Lark. "Some studies have shown that besides replenishing the iron lost through bleeding, a daily iron supplement may actually reduce the amount that a woman will bleed during future periods," she says.

Women with heavy bleeding also benefit from loading up on vitamin C and bioflavonoids, she says. Bioflavonoids are chemical compounds related to vitamin C; they're found in many citrus fruits and included in many supplements.

"Both vitamin C and bioflavonoids reduce bleeding by strengthening the capillary walls, which are at their weakest just before and during the menstrual period," says Dr. Lark. And since bioflavonoids have many of the same chemical properties as estrogen, they can also be helpful in controlling hot flashes, night sweats and mood swings. She recommends a daily supplement that includes at least 1,000 milligrams of vitamin C and 800 milligrams of bioflavonoids.

Because vitamin C helps the body absorb iron more efficiently, Dr. Lark recommends taking these two nutrients together. If you take a multivitamin/multimineral supplement, check to make sure that it contains both vitamin C and iron. Another option is to take an iron supplement, about 15 milligrams, with a glass of orange juice. If you have a juicer, juicing the white pulp of the orange along with the rest of the fruit guarantees an abundant dose of bioflavonoids, Dr. Lark adds.

B-Complex Battles the Blahs

Depression is also common around the time of menopause, though nobody knows for sure how much of it results from hormonal fluctuations and how much is triggered by the everyday stresses that women face at midlife.

Regardless of what's causing it, emotional stress can deplete the body of B vitamins, leaving a woman feeling tired, anxious and irritable, says Dr. Lark.

"High levels of estrogen can also deplete vitamin B_6 and cause depression," says Dr. Lark. "Women who take the Pill or hormone replacement therapy sometimes have this, and some perimenopausal women go through a period of having very high estrogen levels." B_6 also plays an important role in helping the liver to regulate estrogen levels, says Dr. Lark.

Vitamin B_6 should always be taken as part of the B-complex, says Dr. Lark. She suggests a B-complex supplement containing 50 milligrams each of thiamin and niacin and 30 milligrams of B_6.

Coping with Surgical Menopause

While most women experience the gradual progression of natural menopause, others go through "the change" much more abruptly. Each year thousands of women undergo hysterectomy, the surgical removal of the uterus and sometimes the ovaries because of conditions as varied as pelvic infection, endometriosis and cancer.

Prescriptions for Healing

While scientific studies have yet to be done, a number of doctors have found that certain nutrients may help many women avoid problems as they go through menopause. Here's what these doctors recommend.

Nutrient	Daily Amount
B-complex supplement containing . . .	
Niacin	50 milligrams
Thiamin	50 milligrams
Vitamin B_6	30 milligrams
Iron	15 milligrams
Vitamin C	1,000 milligrams
Vitamin E	800 international units

MEDICAL ALERT: *If you're considering taking vitamin E in doses that exceed 600 international units a day, you should discuss it with your doctor first. If you are taking anticoagulant drugs, you should not take vitamin E supplements.*

In most cases, the woman's ovaries are left intact; they continue to produce estrogen until the woman goes through normal menopause. But if a woman's ovaries are removed along with her uterus in what is called a complete hysterectomy, she'll experience surgical menopause, with the same symptoms as any other woman who is going through natural menopause.

Women who experience surgical menopause may actually have more severe symptoms because they go through menopause so abruptly, says Dr. Lark.

A woman who undergoes a hysterectomy can benefit from the same nutritional strategies that help women who are going through natural menopause, says Dr. Lark. "As far as your body is concerned, it's the same process," she says.

Menstrual Problems

Nutrients to Ease Monthly Distress

Imagine you were moving to the North Pole for five years. How would you prepare for your new life? Most likely, you'd learn everything you could about coping with the cold. And if there was anything you could eat or any supplement you could take to make the experience more pleasant, of course you'd want to know about it. It's five years of your life, after all. You might as well be comfortable.

Maybe you never thought about it, but if you add it up—month after month, year after year—you have your period for about five years of your life. And if you're like most women, you'd do anything to sail through those days without feeling crampy and exhausted and swollen up like a baby beluga.

Why You Feel So Bad

Most women have some degree of menstrual discomfort at some point in their lives, says Susan M. Lark, M.D., director of the PMS and Menopause Self-Help Center in Los Altos, California, and author of *Menstrual Cramps: A Self-Help Program* and *PMS: Self-Help Book* and a physician specializing in women's health.

Most menstrual pain is classified as either spasmodic or congestive. Doctors know that spasmodic pain is caused by the female hormones estrogen

Food Factors

When it comes to easing monthly discomfort, supplements are only part of the equation, says Susan M. Lark, M.D., director of the PMS and Menopause Self-Help Center in Los Altos, California, author of *Menstrual Cramps: A Self-Help Program* and *PMS: Self-Help Book* and a physician specializing in women's health. How you feel during your period also depends on what you eat during the rest of the month. Here's what she advises.

Beware of hidden sodium. Most women know that too much salt in the diet can aggravate monthly water retention, says Dr. Lark. But many don't know that much of the salt they're eating is hidden in seemingly healthy foods, such as canned vegetables, frozen dinners and cheeses. Fast foods, pizza and most snacks, such as chips and pretzels, are also heavily salted. Stop adding salt at the table and during cooking, she suggests, and get into the habit of reading food labels for sodium content. Salad dressings, prepared soups and many condiments are loaded with sodium.

Focus on fiber. Constipation is a common complaint of women with menstrual cramps, says Dr. Lark. Solve the problem naturally with a fiber-rich diet that includes plenty of fruits, vegetables, legumes and whole-grain breads and cereals.

Try banishing wheat. Wheat can aggravate monthly symptoms in women who have food allergies, says Dr. Lark. If you suspect that you may be wheat-sensitive, she suggests substituting corn, oatmeal, brown rice and rye bread for wheat products for a month or so to see if it helps.

Steer away from beef. A diet that contains lots of red meats such as beef, lamb and pork may aggravate menstrual cramping, says Dr. Lark. Meats contain saturated fat, which the body uses to produce 2 series prostaglandins. These are chemicals that are responsible for the contraction of the smooth muscles of the uterus, which leads to cramping, she explains.

and progesterone and by prostaglandins, hormonelike substances that control muscle tension. Women with spasmodic cramps generally have an excess of a certain type of prostaglandins called 2 series prostaglandins, which are responsible for contraction of the smooth muscles, including the uterus. Prostaglandin production increases toward the end of your cycle, resulting in cramps that are sometimes accompanied by nausea, constipation or diarrhea.

Probably the best thing that can be said about spasmodic pain is that it tends to improve with age. It's usually most severe in women in their teens and twenties. Spasmodic pain often improves after a woman has children, says Dr. Lark.

The other type of menstrual pain is known as congestive. Women with congestive pain also tend to suffer from bloating, water retention, headaches and breast pain. In addition, they often notice a worsening of their cramps when they eat certain foods, such as wheat and dairy products, or when they drink alcohol, says Dr. Lark. Unfortunately, congestive pain tends to get worse with age, whether or not a woman has children.

While monthly cramps aren't pleasant, they are normal, says Dr. Lark. She cautions that in some cases, the pain can be a symptom of a health problem that requires medical attention, such as endometriosis. "You should always discuss unusual menstrual symptoms with your doctor," she advises.

But most of the time, the cause of cramps is simply menstruation itself. And in such cases, some doctors maintain that a few prudent nutritional changes can do wonders to improve your quality of life during your period, says Dr. Lark. The following nutrients have been shown to help soothe menstrual symptoms.

Calcium and Manganese: A One-Two Punch for Cramps

Scientists at the U.S. Department of Agriculture Grand Forks Human Nutrition Research Center in North Dakota have found that getting enough of certain minerals all month long can make a significant difference in how a woman feels during her period.

In one study, a group of menstruating women were fed a number of different diets over several months and questioned about how they felt at different points in their menstrual cycles. One of the diets was unusually low in calcium and manganese, a trace mineral that's found in nuts, tea, whole-grain cereals and dried peas and beans. The same women also tried a diet that was supplemented with both minerals.

When the researchers analyzed the women's premenstrual symptoms, they noticed a clear pattern: Most women reported much less severe symptoms when they followed the diet high in both calcium and manganese.

It's interesting to note that the diet the researchers considered low in calcium, the one that produced the most uncomfortable menstrual periods, included about 587 milligrams of calcium per day. The high-calcium diet had about 1,336 milligrams of calcium, which is close to the amount experts recommend to prevent osteoporosis, the brittle bone disease.

Just how these minerals fend off menstrual discomfort isn't clear. Researchers know that calcium is involved in the production of prostaglandins. "It may be calcium's role in prostaglandin metabolism that's responsible for the mineral's effect on pain," says James G. Penland, Ph.D., head researcher at the Grand Forks Human Nutrition Research Center.

Manganese's role is even more mysterious. "We do know that manganese is involved in blood clotting, and some research shows that a low intake is associated with a heavier menstrual flow," says Dr. Penland. "This is definitely an area that needs more study."

While researchers continue to try to figure out exactly how these two minerals work their magic on menstrual symptoms, a daily multivitamin/mineral supplement that includes the recommended levels of both calcium and manganese makes good sense for women who want to minimize menstrual discomfort, says Dr. Penland. The Daily Value for manganese is 2 milligrams. Because women of all ages have trouble getting enough calcium through diet, Dr. Penland recommends increasing your intake of low-fat, high-calcium foods such as low-fat yogurt and skim milk. If you still need more calcium, he suggests taking 500 to 1,000 milligrams of supplemental calcium a day.

Vitamin B_6 Keeps Cramps at Bay

The whole B-complex is essential for good health, but when it comes to relieving monthly symptoms, vitamin B_6 and niacin are the stars, says Dr. Lark.

Vitamin B_6 plays a key role in the production of 1 series prostaglandins, the "good" prostaglandins that relax the uterine muscles and keep cramps under control, according to Dr. Lark. But a woman's B_6 stores are easily depleted. Stress and certain medications, such as oral contraceptives, can easily cause a shortage. As a result, your body may not manufacture enough of the right kind of prostaglandins, leaving you feeling tied up in knots when your period comes. And if you're bothered by water retention or monthly weight gain, B_6 can ease those symptoms, too, Dr. Lark says.

Dr. Lark recommends taking vitamin B_6 as part of a B-complex supplement. Look for a B-complex supplement that contains no more than 200 to 300 milligrams of B_6. Large doses can be toxic, she says. It's a good idea to

Prescriptions for Healing

There are a few nutrients that can help make a woman's monthly cycle more comfortable. Here's what some medical experts recommend.

Nutrient	Daily Amount
Calcium	500–1,000 milligrams
Iron	15 milligrams
Manganese	2 milligrams
Niacin	25–200 milligrams, beginning 7–10 days before your period and stopping the day your period starts
Vitamin B_6	200–300 milligrams
Vitamin C	1,000 milligrams

MEDICAL ALERT: Do not take niacin in doses exceeding 100 milligrams without medical supervision. Women with liver disease should use niacin only under medical supervision.

Vitamin B_6 can cause side effects when taken in doses of more than 100 milligrams daily, so it's a good idea to talk to your doctor before supplementing the amount recommended here.

check with your doctor before taking doses of more than 100 milligrams daily.

Equally important in staving off cramps is niacin."Some research shows that niacin is about 90 percent effective for relieving cramps," says Dr. Lark. To head off cramps before they start, she suggests taking between 25 and 200 milligrams of niacin a day, beginning seven to ten days before your period is due and stopping the day that your period starts. This treatment can be repeated every month to prevent menstrual cramps.

Because niacin can cause slight flushing in some women, start with 25 milligrams a day for the first month. "If it doesn't seem to help, you can always increase the dose the following month until you find the level that's right for you," she advises. Women with liver disease should use niacin only under medical supervision, cautions Dr. Lark.

Nutrients to Lessen Bleeding

Next to cramps, heavy bleeding is probably the most common complaint of menstruating women, says Dr. Lark. Besides being inconvenient, heavy bleeding can deplete a woman's iron stores and can even lead to anemia.

It isn't surprising, then, that doctors recommend iron supplements to women with heavy bleeding. What is surprising is that getting extra doses of this mineral doesn't just replace the iron that has been lost. It may actually reduce the amount of bleeding in the future, says Dr. Lark.

"Women need only a small amount of iron. But what they need they really need," she says. She recommends a daily supplement of about 15 milligrams.

Women with heavy bleeding also need plenty of vitamin C and bioflavonoids, says Dr. Lark. Bioflavonoids are chemical compounds related to vitamin C; they're found in many citrus fruits and included in many supplements. Both vitamin C and bioflavonoids reduce bleeding by strengthening the capillary walls, which are at their weakest just before and during the menstrual period, says Dr. Lark. She recommends a daily supplement that includes at least 1,000 milligrams of vitamin C and 800 milligrams of bioflavonoids.

Because vitamin C helps the body absorb iron more efficiently, Dr. Lark recommends taking these two nutrients together.

Migraines

Ending the Pain

The hammering inside your head is utterly horrendous, as if someone were using your brain for a bongo. For what it's worth, you're not the only one with a built-in percussion section: Roughly 45 million Americans reportedly suffer from headaches each year.

Although tension headaches are by far the most common, chronic migraines are much more likely to send a desperate individual to the doctor seeking relief. "I use the term *victim* when I refer to chronic headache sufferers, because it's a very wicked syndrome," says Burton M. Altura, M.D., professor of physiology and medicine at the State University of New York Health Science Center at Brooklyn. "Besides the agonizing pain, these folks often have tremendous sensitivity to light and noise. Just snapping your fingers or clapping around them can be excruciating."

The one-sided, throbbing headache known as a migraine is actually more common in women; roughly 75 percent of those who get migraines are female. But what migraines lack in gender equality they make up for in severity. Some migraines are so extreme that they cause limb numbness, hallucinations, nausea and vomiting.

The good news is that medical research has come up with several vitamin and mineral therapies that might prove helpful for people who have been unable to find relief elsewhere.

"B" Headache-Free

Fifty-two quarts of chocolate syrup. Nine hundred bowls of cornflakes. These might prevent a migraine—if they weren't guaranteed to give you a stomachache first. They add up to a superhigh dose of riboflavin, which research hints may ward off the someone's-put-a-soccer-ball-in-my-head pain.

Fortunately for the 49 people in a Belgian headache study, they were able to take supplements to get the necessary 400-milligram daily dose. The migraine-prone people in the study received this high dose (it's about 235 times the Daily Value) every day for three months. In addition to the riboflavin, 23 of the people in the study took one low-dose aspirin a day.

By the end of the study, migraine severity decreased by nearly 70 percent in both groups compared with what it had been at the study's start. Aspirin had no added value.

Why would something like riboflavin work? Researchers have noticed a deficit in certain energy generators in the brain cells of some people with migraines. They suspect that flooding the system with riboflavin could indirectly help regenerate this flagging energy system and somehow short-circuit migraine pain.

What's attractive about riboflavin, if rigorous scientific studies support these preliminary findings, is that it's likely to have fewer side effects than current headache preventives (although no one knows for sure what the long-term effects of this much riboflavin might be).

"I wouldn't use it as the first line of attack, because we have other agents of proven value," says Seymour Solomon, M.D., professor of neurology at Albert Einstein College of Medicine in New York City. "But since this appears to be a relatively harmless treatment, it would be worthwhile to explore it with patients who haven't responded well to standard therapy."

Food Factors

A host of foods contain chemicals that can cause severe headaches. Here's what nutrition experts say to avoid.

Say no to MSG. A flavor enhancer used in restaurants and in prepared foods such as soups, salad dressings and lunchmeats, monosodium glutamate (MSG), even in small amounts, can provoke severe headaches as well as flushing and tingling in headache-prone people, says Seymour Diamond, M.D., director of the National Headache Foundation and the Diamond Headache Clinic in Chicago. In fact, one study showed that roughly 30 percent of those who eat Chinese food suffer these same symptoms. Although more research needs to be done, MSG seems to act as a vasodilator, which means it opens and then closes the blood vessels in the head. This process is exactly what happens in a migraine.

Because of all of the bad press, spotting MSG on food labels is harder than ever. "Natural flavor" and "hydrolyzed vegetable protein," for example, substitute for MSG in everything from frozen dinners, potato chips and sauces to canned meats.

Nix the nitrites. Commonly used as a preservative in hot dogs, salami, bacon and other cured meats, nitrites have been known to provoke migraines, says Dr. Diamond.

Corral the caffeine. The experts are divided here. Coffee, cola and tea all contain caffeine, which can act as a vasoconstrictor and, as a result, limit blood flow through the blood vessels in your head.

"A little bit of caffeine may help a headache, but you get either withdrawal or a rebound phenomenon from having too much," says Herbert C. Mansmann, Jr., M.D., professor of pediatrics and associate professor of medicine at Jefferson Medical College of Thomas Jefferson University in Philadelphia. Still, even two cups of a caffeine-containing

Although riboflavin generally is quite harmless, it's a good idea to check with your doctor before supplementing with such a high amount.

Making the Magnesium-Migraine Link

An increasing number of doctors believe that a fairly large percentage of the most severe cases of migraines may actually be caused by an imbalance of

beverage a day removes precious magnesium from your system, he says.

The bottom line: If you're having a problem with migraines, try avoiding caffeine and see if it helps, advises Dr. Mansmann.

Consider aspartame. Although few studies show a direct link between this artificial sweetener and headaches, some people do report problems with it, says Dr. Diamond. "My advice to people is that it probably won't bother you, but if you can relate a headache to it, you should not use it," he says.

To test whether this or any other food is causing your headaches, keep a diary of your meals as well as any headaches for a month. If it looks like one of the foods you're eating is causing the problem, cut the food out of your diet and see if it helps, advises Dr. Diamond.

Keep track of tyramine. A whopping 30 percent of migraine sufferers seem to have sensitivity to an amino acid called tyramine. Found in stronger aged cheeses, pickled herring, chicken livers, canned figs, fresh baked goods made with yeast, lima beans, Italian beans, lentils, snow peas, navy beans, pinto beans, peanuts, sunflower seeds, pumpkin seeds and sesame seeds, tyramine means migraine pain for many, says Dr. Diamond. Try eliminating these foods and see if it helps, he suggests.

Cut your kisses. Chocolate contains a chemical called phenylethylamine that, like tyramine, can cause headaches, says Dr. Diamond.

Ban the booze. The alcohol in drinks can dilate the blood vessels in your brain and cause a headache, warns Dr. Diamond. And drinking hard liquor can give you a double whammy. Chemicals known as congeners as well as impurities in scotch and other hard liquors have the same effect, he says.

key minerals such as magnesium and calcium.

"Not all headaches are produced by this imbalance, but we now know that 50 to 60 percent of migraines are magnesium-linked. And that's probably why no prescription therapy on the market successfully treats headaches across the board. They're simply not treating the cause," says Dr. Altura.

"Of the 17 people we've treated with magnesium, 13 have had complete improvement," says Herbert C. Mansmann, Jr., M.D., professor of pediatrics and associate professor of medicine at Jefferson Medical College of Thomas Jefferson University in Philadelphia.

The magnesium-migraine link still is not commonly accepted by headache experts. In fact, Dr. Altura says that one of his magnesium studies was rejected by a prominent medical journal at the suggestion of a top headache researcher. (Shortly thereafter, the study was published by another journal.)

But the weight of evidence for magnesium's use in the treatment of migraines is building. "There's no question that the literature strongly supports it," says Dr. Mansmann. "The so-called headache experts don't believe the data because they don't know anything about the development of magnesium deficiencies within cells."

To understand why magnesium might do the trick, it helps to take a look at how migraines happen.

Migraines are thought to be caused by vascular changes, or changes in the blood vessels, that reduce blood or oxygen flow in the scalp and brain. What causes these vascular changes? Things such as muscle contractions during times of stress and biochemicals called catecholamines and serotonin, which are circulating in the blood. Too much serotonin can cause blood flow to slow; too little can cause blood to move through too rapidly, explains Dr. Altura.

While mainstream researchers have long known that changes in serotonin and catecholamine levels cause migraine pain, stopping these changes has been a hit-or-miss proposition, says Dr. Altura. Aspirin, for example, temporarily inhibits the effects of serotonin but does nothing to prevent a migraine from coming back, he says.

Dr. Altura says he's the first to prove that loss of magnesium from the brain is behind the problem. Without enough magnesium, serotonin flows unchecked, constricting blood vessels and releasing other pain-producing chemicals such as substance P and prostaglandins, he says. Normal magnesium levels not only prevent the release of these pain-producing substances but also stop their effects, says Dr. Altura.

It's very likely that magnesium deficiency is a widespread cause of migraines, maintains Dr. Mansmann. Studies show that many people don't even come close to getting the Daily Value of magnesium, which is 400 milligrams. "On a daily basis, 30 to 40 percent of American people take less than 75 percent of the Daily Value of magnesium," says Dr. Mansmann.

What's more, several different things, from the caffeine in just two cups of coffee a day to the chemicals in most asthma medications, remove some magnesium from your system. "We know that intake is low for a lot of people. We know that a lot of medications, such as diuretics (water pills) and a variety of cardiovascular medications, can increase magnesium losses. We

Prescriptions for Healing

While vitamin and mineral supplements are by no means the first line of treatment for migraines, there are a couple of therapies that just might work when all else fails. Here's what some experts recommend.

Nutrient	Daily Amount
Magnesium	3,000 milligrams (magnesium gluconate), taken as 3 divided doses
Riboflavin	400 milligrams

MEDICAL ALERT: Doses for these two therapies are extremely high. If you wish to try these supplements to treat migraines, you should discuss it with your doctor.

People who have kidney or heart problems should supplement magnesium only under medical supervision.

know that people with diabetes who have high blood sugar lose a lot more magnesium in the urine and, as a result, run the risk of magnesium deficiency," says Karen Kubena, Ph.D., associate professor of nutrition at Texas A&M University in College Station. Even stress, a frequent cause of migraines, can remove magnesium from your system, says Dr. Mansmann.

Based on his records, Dr. Altura says that about 50 to 60 percent of his migraine patients have low magnesium levels. But once they begin treatment, he says, they often experience immediate relief. "We can say that 85 to 90 percent of these patients are successfully treated, and that's pretty miraculous," says Dr. Altura.

So can getting more than your share of magnesium every day prevent migraines? Dr. Altura says it's still unclear. "I'd like to be able to answer that question. I can't at this point, but my guess is that it would," he says.

In Dr. Mansmann's experience, a magnesium gluconate supplement works best. "The advantage is that dose for dose, magnesium gluconate causes one-third of the amount of diarrhea that magnesium oxide produces and one-half of the frequency of diarrhea that magnesium chloride produces," he says. It's also absorbed more quickly, he says.

The difference: Magnesium gluconate is more biologically active. "The active form of magnesium is ionized magnesium. When a substance is chemically bound, it's sort of neutralized, if you want to use a *Star Trek* term. When it's ionized, it is available to do what it is supposed to do, which in this case is possibly prevent constriction of blood vessels in your brain and scalp," explains Dr. Kubena.

Dr. Mansmann's migraine patients take two 500-milligram magnesium gluconate tablets at lunch, two in the afternoon and two at bedtime, upping the dosage each week until their stools become soft, an indication that there is enough magnesium in the body.

If you decide to give this therapy a try, you should be working with a doctor who is willing to monitor your progress. (People who have kidney or heart problems should supplement magnesium only under medical supervision.)

The Calcium Connection

Even if you monitor your magnesium level like a maniac, you're still at risk for migraines if your calcium level is out of whack. The reason: Magnesium and calcium interact with each other.

It seems that higher than normal blood levels of calcium cause the body to excrete the rest, which in turn triggers a loss of magnesium.

"Let's say you have just enough magnesium and too much calcium in your blood. If calcium is excreted, the magnesium goes with it. All of a sudden, you could be low in magnesium," says Dr. Kubena.

In fact, says Dr. Altura, people who have low magnesium and elevated calcium levels are among those who are most successfully treated with magnesium.

Mitral Valve Prolapse

Easing Symptoms of a Troubled Heart

Normally, the valves that regulate blood flow through the heart close neatly, snapping shut with the *lub-dub* sound that we recognize as a heartbeat.

In mitral valve prolapse, however, an additional click—*lub-dit-dub*—is added to the heartbeat. The extra sound occurs because the valve between the two left chambers of the heart is pushed out of shape by high blood pressure in the compressing heart. The valve pops upward, almost like a parachute being snapped in the wind. The condition happens when one of the fibrous cords that hold the valve in place stretches out too far or when either of the two leaflets that make up the valve is elongated, thickened or floppy. If the valve does not seal perfectly, blood may leak backward, causing the swishing noise that's known as a heart murmur.

"Mitral valve prolapse syndrome is considered a hereditary disorder," explains Kristine Scordo, R.N., Ph.D., assistant professor at Wright State University in Dayton, Ohio, director of the Mitral Valve Prolapse Program of Cincinnati and author of *Taking Control: Living with the Mitral Valve Prolapse Syndrome*. "People with the disorder—and there are three times as many women as men—are often tall and slender, with long arms and fingers and thin chests."

Although mitral valve prolapse usually causes no life-threatening problems, it has been associated with an array of disturbing symptoms, including heart palpitations, chest pain, shortness of breath, dizziness, fatigue, anxiety, headaches and mood swings. Doctors refer to these collectively as mitral valve prolapse syndrome. "These symptoms aren't caused by the valve itself," Dr. Scordo says. "But they are often part of the package."

These symptoms seem to be caused by disturbances in the body's autonomic nervous system. That's the nervous system that works without conscious control and governs the glands, the heart muscle and the tone of smooth muscles, such as those of the digestive system, the respiratory system and the skin.

"People with mitral valve prolapse often have overreactive autonomic nervous systems," explains Sidney M. Baker, M.D., a general practitioner in private practice in Weston, Connecticut, with a special interest in mitral valve prolapse. "Their bodies have a hard time adjusting to changes in the environment. They may be sensitive to light and noise, for instance."

"The symptoms are believed to be caused by a number of physiological changes and can often be helped by dietary changes. In fact, dietary changes are often all that's needed to alleviate symptoms," Dr. Scordo says.

Here's what is recommended.

Magnesium Plays a Role

There's no doubt that minerals play important roles in a properly beating heart. Both the nerves that coordinate the heartbeat and the muscles that

Food Factors

The following dietary adjustments won't correct a faulty mitral valve. "But they will help relieve many of the symptoms associated with the disorder," explains Kristine Scordo, R.N., Ph.D., assistant professor at Wright State University in Dayton, Ohio, director of the Mitral Valve Prolapse Program of Cincinnati and author of *Taking Control: Living with the Mitral Valve Prolapse Syndrome*.

These dietary changes are just as important as any vitamin or mineral supplement that you take, experts say. In fact, two dietary recommendations, less caffeine and less sugar, help your body retain the magnesium it needs.

Junk the java. Some of the most bothersome symptoms of mitral valve prolapse—anxiety, chest pain and shortness of breath—worsen when people consume too much caffeine. "Caffeine is a stimulant and has an adrenaline-like effect, which exaggerates the problems of mitral valve prolapse," Dr. Scordo says. "We tell people to avoid coffee, cola, tea and chocolate altogether, if they can."

Ditch the sweets. That sugar high you've heard of is for real, Dr. Scordo says. Foods that contain sugar that's quickly absorbed, such as candy, cookies, soda and the like, make your body pour out insulin. That greatly increases the activity of the sympathetic nervous system, the body's "accelerator," making symptoms worse.

Go for eight a day. Glasses of water, that is. This is to maintain normal blood pressure. "Even slight dehydration can aggravate symptoms of light-headedness and dizziness," Dr. Scordo says. "Most people can alleviate these symptoms in about two weeks just by getting enough fluids and salt."

Diet with care. Crash diets and fad diets aren't just ineffective in the long run. Most of the initial weight loss that's achieved is through water loss, just the opposite of what someone with mitral valve prolapse symptoms needs. If you do need to lose weight, doctors suggest going for a steady one pound a week.

contract to move blood through the heart need magnesium in order to do their jobs.

One mineral that has gotten some attention when it comes to mitral valve prolapse is magnesium. Several studies have found that a high percentage of people with mitral valve prolapse have lower than normal magnesium levels.

And one study by researchers at the University of Alabama School of Medicine in Birmingham found that supplemental magnesium relieved many of the symptoms associated with this disorder.

The study, of 94 people with mitral valve prolapse, found that 62 percent of them had low red blood cell levels of magnesium. Those people were also more likely to have additional symptoms: muscle cramps, migraines and a condition called orthostatic hypotension, in which their blood pressure dropped when they first stood up, making them light-headed.

Fifty of the 94 people took 250 to 1,000 milligrams of magnesium daily, in addition to their regular treatment, for four months to four years.

Overall, there was a 90 percent decrease in muscle cramps, a 47 percent decrease in chest pain and a definite decrease in blood vessel spasms in the people taking magnesium, reports the study's main researcher, Cecil Coghlan, M.D., professor of medicine at the University of Alabama School of Medicine. Palpitations also were markedly less, and a certain kind of heart arrhythmia called premature ventricular contraction was reduced by 27 percent. People taking magnesium also reported fewer migraines and less fatigue.

Magnesium deficiency can be induced by the very drugs meant to help heart problems, such as digitalis and some types of diuretics (water pills). These drugs cause the body to excrete both magnesium and potassium, leaving people in short supply of these nutrients.

Others most likely to come up short on magnesium, in Dr. Scordo's opinion: those who drink a lot of soft drinks or alcohol, those under stress and anyone eating a poor diet with lots of calories from sugar or fat. "The consensus among magnesium watchers is that it is one of the most prevalent and important deficiencies in North America," according to Dr. Baker. Poor diet is to blame.

"We tell people to make sure that they are getting the Daily Value of magnesium, 400 milligrams, through either foods or supplements," Dr. Scordo says. But because people employ a number of dietary changes to relieve their symptoms, "it's very hard for us to know if the magnesium is helpful or not," she adds.

Dr. Baker recommends from 200 to about 800 milligrams of magnesium a day, along with nutrients that work with magnesium, such as vitamin B_6. "People who are going to respond will begin to see improvement in their symptoms within a few days," he says.

Although magnesium is considered to be a fairly safe mineral, even in high doses, people with heart problems or kidney problems should take sup-

Prescriptions for Healing

Only one nutrient, magnesium, is thought to be helpful for symptoms related to mitral valve prolapse. But vitamins that work in conjunction with magnesium, especially vitamin B_6, also are often recommended by some experts.

Nutrient	**Daily Amount**
Magnesium	200–800 milligrams
Vitamin B_6	Up to 100 milligrams

MEDICAL ALERT: *If you have been diagnosed with mitral valve prolapse, you should be under a doctor's care.*

People with heart or kidney problems should take magnesium only under medical supervision.

plements only under medical supervision. Too much magnesium could cause a dangerous buildup of the mineral in the blood.

Note that people can have normal blood levels of magnesium and still have inadequate supplies in their tissues. If you are severely deficient, you may benefit by initially getting intravenous magnesium or high oral doses, Dr. Baker says. This treatment, of course, would have to be administered by your doctor.

Studies show that men get about 329 milligrams of magnesium daily, while women average 207 milligrams. Meats are a good source of magnesium, but if you want heart-healthy sources, try steamed or broiled halibut and mackerel, rice bran, nuts, seeds, tofu and green, leafy vegetables such as spinach and Swiss chard.

"And since the magnesium that's found in plants depends on the amount of magnesium in the soil, I recommend organically grown produce, which contains a better balance of minerals than produce grown with potassium-rich inorganic fertilizers," Dr. Baker adds.

Unlike magnesium, vitamin B_6 can be toxic in large doses. Take B_6 supplements in excess of 100 milligrams per day only under the supervision of your doctor.

Morning Sickness

Taming the Turbulent Tummy

You can be tickled pink at the idea of impending motherhood but still roll out of bed every morning, head straight to the bathroom and heave. Studies show that morning sickness hits 50 to 90 percent of pregnant women. Luckily, some experts believe there is a safe and effective vitamin therapy to reduce stomach-churning symptoms.

Vitamin B_6 to the Rescue

Several studies done back in the 1940s suggested that vitamin B_6 is an effective treatment for morning sickness. More recently, two studies have confirmed this vitamin's effectiveness. Researchers at the University of Iowa College of Medicine in Iowa City found that pregnant women who took 25 milligrams of B_6 every eight hours had significantly less vomiting and nausea than women who took placebos (blank look-alike pills). And in a study that included almost 350 moms-to-be, researchers in Thailand found that 10 milligrams every eight hours reduced symptoms as well.

"This is something more and more obstetricians are hearing about, and it's definitely worth trying," says Jennifer Niebyl, M.D., professor and head of obstetrics and gynecology at the University of Iowa College of Medicine. "It's safe, with no risk of side effects or birth defects at 25 milligrams, and it works for at least half of the women who try it." Both studies found that the vitamin worked best in women with moderate to severe nausea.

No one really knows why pregnant women get nauseated or how vitamin B_6 works, Dr. Niebyl says. "It probably has to do with high hormone levels, but we don't know which hormones cause nausea or how B_6 affects nausea," she says.

She recommends taking vitamin B_6 first thing in the morning, even before getting out of bed, then in midafternoon and before bed. Stick to no more than 75 milligrams of B_6 a day—three doses of 25 milligrams—to be on the safe side, Dr. Neibyl recommends. Amounts higher than 100 milligrams a day have been associated with nerve problems.

Food Factors

What goes down the hatch can make a big difference when it comes to whether or not it comes back up. Some doctors recommend trying these dietary measures the next time you need to steady a pitching stomach.

Eat gingerly. There's good scientific proof that ginger, the popular peppery spice used to flavor cookies, cakes and Asian foods, can calm even supersensitive stomachs.

In one study, 940 milligrams of ginger (about a half-teaspoon) worked as well as the standard dose of Dramamine, a common over-the-counter remedy, in relieving motion sickness. A similar dose kept Danish sailors from turning green during a four-hour jaunt on the high seas.

British researchers found that ginger worked as well as drugs, and without side effects, in relieving the nausea and vomiting common after surgery that involved general anesthesia. And Danish doctors report that one-eighth teaspoon of powdered ginger, given four times a day, relieved morning sickness in pregnant women so seriously stricken that they were hospitalized.

Ginger apparently works directly in the gastrointestinal tract to interfere with so-called feedback mechanisms that send "time to throw up" messages to the brain, explains Daniel Mowrey, Ph.D., director of the American Phytotherapy Research Laboratory in Lehi, Utah.

Although ginger ale or ginger tea may calm your tummy, the powdered stuff packs the most punch, says Jennifer Niebyl, M.D., professor and head of obstetrics and gynecology at the University of Iowa College of Medicine in Iowa City. "The usual dosage is about a half-teaspoon," she says. Ginger has no known adverse side effects, she adds.

Graze and pick. "Eating frequent light meals that are rich in carbohydrates and low in fat may help your nausea, so it's worth a try," says Dr. Niebyl. "The idea is to always have some easy-to-digest food in your stomach, but not to have a full stomach." That's why eating a few crackers before you get out of bed in the morning helps, she adds.

Prescriptions for Healing

Here's what some doctors recommend for nausea associated with pregnancy.

Nutrient	Daily Amount
Vitamin B_6	75 milligrams, taken as 3 divided doses (every 8 hours)

MEDICAL ALERT: *As a general rule, pregnant women should get a doctor's okay before taking any supplements. More than 100 milligrams of vitamin B_6 a day has been associated with nerve damage.*

If vitamin B_6 is going to help your symptoms, you should feel relief after the first few doses, Dr. Niebyl says. If it hasn't worked by then, you may need to ask your doctor about other forms of treatment.

As a general rule, pregnant women should never take any drugs or supplements without first discussing it with their physicians.

Multiple Sclerosis

Slowing a Nerve-Racking Disease

Leonard Flynn of Morganville, New Jersey, considers himself lucky. Diagnosed with multiple sclerosis (MS) in 1988, the organic chemist believes he is healthier now than he has been in years. To prove it, he climbed Mount Scenery, a peak on the island of Saba in the West Indies that has more than 1,000 stony steps cut into its steep side. "If there's one thing that people with MS have problems with, it's steps," he says. "I wouldn't have been able to do that earlier."

He attributes his improved health to a low-saturated-fat diet that some studies suggest slows the course of this disease. He also takes the same antioxidant nutrients thought to protect against cancer and heart disease: vitamins C and E, selenium and beta-carotene, the yellow pigment found in carrots, cantaloupe and other orange and yellow fruits and vegetables. Plus he eats lots of fatty fish, mostly sardines, salmon and water-packed tuna, and relies on sunflower oil and safflower oil for additional fat.

This is not to say that MS isn't a serious condition or that it can be cured by a particular diet. But there are ways to make life with MS easier. Doctors are especially excited about three new drugs, all of which have been shown in large studies to significantly reduce the relapse rate. The studies also show that two of these drugs slow the disease's progression and delay the onset of physical disability.

Fending Off the Immune System

In MS, certain cells in the immune system attack the nerves, causing a breakdown in the fatty sheath that surrounds and insulates a nerve cell. The breakdown occurs mostly in the brain and spinal cord. Once the fatty sheath starts to go, messages traveling to and from the brain are blocked. A message from the brain to "shake a leg," for instance, may simply dead-end while it's still in the brain, never reaching the muscles in the leg that could perform the task.

"No one knows for sure what sets off the immune system to attack nerves," says Timothy Vollmer, M.D., medical and research director of the Rocky Mountain Multiple Sclerosis Center in Englewood, Colorado. "There are good data to suggest that genetics plays a role in determining risk and that other risk factors include some sort of outside trigger, possibly exposure to a virus, that apparently sets off immune system changes."

Depending on which nerves lose their fatty sheaths, symptoms may include blurred or double vision, numbness, loss of bladder control and fatigue or tremors in the arms or legs. Fatigue so extreme that it has been called paralyzing also strikes some. Most symptoms wax and wane, with problematic conditions and remissions occurring over the years.

Dr. Vollmer believes most doctors think that nutrition has little, if anything, to do with the development or progression of MS and that no dietary measure can repair damaged nerve cells.

"Many of us do, however, think that a healthy diet is important to maximize function and to decrease the disability that occurs in MS," Dr. Vollmer says. "We want to avoid nutritional deficiencies and keep our patients as healthy as possible so that they don't develop some additional chronic ailment such as heart disease or diabetes, which can magnify the symptoms of MS." Even an infection that raises body temperature as little as 1°F can worsen symptoms of MS, Dr. Vollmer says.

Here's what nutritional research suggests may play a role in controlling the symptoms of MS. Keep in mind that even the doctors who recommend nutritional therapy use it along with other medical care, including physical therapy. Dr. Vollmer suggests that you enlist your doctor to work with you in devising a treatment plan that is best for your particular case.

Antioxidant Nutrients May Help

There's some evidence that the damage to a nerve's fatty sheath that is associated with MS is caused by what is known as oxidative injury. That damage, also called lipid (fat) peroxidation, occurs because unstable molecules called free radicals steal electrons from the healthy molecules in this fatty covering, causing breakdown and scarring that eventually destroys the nerve. Free radicals can be generated by attacking immune cells. They also occur when the body is exposed to certain toxic chemicals.

Researchers at Cook County Hospital in Chicago found that people experiencing MS attacks had significantly higher levels of pentane, a by-product of lipid peroxidation, in their breath than they did when their symptoms were in remission.

"Our findings very much support the theory that the mechanism for destruction in MS is associated with free radicals," says Edwin Zarling, M.D., associate professor of medicine at Loyola University of Chicago Stritch School of Medicine in Maywood, Illinois, and a researcher for the Cook County Hospital study. "Our work shows that antioxidants should be tried for MS." Studies have yet to be done that show antioxidants help people with MS, he adds.

Because of these findings, some doctors recommend that their patients with MS take the array of so-called antioxidant nutrients, which neutralize free radicals by offering up their own electrons, protecting your body's healthy molecules from harm. These nutrients include vitamins C and E, beta-carotene and the mineral selenium. Amounts recommended can vary widely.

"I recommend taking at least 500 milligrams of vitamin C two to four times a day and 100 micrograms of selenium and 800 international units of vitamin E once a day," says Mary Dan Eades, M.D., medical director of the Arkansas Center for Health and Weight Control in Little Rock and author

Food Factors

Dietary changes are not the mainstay of traditional treatment for multiple sclerosis (MS). Still, some say dietary changes can make a difference in the course of the disease, says Mary Dan Eades, M.D., director of the Arkansas Center for Health and Weight Control in Little Rock and author of *The Doctor's Guide to Vitamins and Minerals*.

Switch fats. Some evidence suggests that trimming saturated fat and increasing intake of two essential fatty acids, gamma-linolenic acid (GLA) and eicosapentaenoic acid (EPA), can help people with MS, says Dr. Eades.

Doctors who recommend this sort of diet may have their MS patients cut their saturated fat intakes to about 10 percent of calories by eliminating fatty meats, butter, mayonnaise, whole milk and cheeses, according to Dr. Eades. Then to keep fat intake at about 25 to 30 percent of calories, doctors have their patients add supplements of GLA (from evening primrose oil or borage oil) and EPA (from fatty fish), she says.

Dr. Eades prescribes one part GLA to four parts EPA, a ratio that's found in a product called EicoPro. EicoPro, manufactured by Eico-Tech of Marblehead, Massachusetts, is an essential fatty acid product that contains ultrapure sources of GLA and EPA.

In the United States, the main proponent of the low-fat diet is Roy L. Swank, M.D., Ph.D., of the Swank Multiple Sclerosis Clinic in Beaverton, Oregon. Dr. Swank has his patients stick to 10 to 15 grams of saturated fat and 20 grams of unsaturated oils (such as safflower oil, sunflower oil, olive oil and cod liver oil) daily. He has had 150 patients who have been on this diet for more than 35 years.

"We've been following patients for 40 years, and without question, animal fat is the real culprit in this disease," Dr. Swank contends. "This diet has helped more than 3,000 MS patients worldwide. It helps anyone at any stage of the disease but prevents disability in 95

of *The Doctor's Guide to Vitamins and Minerals*. It's a good idea to check with your doctor before taking more than 600 international units of vitamin E a day. Vitamin C in doses exceeding 1,200 milligrams a day can cause diarrhea in some people.

percent of patients when it's started before disability has developed."

Bulk up with bran. To coax the sluggish bowel associated with MS, get plenty of fiber every day, urges Timothy Vollmer, M.D., medical and research director of the Rocky Mountain Multiple Sclerosis Center in Englewood, Colorado. Whole grains, fruits, vegetables and beans can all help keep you regular.

Drink plenty of water. Getting lots of water relieves constipation, too. And it can ward off the bladder infections that can plague people with MS, Dr. Vollmer says. (Try cranberry juice for extra infection-fighting power.)

Find your food foes. The idea that food allergies or intolerances can contribute to symptoms of MS remains entirely unproven. Still, some doctors believe that for some people, certain foods can trigger or worsen symptoms.

Two Dutch doctors cite several reports of people whose symptoms worsened after chocolate binges, which suggests that chemicals in cocoa, coffee and cola can be toxic to nerve cells in large amounts. (It's true that large amounts of chocolate can be toxic to some animals. For instance, a dog that gobbles up a box of chocolates might develop twitching and muscle and heart weakness and lose control of bowel and urinary functions, the same symptoms associated with MS.)

One case report implicates fresh pineapple as the cause of a woman's muscle weakness and loss of vision. And in the United States and 21 other countries, the incidence of MS correlates most strikingly with milk consumption, according to one survey.

While most doctors pooh-pooh these possible connections, common sense suggests that if your symptoms seem to worsen after eating a particular food, drop that food from your diet for a least a few weeks to see if you notice improvement.

Check Out Vitamin B_{12}

Most doctors in the United States say there is no proof that a vitamin B_{12} deficiency contributes to the development of MS or that taking B_{12} helps re-

Prescriptions for Healing

Drugs are the mainstay of treatment for multiple sclerosis. There are, however, a few nutrients that may prove helpful. Here's what some doctors recommend.

Nutrient	Daily Amount
Selenium	100 micrograms
Vitamin B_{12}	500 micrograms
Vitamin C	1,000–2,000 milligrams, taken as 2–4 divided doses
Vitamin E	800 international units

Plus a multivitamin/mineral supplement containing the Daily Values of all essential vitamins and minerals

MEDICAL ALERT: *If you have been diagnosed with multiple sclerosis, you should be under a doctor's care.*

Injections of vitamin B_{12} are required for people who have problems absorbing this nutrient.

Vitamin C in doses exceeding 1,200 milligrams a day can cause diarrhea in some people.

It's a good idea to check with your doctor before taking more than 600 international units of vitamin E a day. If you are taking anticoagulant drugs, you should not take vitamin E supplements.

duce symptoms. Nevertheless, there appear to be some potential links between the nutrient, which is so essential for proper nerve function, and this debilitating disease.

For instance, vitamin B_{12} deficiency can mimic some of the symptoms of MS, such as numbness and tingling in the arms and legs, loss of balance and fatigue, says Donald W. Jacobsen, Ph.D., director of the Department of Cell Biology at the Cleveland Clinic.

"A severe vitamin B_{12} deficiency can cause breakdown of the myelin sheath, similar to what occurs in MS," Dr. Jacobsen says. That's why many doctors test for B_{12} deficiency if you have symptoms of MS. Although most people get enough B_{12} in their diets, absorption problems can cause a B_{12} shortage, especially in people ages 60 and older. If you have absorption problems, you'll probably have to get B_{12} shots or possibly include daily supplements in your diet for the rest of your life, depending on your particular case.

Studies are mixed as to how many people diagnosed with MS or with MS-like symptoms have low blood levels of vitamin B_{12}, Dr. Jacobsen says. For example, a study by British researchers found that a fairly high number of people with MS have low blood levels of B_{12}. On the other hand, researchers at the Cleveland Clinic, using tests that measure blood levels of B_{12} and two B_{12}-related compounds, homocysteine and methylmalonic acid, found fewer B_{12}-deficient people than did the British.

"At this point, we just don't know what to make of all of this," Dr. Jacobsen says. "We still feel like we are missing major pieces of the puzzle. It's still an open question whether true, functional vitamin B_{12} deficiency exists in MS."

To complicate matters further, people with MS often have what's called mild macrocytosis. They have some larger than normal but immature red blood cells in their blood that resemble a budding case of pernicious anemia, a disease that is associated with severe vitamin B_{12} deficiency. Most, however, never go on to develop a full-blown case of pernicious anemia.

Your doctor can determine with a few tests whether you're having absorption problems. If it turns out that you do have an absorption problem, you'll need to get injections of vitamin B_{12} from your doctor. If you don't have absorption problems, you can safely take oral doses of up to 500 micrograms of B_{12} a day, Dr. Jacobsen says. (This amount is many times the Daily Value of B_{12}, which is only 6 micrograms.)

It's also important to have your doctor check your blood levels of the B vitamin folate (the naturally occurring form of folic acid), Dr. Jacobsen says. That's because folate deficiency can cause symptoms similar to vitamin B_{12} deficiency, although its neurological consequences are much less severe. If you're found deficient, you'll have to take oral folic acid supplements to get your blood level back to normal. You shouldn't take folic acid unless your doctor recommends it, says Dr. Jacobsen.

Night Blindness

Eyes Need Vitamin A

Night blindness is a complex subject. Doctors now know that it can result from nutritional factors, genetics, uncorrected nearsightedness or an eye disease such as cataracts, macular degeneration or retinitis pigmentosa. And anything that affects vitamin A metabolism, such as liver disease, intestinal surgery, malabsorption or alcoholism, can also cause the problem.

Some forms of night blindness can be corrected with a pair of new glasses, according to Mitchell Friedlaender, M.D., director of cornea and refractive surgery at the Scripps Clinic and Research Foundation in La Jolla, California. Other forms require surgery. Still other forms of night blindness respond to something as simple as vitamin A.

The Vitamin Connection

What does vitamin A have to do with vision?

The answer is complex, says Elias Reichel, M.D., assistant professor of ophthalmology at Tufts University School of Medicine in Boston. But it involves the part of the eye called the retina.

"The retina is that part of the eye that acts like the film in a camera," he explains. "It's used to perceive light." On the retina there are structures called rods and cones. These house four kinds of pigments, one of which binds to an eye-friendly form of vitamin A. When you enter a sunny room and light enters your eye, the pigment transforms. Instantly, the vitamin A in your eye changes shape and, in that process, excites nerve endings to start transmitting electrical impulses to your brain to let it know what's going on—that you've entered a sunny room.

When you enter a dark room, the vitamin A changes shape again and helps your eyes realize that you've entered a dark room.

But nothing is ever completely light or completely dark. That's why you have more than 130 million light- and dark-sensing eye structures that make the minute adjustments necessary to perceive light and dark. And they're all dependent on vitamin A to do their jobs.

Despite this heavy demand for vitamin A, it still is pretty hard to develop

Getting the Right Stuff

What's in a name? Plenty, if you have retinitis pigmentosa, a genetic disease in which light-sensing structures within the eye are destroyed. That's because only the form of vitamin A known as palmitate, taken in a daily dose of 15,000 international units, has been found to slow the course of the disease.

But vitamin A palmitate in such a high dose is generally not sold in pharmacies, supermarkets or health food stores. So here are four companies that sell the product by mail order.

If you have retinitis pigmentosa and want to try vitamin A palmitate, be sure to check with your doctor first. *Note:* The products available from the companies listed below have not been tested or evaluated to determine their safety or effectiveness for children or adolescents with retinitis pigmentosa.

Akorn, Inc.
100 Akorn Drive
Abita Springs, LA 70420
1-800-535-7155

Chronimed
13911 Ridgedale Drive
Minnetonka, MN 55305
1-800-787-5577

Freeda Vitamins, Inc.
36 East 41st Street
New York, NY 10017
1-800-777-3737

J. R. Carlson Laboratories, Inc.
15 College Drive
Arlington Heights, IL 60004
1-800-323-4141

a deficiency of this nutrient in the United States, where the foods in which it is contained are plentiful. Common staples such as milk and margarine are fortified with vitamin A, and orange and yellow foods such as sweet potatoes and carrots are rich sources of beta-carotene. (Beta-carotene is a precursor of vitamin A and converts to vitamin A in the body.) We need to depend on outside sources for vitamin A because the body can't make its own.

Besides, since a healthy liver is usually able to store up to a year's supply of vitamin A, you'd have to be chronically deprived of vitamin A food sources for quite a while for it to affect your sight, as is the case with millions of children in developing nations.

"Night blindness resulting from vitamin A deficiency is very, very, very, very rare in individuals who live in America," says Dr. Reichel. And even if it does develop, it can frequently be reversed within an hour by injections of vitamin A.

Most people with night blindness have eyes that mobilize vitamin A so slowly that it takes a while to adjust to the dark, says Dr. Reichel. People notice it most often when they're going into theaters or driving at night.

Slowing Genetic Damage

Not only is vitamin A an effective treatment for deficiency-induced night blindness, but it may also slow night blindness that is induced by several hereditary conditions, usually grouped under the name retinitis pigmentosa.

Retinitis pigmentosa is considered rare in the United States, occurring in somewhere between 50,000 and 100,000 people. But it is the most common genetic eye disease, striking those who have a genetic mutation that slowly destroys the light-sensing structures in their eyes. The mutation is inherited from a parent, who frequently is unaware that he carries a gene that can imperil his child's vision.

Unfortunately, it does. People with retinitis pigmentosa usually begin to develop a loss of daytime side (peripheral) vision in young adulthood that progresses to tunnel vision and eventually to loss of vision in midlife. Without treatment, most people with retinitis pigmentosa will have significantly reduced day vision between the ages of 50 and 80.

Fortunately, research has shown that vitamin A can slow the retinal damage that can cause night blindness in adults with retinitis pigmentosa.

In a study of nearly 600 people between the ages of 18 and 49, researchers at the Massachusetts Eye and Ear Infirmary in Boston reported that 15,000 international units of vitamin A in supplement form each day, added to the approximately 3,000 international units a day generally available in a well-balanced diet, could slow the progression of retinal degeneration that can cause night blindness as a result of retinitis pigmentosa. The study was led by Eliot L. Berson, M.D., professor of ophthalmology and director of the Berman-Gund Laboratory at Harvard Medical School.

The study showed that those who had the lowest intakes of vitamin A had the most progression of retinal degeneration, while those who had intakes of 18,000 international units a day had the least retinal degeneration. The 18,000 international units came from both supplements and foods: 15,000 international units from a supplement, plus a regular dietary intake of 3,000 international units.

Although it isn't a cure, the daily supplement of 15,000 international units of vitamin A is estimated to provide seven additional years of useful vi-

Prescriptions for Healing

Night blindness caused by deficiency of vitamin A can be reversed by adding vitamin A to the diet or by taking vitamin A supplements, according to medical experts.

The genetic eye disease known as retinitis pigmentosa is associated with night blindness as well as with the loss of day vision. This condition can be slowed with vitamin A supplements, according to Eliot L. Berson, M.D., professor of ophthalmology and director of the Berman-Gund Laboratory at Harvard Medical School.

Nutrient	Daily Amount
Vitamin A	15,000 international units (vitamin A palmitate)

MEDICAL ALERT: *If you have symptoms of night blindness, you should see your doctor for proper diagnosis and treatment.*

Vitamin A has been linked to birth defects when taken in doses of 10,000 international units in early pregnancy. If you are a woman of childbearing age, you should talk to your doctor before taking the amount of vitamin A recommended here. Women who are pregnant should not use this therapy. Vitamin A can also cause liver damage when taken in doses exceeding 25,000 international units a day.

sion to the average person with retinitis pigmentosa who starts this therapy at age 32.

But not all types of vitamin A will do the job, says Dr. Berson. Although there are several forms of vitamin A, they all have different functions in the body and cannot be used interchangeably. The form used in the study was vitamin A palmitate.

There are no reports of otherwise healthy adults with retinitis pigmentosa becoming ill from 15,000 international units of vitamin A palmitate daily, says Dr. Berson. But that doesn't mean that it's okay to take more than this amount or that more is better. Vitamin A can cause liver damage when taken in doses exceeding 25,000 international units a day. And doses of 10,000 international units in early pregnancy have been linked to birth defects.

The therapeutic dose of 15,000 international units greatly exceeds the Daily Value of vitamin A, which is 5,000 international units. If you'd like to try this therapy, discuss it with your doctor first, especially if you are a woman of childbearing age. Women who are pregnant should not use this therapy.

Vitamin E Accelerates Vision Loss

Although vitamin A has been shown to slow the course of retinitis pigmentosa, researchers have data to suggest that vitamin E does exactly the opposite: In high doses, it destroys light-sensing cells by inhibiting the transport of vitamin A in the retina.

In Dr. Berson's study, for example, people with retinitis pigmentosa who took 400 international units of vitamin E every day appeared to lose their vision faster than those not taking this dose of vitamin E. Based on this information, the researchers estimated that if vitamin E supplements were started in someone with retinitis pigmentosa at age 32, the course of the condition could be accelerated by as much as five years.

The researchers noted that they had no evidence to suggest that small amounts of vitamin E, such as those found in multivitamin/mineral supplements, affect those with retinitis pigmentosa.

Osteoarthritis

Slowing Joint Wear and Tear

Check out a chicken drumstick the next time you bake a bird. You'll note that the knobby end of the thighbone is covered with a tough, rubbery coating. That's cartilage, a tissue designed to cushion joints and ensure smooth motion.

In osteoarthritis, cartilage breaks down. It becomes frayed, thin, perhaps even completely worn away in areas. The underlying bone disintegrates, while painful bone spurs may grow around the edges of the joint. A formerly smooth, quiet joint may feel like it's grinding. It might even sound rough, like crinkling cellophane, when it's moved.

No one really knows why cartilage breaks down. Heavy use of a joint is sometimes a contributing factor. Also, a joint injured in the past tends to develop osteoarthritis sooner than a normal joint, perhaps because misalignment causes cartilage wear.

Osteoarthritis usually develops slowly, over many years. Some people never have more than a mild ache. Others develop crippling pain, and a few even end up trading in a creaky old hip or knee for a shiny new titanium-alloy model.

Many doctors who treat osteoarthritis consider it pretty much an unavoidable part of growing older. In fact, more than half of people ages 65 and older can expect to have at least a touch of osteoarthritis. Those same doctors think there's not a whole lot that can be done for this disease, except to nurse aching joints with mild painkillers such as acetaminophen or aspirin, heat and a careful balance of exercise and rest.

The relatively few doctors who treat osteoarthritis with nutritional therapy take a different stance, however. They contend that osteoarthritis is a metabolic disorder, a breakdown in the body's ability to regenerate bone and cartilage. Although they concede that the breakdown is partly the result of old age, they also believe that providing the proper nutrients, in proper amounts, can help stop the process of deterioration and reduce pain and swelling.

Unfortunately, while there is some sketchy evidence that certain nutrients can help osteoarthritis, the kind of large scientific studies that would confirm these benefits have yet to be done.

Until then, here's what doctors say may be helpful.

B_{12} Gives Bones a Boost

Vitamin B_{12} is best known for its role in maintaining a healthy blood supply. In the bone marrow, B_{12} stimulates stem cells, a certain type of bone cell, to make red blood cells. When B_{12} levels are low, people develop anemia.

But that's not the only role vitamin B_{12} plays in bone. A few years ago researchers at the University of Southern California School of Medicine in Los Angeles discovered that B_{12} also stimulates osteoblasts, another type of bone cell that generates not red blood cells but bone. That could be important to people with osteoarthritis, because underneath degenerating cartilage, bone also deteriorates, causing additional pain and further cartilage erosion.

This finding about vitamin B_{12} led researchers at the University of Mis-

Food Factors

Taming osteoarthritis may well be a matter of adding nutrients while subtracting calories.

Drop some pounds. Research shows that people who maintain their proper weight or stay close to it are much less likely to develop osteoarthritis in certain joints than people who are overweight.

Staying slim spares weight-bearing joints such as the knees and hips. Joints can be so compressed by excess body weight that the fluid-filled space normally found between the cartilage-covered surfaces of bone ends becomes obliterated, says Robert McLean, M.D., clinical assistant professor of medicine at Yale University School of Medicine and an internist in New Haven, Connecticut.

"If you already have osteoarthritis, losing some weight can help decrease stress on some of the joints and thereby reduce pain," Dr. McLean says. Your doctor can recommend specific exercises, designed to strengthen the muscles supporting the joints (especially around the knees), to help reduce the pain of osteoarthritis, he adds.

souri in Columbia to try giving B_{12} to people with osteoarthritis in their hands. They found that people who took 20 micrograms of B_{12} (3.3 times the Daily Value of 6 micrograms) and 6,400 micrograms of folic acid, another B vitamin that works in concert with B_{12}, for two months had fewer tender joints and better hand strength and took less medicine for pain than people not getting this B vitamin combo. (This amount of folic acid is 16 times the Daily Value and should be taken only under medical supervision, as excess folic acid can actually mask signs of B_{12} deficiency.)

"This doesn't necessarily prove that vitamin B_{12} deficiency causes osteoarthritis or that getting extra B_{12} will cure it, but I'd say it is definitely worth discussing with your doctor," says Margaret Flynn, R.D., Ph.D., a medical nutritionist at the University of Missouri–Columbia School of Medicine, the study's main researcher. She notes that the people in her study were not B_{12}-deficient. They were getting enough of the vitamin in their diets, and they had blood levels that are considered normal. Still, they benefited from getting more.

"Older people often have trouble absorbing vitamin B_{12}, and that accounts for about 95 percent of B_{12} deficiencies in the United States," she says. Taking large doses of vitamin B_{12} supplements may help overcome the absorption problem. Or your doctor may recommend B_{12} injections, she says.

Vitamin E Eases Painful Joints

Joints damaged by osteoarthritis don't get as hot and swollen as joints hit with rheumatoid arthritis, but they are somewhat inflamed. That's one reason doctors sometimes recommend vitamin E for osteoarthritis. Vitamin E fights inflammation by neutralizing the biochemicals that are produced during inflammation. These biochemicals, released by immune cells, contain free radicals, unstable molecules that grab electrons from your body's healthy molecules, damaging cells in the process. Vitamin E offers up its own electrons, protecting cells from damage.

In a study by Israeli researchers, people with osteoarthritis who took 600 international units of vitamin E every day for ten days had significant reductions in pain compared with when they were not taking vitamin E. "Vitamin E also apparently stimulates the body's deposit of cartilage-building proteins called proteoglycans," says Joseph Pizzorno, Jr., N.D., a naturopathic physician and president of Bastyr University in Seattle.

Doctors recommend 400 to 600 international units of vitamin E, amounts that are considered safe, says Jonathan Wright, M.D., a doctor in Kent, Washington, who specializes in nutritional therapy and is the author of *Dr. Wright's Guide to Healing with Nutrition*. These large amounts are available only by supplementation. To get some vitamin E from foods, try sunflower oil, almond oil and wheat germ. Most people get about 10 international units a day.

Selenium, a mineral that increases the effectiveness of vitamin E, is often added to the osteoarthritis formula in amounts of about 200 micrograms a day. "That amount is considered safe, but you won't want to take much more than that without medical supervision," says Dr. Wright.

Vitamin C Stimulates Cartilage Repair

Most of us know vitamin C as an infection fighter and an immunity builder. But vitamin C is also used throughout the body to manufacture a variety of tissues, including collagen. Collagen forms a network of protein fibers that lay down the structural foundation for many tissues, including cartilage, bone, tendons and muscles, all necessary to keep joints strong and operating smoothly.

"It's well-known that animals deficient in vitamin C develop an array of health problems associated with collagen breakdown, including joint pain and cartilage breakdown," Dr. Pizzorno says.

Guinea pigs, one of few animals besides humans that can't make vitamin C in their bodies, show the classic symptoms of osteoarthritis—cartilage erosion and inflammation—when put on a diet containing only a small amount of vitamin C.

And one study suggests that large amounts of vitamin C encourage the growth of cartilage cells (chondrocytes) by stimulating synthesis of these cells' genetic material, report researchers at the State University of New York at Stony Brook.

"Although there are no human studies confirming a benefit, there's enough evidence out there, I think, to include vitamin C in a program to slow osteoarthritis," Dr. Pizzorno says. And there's some evidence that vitamins C and E work together to protect cartilage from breakdown. You can get sufficient vitamin C for this purpose in a multivitamin/mineral supplement, he says.

Niacinamide Could Be Worth a Try

You may not have heard of niacinamide. It's a form of niacin, one of the B-complex vitamins.

Prescriptions for Healing

Many doctors do not make dietary recommendations for the treatment of osteoarthritis beyond maintaining normal weight. Some nutrition-oriented doctors, however, recommend an array of nutrients, including these.

Nutrient	Daily Amount
Folic acid	6,400 micrograms
Niacinamide	1,000–3,000 milligrams, taken as 2 or 3 divided doses
Selenium	200 micrograms
Vitamin B_{12}	20 micrograms
Vitamin E	400–600 international units
Plus a multivitamin/mineral supplement containing the Daily Values of all essential vitamins and minerals	

MEDICAL ALERT: *If you have symptoms of osteoarthritis, you should see your doctor for proper diagnosis and treatment.*

This amount of folic acid should be taken only under medical supervision, as excess folic acid can actually mask signs of vitamin B_{12} deficiency.

Large amounts of niacinamide can cause liver problems. Doses significantly above 100 milligrams a day require careful medical supervision. If you have liver disease, you should not use this treatment.

The amount of selenium recommended here exceeds the Daily Value for this mineral. While some doctors consider this dosage to be safe, you may want to talk to your physician before taking supplements.

If you are taking anticoagulant drugs, you should not take vitamin E supplements.

Some nutrition-oriented doctors have been recommending large doses of niacinamide for osteoarthritis since the 1940s, when William Kaufman, M.D., Ph.D., a pioneer in nutrition research for the treatment of osteoarthritis, found it helpful in relieving swelling and joint pain and improving muscle strength.

"I've treated more than 1,000 patients for joint dysfunction using niacinamide alone or combined with other vitamins," says Dr. Kaufman, now retired, of Winston-Salem, North Carolina. Improvement is usually noticeable after the first few weeks and becomes even more pronounced with continued treatment, he says. Very severely damaged arthritic joints respond slowly, or don't respond at all, to niacinamide treatment, however.

No one really knows why niacinamide seems to help osteoarthritis, Dr. Kaufman admits. "The vitamin is thought to somehow improve the metabolism of joint cartilage," he says. No further studies of niacinamide have been published since Dr. Kaufman's work, but reports of its clinical use remain positive.

"As a practitioner who has been doing this for more than 20 years, I can tell you that niacinamide is extremely effective in a large majority of cases at taking the pain out of osteoarthritis and in most cases at taking out the swelling, too, and apparently stopping the process," Dr. Wright says.

Niacinamide is often recommended as an alternative to niacin because it produces fewer side effects. This is one remedy, however, for which medical supervision is essential. The large amounts of niacinamide used in this treatment, from 500 milligrams twice a day to 1,000 milligrams three times a day, have the potential to cause liver problems.

"Anyone taking more than 1,500 milligrams of niacinamide a day should have a blood test for liver enzymes after three months of treatment, then annually thereafter," Dr. Wright says. "If the levels are elevated, the dose should be reduced." Nausea is an early warning sign of stress on the liver.

If you have liver disease, you should not use this treatment.

Adding a Bit of Insurance

Doctors who treat osteoarthritis make an additional recommendation that's designed to cover all bases. They recommend a multivitamin/mineral supplement that provides the Daily Values of all of the essential vitamins and minerals.

That recommendation might not be such a bad bit of advice. There's a scattering of evidence that a host of nutrients—pantothenic acid, vitamin B_6, zinc and copper and other trace minerals—play roles in maintaining healthy bones and cartilage. "And these nutrients interact in many ways that we still don't understand," Dr. Wright points out.

Osteoporosis

Walking Tall into Your Golden Years

Imagine a bank that never let you know how much (or how little) money you have in your account. Unless you were a diligent bookkeeper, chances are that sooner or later, you'd start bouncing checks. Well, your bones are that bank, only instead of money, you're withdrawing calcium.

Essentially, that's what happens when people get osteoporosis, a disease causing porous bones: Their skeletons become bankrupt. Their bodies have withdrawn more calcium from the bones than has been deposited over the years, and all that's left is a fragile shell.

Osteoporosis is responsible for 1.5 million fractures each year, most notably fractures of the vertebrae (these cause the hunched appearance often seen in elderly women), forearms, wrists and hips (these are often crippling and sometimes fatal).

That's the bad news. The good news is that osteoporosis is both preventable and treatable.

"There is no reason this disease should exist. It's so preventable just through nutrition and exercise, if a woman starts young enough," says Ruth S. Jacobowitz, former vice-president of Mount Sinai Medical Center in Cleveland, a member of the board of trustees of the National Council on Women's Health and author of *150 Most-Asked Questions about Osteoporosis*. "It is never too early and never too late to build bone. Even very elderly women can still build some amount of bone density."

Making Deposits into the Bone Bank

The first step in building bone is understanding how bones work. Even after we've stopped growing, our bones undergo constant remodeling. *Remodeling* is the actual term that doctors use to describe the body's ongoing process of removing old bone and forming new bone. Generally, the formation of new bone stays ahead of, or even with, the removal of old bone during the first 20 to 30 years of our lives.

Sometime after age 30, our bones begin operating in the red, and both men and women lose slightly more bone than they form—that is, until women hit menopause and stop producing estrogen, one of the hormones that regulate remodeling. Then they lose significantly more bone than men, up to 2 to 5 percent a year during the first five to seven years after menopause. For this reason, osteoporosis is much more common among women, though it does occur in elderly men.

That is why it's particularly important for women to build and maintain peak bone mass, the maximum amount of bone you can form during your lifetime. And you form peak bone mass by taking in calcium and getting plenty of exercise, explains Clifford Rosen, M.D., director of the Maine Center for Osteoporosis Research and Education at St. Joseph's Hospital in Bangor. The earlier you start, the better, because the majority of peak bone mass is achieved by your midtwenties, though some researchers believe you can build bone until age 35.

Does that mean you're doomed if you're already past age 30 and just learning what peak bone mass is? "Absolutely not," says Dr. Rosen. Calcium and exercise can prevent the bone loss that occurs in your thirties and forties. "And slowing bone loss is enough to keep you from having osteoporosis, no matter how low your peak bone mass," he says.

One of the most effective ways of preventing bone loss and osteoporotic fractures is hormone replacement therapy, says David Dempster, Ph.D., director of the Regional Bone Center at Helen Hayes Hospital in West Haberstraw, New York, and associate professor of clinical pathology at Columbia University in New York City. Hormone replacement therapy is not appropriate for all women, however. You should discuss the pros and cons of this treatment with your doctor.

And medical experts agree that for both women and men, a healthy diet plays an important role in preventing and treating osteoporosis.

In addition to calcium, the nutrients shown by research to have the best bone-building potential include vitamin D, boron, magnesium, fluoride, manganese, copper, zinc and vitamin K. Here's what we know so far.

Straight from the Cow

Mom always said "Drink your milk, or you won't have strong teeth and bones." As usual, she was right.

"Far and away, the biggest problem with osteoporosis is a lack of calcium in people's diets," explains Paul Saltman, Ph.D., professor of biology at the University of California, San Diego.

Calcium, a mineral abundant in milk, is essential for strong, healthy bones. In fact, 99 percent of the body's calcium is stored in the skeleton. But you also need a stable level of serum calcium (calcium in your blood) for normal heartbeat, nerve and muscle function and blood coagulation. It's your bones that suffer when there isn't enough to go around.

Maintaining enough calcium in the blood is the body's ultimate priority, explains Dr. Rosen. "If it doesn't have enough, it goes to the reservoir and takes it," he says. The reservoir, in this case, is your bones.

To keep that reservoir full and calcium-rich, Dr. Saltman recommends that all people, beginning in their teens, take supplements and eat a good diet to ensure that they receive between 1,200 and 1,500 milligrams of calcium daily.

According to researchers at the University of California, San Diego, every little bit of calcium counts. Of the 581 60- to 79-year-old women they studied, those who had drunk one or more glasses of milk daily as adolescents and young adults had significantly higher bone mineral density at the midforearm (3 to 4 percent), spine (5 percent) and hip than those who had not. The effect of drinking milk on bone mineral density was even greater at the hip (4 percent) and spine (7 percent) for adults ages 20 to 50.

Calcium can also be helpful in treating osteoporosis once the disease has developed. Investigators at Winthrop-University Hospital in Mineola, New York, studied 118 women past the age of menopause. Over a three-year period, they gave the women 1,700 milligrams of calcium, 1,700 milligrams of calcium plus the female hormones estrogen and progesterone or placebos (medically ineffective pills). Though the calcium-hormone mix was most effective, calcium alone significantly slowed bone mineral loss. Researchers measured bone mineral loss in the upper thighbone, noting a 0.8 percent decline a year in the women taking calcium versus a 2 percent decline a year in those taking the placebos.

When it comes to getting enough calcium, however, drinking more milk is by no means the final word. Calcium from dairy products can be difficult to absorb, and many people have difficulty digesting dairy products, says Neal Barnard, M.D., president of the Physicians Committee for Responsible Medicine in Washington, D.C., and author of *Eat Right, Live Longer*. He recommends foods such as beans, broccoli and fortified orange juice as calcium sources instead. Other calcium-rich foods include collard greens, kale, mustard greens, butternut squash, tofu and sweet potatoes.

The Daily Value for calcium is 1,000 milligrams. And the National Institutes of Health in Bethesda, Maryland, recommends the following intakes:

(continued on page 434)

Food Factors

There is an abundance of vitamins and minerals that build and maintain a healthy skeleton, but there are also plenty of everyday foods that are nothing less than bad to the bone. Here are some to avoid.

Drink a little less java. Though controversy still brews on how much caffeine is too much, experts agree that caffeine consumption increases the urinary excretion of calcium.

The Rancho Bernardo Study, a three-year study of 980 women past the age of menopause, found that coffee drinkers had less bone. The study noted a significant decrease in hip and spinal bone mass associated with lifetime caffeine intake equivalent to only two cups of coffee per day among women who did not drink milk on a daily basis.

Although drinking at least one glass of milk per day offset the bone loss in this study, it's wise to limit caffeine, since most women are not taking in enough calcium to begin with, says Ruth S. Jacobowitz, former vice-president of Mount Sinai Medical Center in Cleveland, a member of the board of trustees of the National Council on Women's Health and author of *150 Most-Asked Questions about Osteoporosis*.

Can the cola. Phosphorus may be a necessary component of bone, but many experts agree that excessive phosphorus intake blocks calcium absorption and wreaks havoc on bone health. Cola, which is high in phosphorus, sugar and caffeine, is "among the worst foods for people trying to avoid osteoporosis," says Alan R. Gaby, M.D., a doctor in Seattle specializing in natural and nutritional medicine, past president of the American Holistic Medical Association and author of *Preventing and Reversing Osteoporosis*.

Too much phosphorus, it seems, sends your body into double jeopardy. Not only does the excess phosphorus bind with calcium in your blood, thus making calcium unavailable for your body's functions, but your body, as a result, senses that it doesn't have enough calcium and takes it from your bones.

If you can't cut the cola from your diet completely, it's a good idea to restrict it to no more than one can per day.

Think greens and beans. While protein is an important part of your diet for both bone formation and overall health, there is evidence that protein from meats and other animal products increases calcium loss and thereby weakens bones, says Neal Barnard, M.D., president of the Physicians Committee for Responsible Medicine in Washington, D.C., and author of *Eat Right, Live Longer*.

"The majority of the problem with osteoporosis in this country is the result of calcium loss," Dr. Barnard says. He advocates getting protein from grains, beans and vegetables and getting calcium from greens such as broccoli, kale, collards and beans to avoid the animal protein found in milk (one gram per fluid ounce).

Pass on the salt. High salt intake increases urinary excretion of calcium, says Dr. Barnard. "It is well-documented that cutting your daily sodium intake to 1,000 to 2,000 milligrams can save 160 milligrams of calcium per day," he says. That means keeping your salt intake to a teaspoon or less a day.

Go easy on the spirits. "You can't get calcium from beer or chardonnay," says Paul Saltman, Ph.D., professor of biology at the University of California, San Diego. And too much imbibing may inhibit calcium absorption as well as bone formation.

Researchers have found reduced bone mass and osteoporotic fractures in a significant percentage of men with chronic alcoholism. The effects of moderate drinking, however, are unknown.

Nix the aluminum. Although more research is needed, there is evidence that too much aluminum may also cause bone loss, says Jacobowitz. She notes that aluminum not only can bind with phosphorus and calcium, drawing them into the urine, but also deposits on bones, causing osteomalacia (soft bones).

"It's a bad idea to use aluminum-based antacids for calcium supplementation. Not only will it do you no good, it could do you harm. Read labels," she warns.

- Men, ages 25 to 65: 1,000 milligrams
- Women, ages 25 to 50: 1,000 milligrams
- Pregnant and nursing women: 1,200 to 1,500 milligrams
- Women at menopause (ages 51 to 65) who are taking estrogen: 1,000 milligrams
- Women at menopause (ages 51 to 65) who are not taking estrogen: 1,500 milligrams
- Men and women over age 65: 1,500 milligrams

Since many people fall short of getting these amounts from foods, doctors often recommend supplements of between 500 and 1,200 milligrams of calcium per day to make up the difference.

Play in the Sunshine for Vitamin D

Often referred to as the sunshine vitamin, vitamin D is a must if you want all of that calcium to do any good. Vitamin D, which your skin makes whenever it's exposed to sunlight (except during the winter at northern latitudes), helps your body absorb calcium and build good bones.

There are no conclusive studies pointing to vitamin D deficiency as a direct cause of osteoporosis. It is well-documented that vitamin D deficiency causes osteomalacia, or soft bones, in adults, which could contribute to fractures.

Vitamin D might also be useful as an osteoporosis treatment. In one study, Finnish researchers found that 341 elderly people (mostly women ages 75 and older), given annual large-dose injections of vitamin D during a five-year period, experienced fewer fractures than 458 people who did not receive the vitamin.

"Research here in Boston and in Europe has found that up to 40 percent of elderly men and women with hip fractures are vitamin D–deficient," says Michael F. Holick, M.D., Ph.D., director of the General Clinical Research Center and chief of the Section of Endocrinology, Diabetes and Metabolism, both at Boston University Medical Center.

Unfortunately, your skin's ability to manufacture vitamin D decreases with age, says Dr. Holick. Matters are even worse for those living where the days are short and the winters are long. You can't make any vitamin D in the wintertime at northern latitudes such as Boston. "During the months from November through February in Boston, even if you exposed your entire body to sunlight from sunrise to sunset, you would not be able to make enough vitamin D to satisfy your body's requirement," Dr. Holick says. And the closer your abode to the polar ice caps, the longer that stretch.

"This problem is compounded by the use of sunscreen in the summer," adds Dr. Holick. "Sunscreen with an SPF (sun protection factor) of eight is enough to markedly diminish your ability to make vitamin D. Clothing completely prevents it."

Although it's okay to drink fortified milk, you shouldn't count on it as your primary source of vitamin D, notes Dr. Holick. "It is difficult to fortify milk with vitamin D, and our research has shown that only 30 percent of milk samples contain the amount of vitamin D shown on the label. That percentage is even lower in skim milk samples."

That makes it rather difficult to get adequate amounts of vitamin D from your diet alone. Fortunately, the answer to the vitamin D dilemma is as close as your local drugstore, especially if you walk there on a sunny day.

Vitamin D can be toxic in large doses. For that reason, you should never take supplements in excess of 600 international units daily unless your doctor specifically recommends it. Many multivitamin/mineral formulas contain adequate amounts of vitamin D, however. "Taking a multivitamin/mineral supplement that contains 400 international units of vitamin D essentially guarantees that you get at least the adult Daily Value of vitamin D, which is also 400 international units," says Dr. Holick. "We also recommend that people, particularly the elderly, go outside for five to ten minutes, two or three times a week, during the spring, summer and fall for sun exposure on their hands, faces and arms. It is casual exposure to sunlight that provides us with more vitamin D."

Take Magnesium to Regulate Calcium

Magnesium, an essential mineral used to treat almost everything from depression to heart attack, is also crucial to bone health. Magnesium helps calcium get into the bones and also converts vitamin D to its active form in the body. Nearly half of the body's magnesium is found in the skeleton.

"We don't have enough research, but if I had to guess which nutrient is most important to bone health, I would say magnesium," says Alan R. Gaby, M.D., a doctor in Seattle specializing in natural and nutritional medicine, past president of the American Holistic Medical Association and author of *Preventing and Reversing Osteoporosis*.

Magnesium may also help in the treatment of osteoporosis. Researchers in Israel studied 31 women with osteoporosis who were past the age of menopause. They gave the women daily magnesium supplements of 250 to 750 milligrams for 6 months and then 250 milligrams for 18 months. At the end of that period, 22 women increased their bone density by 1 to 8 percent, and 5 women experienced decreases in their rates of bone loss. Conversely, bone density decreased markedly in 23 women who did not receive magnesium supplements during the same period.

Here in the United States, the U.S. Department of Agriculture continues to study magnesium's role in osteoporosis, says Forrest H. Nielsen, Ph.D., center director for the U.S. Department of Agriculture Grand Forks Human Nutrition Research Center in North Dakota. "Based on what we know about magnesium regulating calcium, we can say that an adequate magnesium diet is necessary to maintain healthy bones," he says.

The Daily Value for magnesium is 400 milligrams. Since many Americans lack sufficient magnesium in their diets, doctors who recommend magnesium supplements advise taking 200 to 400 milligrams daily. (If you have heart or kidney problems, you should talk to your doctor before taking magnesium supplements.) Magnesium-rich foods include wheat germ, sunflower seeds, seafood, nuts, dairy products and green, leafy vegetables.

Boron Plugs the Calcium Leak

Researchers have speculated that boron, a trace mineral found mostly in fruits and vegetables, may reduce urinary excretion of both calcium and magnesium and therefore help prevent osteoporosis.

"It's still too early to tell how much of a benefit boron is," says Curtiss Hunt, Ph.D., a research biologist at the Grand Forks Human Nutrition Research Center. In one study, Dr. Hunt and his fellow researchers found marginal differences in the amounts of calcium and magnesium excreted in the urine of 12 women past the age of menopause who were given first a low-boron diet and then daily supplements of three milligrams of boron.

"So far, we've found that boron has a slight effect in decreasing urinary excretion of calcium and magnesium as well as in increasing the production of estrogen and testosterone, but the results haven't been dramatic," says Dr. Hunt. "It's still important to eat a boron-rich diet, however. Beyond a shadow of a doubt, boron affects bone and mineral metabolism, especially in animals. But it would be foolhardy to take boron supplements at this time. People should eat their fruits and vegetables. You can get 0.5 milligram of boron just by eating one good-size apple."

Something in the Water Could Help

Fluoride, the electrically charged form of fluorine, has long been touted for its cavity-fighting ability. Now some researchers believe it can build bones as well.

"The women in our study had a 70 percent reduction in spinal fractures over a 30-month period and close to a 5 percent increase in spinal bone density every year for almost three years," says Khashayar Sakhaee, M.D., professor of internal medicine at the Center for Mineral Metabolism and Clinical Research of the University of Texas Southwestern Medical Center at Dallas.

In the study, Dr. Sakhaee gave 48 women who were past menopause 25 milligrams of slow-release fluoride and 800 milligrams of calcium (as calcium citrate) twice a day for three 12-month cycles, with a 2-month break from fluoride between cycles. With this new method of delivery, Dr. Sakhaee says, fluoride treatment is safe and effective.

"Other researchers used to use a rapid-release fluoride that went right to the skeleton, and the patients were getting toxic levels," says Dr. Sakhaee. The rapid-release formula did create dense bones, he explains, but the bone material it formed was brittle and weak. The new slow-release formula is creating strong bones.

Researchers remain leery about rapid-release sodium fluoride. Very high doses of fluoride, from 2,500 to 5,000 milligrams, can be fatal, though amounts needed for bone health are nowhere near that level, says Dr. Sakhaee.

"People really aren't getting enough fluoride to do their bones any good," says Dr. Sakhaee. He notes that soil and well water are rich in fluoride, but in towns and cities where the water is fluoridated, government standards prohibit more than one milligram of fluoride per liter of water. And many communities don't have fluoridated water at all.

Fluoride supplements are available only with a doctor's prescription. If you want to try fluoride, you'll have to discuss these supplements with your doctor. If your water isn't fluoridated, good food sources of fluoride include tea, mackerel and canned salmon with bones. Daily intake of up to ten milligrams of fluoride from foods and water is considered safe for adults.

Zinc, Copper and Manganese: Working Together for Stronger Bones

For years, researchers have looked for connections between osteoporosis and the minerals zinc, copper and manganese. While it's well-documented that deficiency of any one of these nutrients has a negative impact on bone health, research shows that they may work best when taken together.

"The diets of many elderly people are lacking in essential nutrients, including zinc. And certainly, zinc deficiency leads to problems with bone metabolism," says Joseph Soares, Ph.D., professor of nutrition in the nutritional sciences program at the University of Maryland at College Park. It's not known, however, whether zinc deficiency plays a role in the development of osteoporosis, he says.

The story is the same for copper. Experiments with copper deficiency in animals have been reported to produce bone abnormalities, and severe copper deficiency has been reported to result in osteoporosis in malnourished premature infants, says J. Cecil Smith, Ph.D., research chemist at the U.S. Department of Agriculture Beltsville Human Nutrition Research Center in Maryland. "But there are no conclusive studies on copper and osteoporosis," he says.

Manganese is also essential to bone formation, and manganese deficiency has been reported in women with osteoporosis. Dr. Nielsen maintains that like zinc and copper, manganese probably works best in concert with other vitamins and minerals.

Recognizing the importance of each of these minerals, investigators at the University of California, San Diego, studied the effects of zinc, copper and manganese when taken together. During a two-year study of 59 women past the age of menopause, the researchers found that 1,000 milligrams of calcium slowed spinal bone mineral loss. Adding a "mineral cocktail" of 15 milligrams of zinc, 2.5 milligrams of copper and 5 milligrams of manganese, however, actually stopped bone mineral loss in these women.

"For the best results, I recommend that people take a multivitamin/mineral supplement that supplies 100 percent of the daily requirements of zinc, copper and manganese as well as a separate calcium supplement," says Dr. Saltman, a leading investigator in the study.

The Daily Value for zinc is 15 milligrams; for both copper and manganese, it's 2 milligrams. Since too much zinc can block the absorption of copper, it is important to keep them in balance.

Vitamin K: The Unsung Hero

If you were to tell someone to get vitamin K, their response would probably be "Vitamin what?" Yet vitamin K, abundant in the food chain and produced by intestinal bacteria, plays a key role in bone formation. And vitamin K deficiency, which previously thought to be very rare, may be a factor in osteoporosis.

"Research shows that people with osteoporosis have low blood levels of vitamin K," says Dr. Gaby, who believes that vitamin K deficiency may not be all that rare. When medical scientists deemed vitamin K deficiency a rarity, they were using crude measuring techniques, he says. "And our overuse of antibiotics today may be inhibiting intestinal vitamin K production," he adds.

One study done in the Netherlands, in fact, showed that vitamin K may help protect the body's calcium stores. Seventy women past the age of menopause were given one milligram (1,000 micrograms) of vitamin K daily for three months. They experienced "significant" decreases in urinary calcium loss.

The Daily Value for vitamin K is 80 micrograms, and it's easy to get this vitamin in your diet. Fruits, leafy greens, root vegetables, seeds and dairy products are all good sources. For those who wish to take supplements, 100

Prescriptions for Healing

Doctors agree that good nutrition is essential for bone health. Experts recommend these nutrients to help prevent osteoporosis or slow its progression.

Nutrient	Daily Amount
Boron	3 milligrams
Calcium	1,200–1,500 milligrams
Copper	2 milligrams
Fluoride	Up to 10 milligrams
Magnesium	200–400 milligrams
Manganese	5 milligrams
Vitamin D	400 international units
Vitamin K	Up to 100 micrograms
Zinc	15 milligrams

Plus a multivitamin/mineral supplement containing the Daily Values of all essential vitamins and minerals

MEDICAL ALERT: *If you have been diagnosed with osteoporosis, you should be under a doctor's care.*

If you have heart or kidney problems, you should talk to your doctor before taking magnesium supplements.

micrograms daily is a safe limit, says Dr. Gaby, although he often prescribes larger amounts in specific cases.

The Grab Bag

In addition to these vitamins and minerals, some doctors have suggested the possible benefits of vitamin C, vitamin B_6 and folic acid. Researchers don't recommend individual supplements of these nutrients for osteoporosis, but they don't hesitate to recommend a little multivitamin/mineral insurance.

"It wouldn't hurt to take your calcium supplement as well as a multivitamin/mineral to make sure that you're getting the Daily Values of all of the essential vitamins and minerals," advises Dr. Saltman.

Overweight

Nourishing Yourself Thin

Shakes, puddings, powders and grapefruit: Name the diet, and you've tried it, each time hoping it would be the one that works. Then you watched that dreaded needle on that dreadful scale drift right back up to where you started.

Despite sage advice against dieting from physicians and national experts, we're still doing it. National surveys indicate that 84 percent of women and 77 percent of men "go on diets" when they want to lose weight. And regardless of all of that calorie counting, our national waistline continues to expand, with 33.4 percent of Americans now overweight.

Could it finally be time to throw in the towel and pick up the fork? "No," says Judy Dodd, R.D., past president of the American Dietetic Association. "We just have to be sensible about our diets. Even people who are genetically predisposed to putting on weight do not have to be overweight. There are steps you can take to beat it, such as exercise and nutrition."

Multivitamins May Lend a Hand

And what about vitamins and minerals? What role do they play in a sensible no-diet weight-loss plan? Although the topic is controversial, some doctors believe that multivitamin/mineral supplements, combined with a healthy food and exercise plan, can help. They find that the struggles of overweight people are often brought on by a combination of poor general nutrition and dieting that leaves them feeling fatigued and craving food.

"It becomes like a dog chasing its tail," says Michael Steelman, M.D., vice-president of the American Society of Bariatric Physicians. "When people don't feel good mentally and physically, they often eat sweets to try to feel better, only to find themselves feeling worse. The first line of defense is getting proper exercise and nutrition."

Unfortunately, given the wide appeal of fad diets, that's easier said than done, says Dodd. "Some of the old fad diets, such as the high-protein diet, are popular again, and people tend to skimp on important dietary elements such as fruits, vegetables and dairy."

According to diet research, the most popular diets—those emphasizing high or low levels of protein, carbohydrates and fat—all lead to deficiencies in important vitamins and minerals, particularly vitamins A and C, thiamin, iron and calcium. And low-calorie diets, even those that are well-balanced, typically lack folate, vitamin B_6, magnesium and zinc.

"Nutrition is a problem when people restrict calories," says Dodd. "I encourage people to get their vitamins and minerals from natural food sources, but if they go below 1,200 calories, they should consider a multivitamin/mineral supplement with 100 percent of the Daily Values."

In fact, multivitamin/mineral supplements are good for anyone who is overweight, dieting or not, says Donald Robertson, M.D., medical director of Southwest Bariatric Nutrition Center in Scottsdale, Arizona. "Too many overweight people are nutritionally deficient. Supplementation helps keep them healthier."

Aside from multivitamin/mineral supplements, here are some of the nutrients that many experts believe can help you stay healthier and feel better and may even promote weight loss.

Nutrients to Build Immunity

As if the well-documented health risks associated with overweight, such as heart disease and diabetes, weren't bad enough, some researchers now believe that overweight people have lowered immunity, perhaps because of deficiencies of vitamins and minerals, especially the antioxidants.

Antioxidants such as vitamins C and E are important because they protect our bodies against free radicals, unstable oxygen molecules that damage

Food Factors

When it comes to weight loss, selecting your foods can be a real balancing act. You have to lose some of what you've grown accustomed to and add some items that may be new to you. Here's what experts recommend to promote weight loss.

Reduce fat. With regard to fat, the research is clear: Diets too high in fat promote overweight. You should strive to consume no more than 25 percent of your calories from fat.

Don't be so sweet. Numerous studies have linked table sugar to increased calorie consumption. While sugar doesn't do as much dietary damage as fat, you'll find that when you eat sweets, you simply want to eat more . . . of everything. Not only that, but sugar also makes your body excrete chromium, and chromium is a mineral that helps your body build calorie-burning lean tissue.

Drink up. "If people want to keep their nutrients in balance, they need to drink plenty of plain, unflavored water every day," says Judy Dodd, R.D., past president of the American Dietetic Association. Water not only acts as a solvent for many vitamins and minerals but also is responsible for carrying nutrients into and wastes out of cells, so the body functions properly. As a rule of thumb, you

your body's cells by stealing electrons from healthy molecules. Antioxidants offer their own electrons, neutralizing free radicals and protecting cells.

According to a study done in Poland, overweight people may not be reaping antioxidant benefits. Researchers at the National Institute of Food and Nutrition in Warsaw studied 102 overweight women and found that the women had significantly lower levels of the antioxidant vitamins C and E, as well as of vitamin A, and a higher prevalence of overall vitamin deficiency than those of normal weight.

These deficiencies are at least partially responsible for depressing immunity in overweight individuals, leaving them more susceptible to cancer and infectious illness, say some researchers.

And because of abnormal hormone activity, overweight people may also have greater need for antioxidants than people who are not overweight. Studies show that the excess fat in people who are very overweight drives es-

should drink a half-ounce of water for every pound of body weight daily, unless you're very active, in which case you should increase your water intake to two-thirds of an ounce per pound of body weight daily.

Fill up on fiber. You can curb your hunger by increasing your intake of dietary fiber, which is filling, so you feel full but eat less. To do that, experts recommend eating more fruits, vegetables and whole-grain cereals.

Get treatment for food allergies. Some researchers believe that overweight is the result of people craving foods that they are allergic to. For these people, weight loss is extremely difficult until they figure out what those trigger foods are and eliminate them from their diets. "There are specific food allergies that trigger uncontrollable craving and bingeing," says Joseph D. Beasley, M.D., director of Comprehensive Medical Care in Amityville, New York, and co-author of *Food for Recovery*. "It's a common problem in overeaters."

If you suspect that food allergies might be part of your problem, ask your doctor to help you identify the offending items. Your doctor may recommend that you see an allergy specialist.

trogen production up and testosterone down, a deadly combination that scientists believe could be a major factor in certain female reproductive cancers.

"Overweight people probably need antioxidants more than anybody," says Dr. Robertson, who recommends daily supplements of 1,000 milligrams of vitamin C and 400 international units of vitamin E, along with 25,000 international units of vitamin A. These doses greatly exceed the Daily Values of these nutrients, and vitamin A in particular can be toxic in high doses. Research has found that taking 10,000 international units of vitamin A daily in early pregnancy can cause birth defects. For this reason, this much vitamin A should be taken only under medical supervision, especially if you are a woman of childbearing age. And pregnant women should not use this therapy.

To get more antioxidants through your diet, reach for fruits and vegetables. Those with bright orange coloring, such as sweet potatoes, carrots and cantaloupe, are rich in beta-carotene (a precursor of vitamin A); broccoli,

Prescriptions for Healing

Some nutrition experts find that overweight people have special vitamin and mineral needs, especially if they're trying to lose weight. Here's what these experts recommend.

Nutrient	Daily Amount
Calcium	1,000 milligrams 1,500 milligrams for postmenopausal women
Chromium	50–200 micrograms (chromium picolinate)
Copper	1.5–3 milligrams (1 milligram for every 10 milligrams of zinc)
Iron	15 milligrams
Magnesium	250–500 milligrams
Vitamin A	25,000 international units
Vitamin C	1,000 milligrams
Vitamin E	400 international units
Zinc	15–30 milligrams

Plus a multivitamin/mineral supplement containing the Daily Values of all essential vitamins and minerals

MEDICAL ALERT: *People with diabetes who take chromium should be under medical supervision, since their insulin dosage may need to be reduced as their blood sugar levels drop.*

If you have heart or kidney problems, you should talk to your doctor before taking magnesium supplements.

Vitamin A in the amount recommended here should be taken only under medical supervision, especially if you are a woman of childbearing age. Women who are pregnant should not use this therapy.

If you are taking anticoagulants, you should not take vitamin E supplements.

Doses of zinc in excess of 15 milligrams daily should be taken only under medical supervision.

brussels sprouts and citrus fruits will give you a burst of vitamin C; and wheat germ and kale are good sources of vitamin E.

Chromium Can Help

It might not be the waist-whittling miracle mineral that some advertisements tout it as, but according to the latest research, chromium picolinate (a supplemental form of chromium) may indeed help build lean tissue and reduce fat in adults who exercise.

In one study of 59 college-age students at Louisiana State University in Baton Rouge, researchers found that women taking 200 micrograms of chromium picolinate a day gained almost twice as much lean body mass as those who did not take the supplements, an effect that could result in long-term reductions in body fat, since lean body mass burns more calories than fat.

"What makes the effectiveness of chromium more and more believable is that the results we see in humans are so well-documented in animal studies," says Richard Anderson, Ph.D., lead scientist in the nutrient requirements and functions laboratory at the U.S. Department of Agriculture Beltsville Human Nutrition Research Center in Maryland and a leading chromium researcher. And although chromium will benefit only those who are deficient, Dr. Anderson reports that most people in Westernized countries receive only 25 percent of the Daily Value of 120 micrograms. So a lot of people are deficient.

Chromium also improves the effectiveness of insulin, the hormone that allows cells to pick up glucose (a simple sugar that your body uses for fuel) from the bloodstream. For this reason, chromium may also be helpful in preventing diabetes, which is common in people who are overweight. People with diabetes who take chromium should be under medical supervision, since their insulin dosage may need to be reduced as their blood sugar levels drop.

Doctors who recommend chromium picolinate supplements suggest daily doses ranging from 50 to 200 micrograms. If you'd like to increase chromium through your diet, try whole-grain cereals, black pepper, cheeses and brewer's yeast.

Think Zinc

It's well-documented that zinc, a mineral found in wheat germ, seafood and whole grains, frequently gets left by the wayside when calorie intake dips below 1,200.

Most experts do not recommend such low-calorie regimens. If you're among those who keep a too-tight daily calorie tally anyway, you should know that zinc deficiency not only depresses the immune system but also can be a barber's nightmare, causing brittle, dry hair and hair loss.

"When overweight people show any problems with their hair, nails, gums or skin, I recommend supplementing 20 milligrams of zinc a day," says Dr. Robertson.

Experts usually recommend between 15 and 30 milligrams of zinc daily. Since zinc competes with other metals in the body, however, daily doses of more than the Daily Value of 15 milligrams warrant medical supervision. For the best results, you should take 1 milligram of copper for every 10 milligrams of zinc.

Minerals Make a Difference

Magnesium and iron are the major minerals that doctors find deficient in people who are overweight, particularly in those who are trying to slim down.

Magnesium is essential for every major biological function, including your heartbeat. According to research, even marginal magnesium deficiency is not to be taken lightly, especially when you are dieting and losing weight, as it can lead to potentially fatal heart abnormalities.

"In general, magnesium supplementation helps for a lot of things," says Dr. Steelman. "I use it to treat the muscle cramps that people get when they're trying to lose weight, and it also seems to curb sweet cravings."

Doctors who recommend magnesium supplements call for between 250 and 500 milligrams daily, which is right around the Daily Value of 400 milligrams. (If you have heart or kidney problems, you should check with your doctor before taking magnesium supplements.) Good dietary sources of magnesium include seafood, green vegetables and low-fat dairy products.

Iron is another frequent victim of low-calorie dieting, says Dr. Steelman. "In fact, it's the most common nutrient deficiency I see, especially in premenopausal women."

The most common complication arising from a lack of iron is iron-deficiency anemia, which can cause headaches, shortness of breath, weakness, heart palpitations and fatigue.

Doctors who recommend supplementing iron suggest 15 milligrams a day, particularly for adults who are following a low-calorie diet to lose weight. To pump some iron into your diet, try steamed clams, Cream of Wheat cereal, tofu and soybeans.

Calcium is another mineral that's often in short supply in those who are trying to shed extra pounds. Experts suggest making sure that you're getting the Daily Value of calcium, which is 1,000 milligrams; women who are past menopause should aim for 1,500 milligrams daily.

Parkinson's Disease

Smoothing Out the Tremors

It's like going from automatic to manual.

That description of Parkinson's disease, from someone who has had first-hand experience, sums it up neatly. As this disease of the central nervous system progresses, movements that were once second nature, such as walking and writing, take on a ponderous and deliberate quality. And hand tremors can complicate simple tasks such as buttoning clothes. Frequently, it's tremors that send people to their doctors for diagnosis, but most people with the disease can recall years of vague symptoms before doctors pinpointed the cause.

"I was very slow and sluggish; I just didn't have the old pizzazz. But I didn't know if it was normal old age or not," explains Michael Locoputa, a retired electronics specialist from Syracuse, New York, who has had Parkinson's disease for about ten years.

He especially recalls problems with public speaking, something that gives most people the willies anyway. "I'd have to anchor my arms to the podium and lock my elbows and knees to keep my body still," he says.

It wasn't until he read an article about Muhammad Ali, also a Parkinson's sufferer, that Locoputa began to put the pieces together. "I told my wife 'That's what I have,' " he recalls. His suspicion was later confirmed by a doctor.

Parkinson's disease is caused by damage to brain cells in the substantia nigra, an area deep in the center of the brain that helps coordinate muscle movement. These cells produce a chemical called dopamine, a neurotransmitter that's essential for the brain to send messages to the muscles. As the cells die and dopamine levels drop, muscle control suffers.

Nobody knows for sure why the cells die, but a combination of exposure to environmental toxins and genetic susceptibility, along with normal wear and tear, seems to be the most likely reason, says Caroline M. Tanner, M.D., a researcher with the Parkinson's Institute in Sunnyvale, California. "Certain chemicals can cause symptoms similar to Parkinson's in both animals and humans," Dr. Tanner says. Locoputa, for instance, recalls years of exposure to the solvents used to make electronics components.

Getting the Rust Out

One aspect of nutritional therapy for Parkinson's is directly related to the disease's probable causes, says J. William Langston, M.D., president of the Parkinson's Institute.

"Both normal aging and possible exposure of this part of the brain to toxins may cause oxidative chemical reactions that allow the release of free radicals, molecular particles that steal electrons from other molecules, setting off a chain reaction of cell damage," Dr. Langston explains.

Even dopamine, the neurotransmitter highly concentrated in this part of the brain, is oxidized as part of the message-sending process, Dr. Langston explains. "It's as if dopamine were too hot to handle, and over many years, as it's oxidized, it may eventually kill the very same cells that make it and use it to cause normal motor function," he says.

Vitamin E and sometimes vitamin C have been recommended for people with Parkinson's because these two nutrients act as antioxidants. They stop the chain reaction of free radicals by offering their own electrons, sparing healthy molecules from harm. Most attention has been on vitamin E, since it acts in the fatty parts of cells (brain and nerve tissues contain lots of fatty membranes). Here's what research shows.

Vitamin E: Promise and Disappointment

"The theory behind giving vitamin E for Parkinson's disease is that this nutrient is a free radical scavenger and therefore can protect against free radical damage to the brain," Dr. Langston says. "If you have excessive production of all of these potentially damaging, reactive chemicals over time, and if you put in something like a sponge, something that can soak up or block their effects, you might protect against further damage to the brain."

That's the theory, anyway. In practice, research results so far have been mostly disappointing.

It's true that one study found that people with early Parkinson's disease who took vitamins E and C were able to postpone taking medication for symptoms for 2½ years longer than people not getting these vitamins. (The vitamin takers gradually increased to 3,200 international units of vitamin E and 3,000 milligrams of vitamin C daily, taken in four divided doses.)

But a large nationwide study that followed, the DATATOP study, found that 2,000 international units of vitamin E, taken for up to two years, offered no apparent benefit to people with Parkinson's.

"I would say vitamin E is down but not out," Dr. Langston says. "This is the type of study where if we had gotten positive results, it would have been considered important and well-accepted. Negative results, unfortunately, don't tell us much of anything. It could be that the dose was wrong, that we weren't getting enough vitamin E into the brain, that people were getting it too late in the course of the disease to help much. This negative finding certainly does not rule out the possibility that vitamin E and other antioxidants might be helpful in treating Parkinson's disease."

His research is looking at "prescription antioxidants," chemically engineered varieties not found in nature that get into the brain more easily than vitamin E.

Certainly, fewer neurologists now recommend vitamin E to their patients than before the disappointing results of the DATATOP study, but those who suggest it seem to be taking a can't-hurt-and-may-help position, says Jean Lee, education director for the United Parkinson Foundation in Chicago. "People with Parkinson's disease often don't eat well to begin with, so a complete nutritional supplement program may be appropriate for some of them," she says.

Dr. Langston doesn't recommend vitamin E, but he doesn't discourage his patients from taking it, either. He takes it himself to prevent heart disease.

One doctor who believes that vitamin E may have antioxidant effects, Robert G. Feldman, M.D., professor and chairman of the Department of Neurology at Boston University Medical Center, suggests that people take 400 international units three times a day.

Michael Locoputa takes 800 international units of vitamin E daily. "I was in a vitamin study, but I found out later that I was in a placebo (blank pill)

Food Factors

The amount of protein you eat each day can have a major impact on the symptoms of Parkinson's disease. Here are the dietary changes that doctors are most likely to recommend.

Go high-carb, low-protein. People who are taking levodopa need to limit the amount of protein they eat. Protein is made up of amino acids, and the amino acids in foods interfere with levodopa getting into the brain. (Levodopa is also an amino acid.) *Note:* You should not go below the minimum daily requirement of protein that your doctor determines is right for you.

Your doctor will provide you with detailed instruction on which foods contain carbohydrates and which contain protein. You should aim for a ratio of seven grams of carbohydrates to one gram of protein, spread throughout the day.

That's 47 grams of protein per 2,000 total calories, which translates into about half of the protein that people normally eat. That's the amount that researchers at Boston University have found produces optimum brain levels of amino acids for people with Parkinson's. "If you eat too little protein, too much medication travels to the brain, causing uncontrolled muscle movement and tremors," explains Robert G. Feldman, M.D., professor and chairman of the Department of Neurology at Boston University Medical Center.

On the other hand, if you eat too much protein, you don't get enough dopamine effect in your brain cells, and you end up with Parkinson's characteristic rigidity.

A typical day's menu for such a diet might look something like this.

group, not a vitamin group," he says. "I figured that if they had enough reason to try vitamin E in a big study, then it's worth trying. I had used it for burns and cuts and was impressed with how well it heals. I had also heard that it is helpful in preventing heart disease and cancer. So I thought, why not?"

He has been taking vitamin E for about five years. "I can't say that I've noticed a difference," he says. "I can still play tennis, but I don't have the kind of coordination I used to."

Breakfast

½ cup canned peaches
2 large waffles
2 teaspoons margarine
2 tablespoons syrup
6 ounces 2 percent low-fat milk
Coffee or tea

Lunch

¾ cup vegetarian chili
1 tablespoon grated cheese
1 square cornbread
12 ounces juice
2 small plums

Dinner

2 ounces ham
3 slices canned pineapple
1 medium candied yam
3 brussels sprouts
8 ounces 2 percent low-fat milk
16 ounces juice or lemonade
½ cup sorbet

Beware the fava bean. This flat, tan bean, used in Mediterranean and Middle Eastern dishes, contains dopamine. Eating more than a half-cup or so of beans, along with your daily dose of levodopa, can cause symptoms of dopamine overdose, including agitation and extra involuntary movements, Dr. Feldman says.

The high amounts of vitamin E that are sometimes recommended for Parkinson's disease are not available from normal amounts of even the best food sources, such as hazelnut oil, sunflower oil, almond oil, wheat germ, nuts, whole grains and leafy greens. According to Dr. Feldman, no adverse side effects have been reported in people taking up to 1,600 international units of vitamin E daily. Also, many experts believe that taking up to 600 international units a day is safe without medical supervision. If you want to take high

Prescriptions for Healing

Drugs, not vitamins and minerals, are the mainstay of treatment for Parkinson's disease. Doctors who also offer nutritional guidance are most likely to make these recommendations.

Nutrient	Daily Amount
Thiamin	50 milligrams
Vitamin E	1,200 international units, taken as 3 divided doses

Plus a multivitamin/mineral supplement containing the Daily Values of all essential vitamins and minerals, including the trace minerals

MEDICAL ALERT: *If you have Parkinson's disease, take supplements only under the supervision of your doctor.*

Vitamin E in doses exceeding 600 international units daily can cause side effects in some people. Also, if you've had a bleeding disorder or a stroke, check with your doctor before taking vitamin E supplements in any amount. If you are taking anticoagulant drugs, you should not take vitamin E supplements.

amounts of vitamin E, however, you should check with your doctor first.

If you have had a bleeding disorder or a stroke or have a family history of stroke, you should use large-dose supplements of vitamin E only under medical supervision. If you are taking anticoagulants, you should not take supplements of vitamin E. It's possible that these large amounts of vitamin E may interfere with the absorption and action of vitamin K, which is involved in blood coagulation, says James Sadowski, Ph.D., research leader at the Jean Mayer USDA Human Nutrition Research Center on Aging at Tufts University in Boston.

Add a Little Insurance

Dr. Feldman recommends that his patients take a multivitamin/mineral tablet that includes the Daily Values of all of the essential vitamins and minerals, including the trace minerals. There's a bit of evidence that selenium, a mineral with antioxidant properties, may play a role in Parkinson's. In people with this disease, the part of the brain that's involved, the substantia nigra, is low in a selenium-based antioxidant called glutathione peroxidase. Some experts speculate that low levels of this substance may help set the stage for cell damage.

Dr. Feldman also recommends a supplement that offers up to a 50-milligram dose of thiamin in a B-complex vitamin preparation. "I give it because the patients I see who take it tell me that they feel much more alert and energetic," he explains. In fact, there's a bit of evidence that people with Parkinson's may be low in the B vitamins and may benefit from getting additional amounts.

People taking levodopa should check with their doctors before taking vitamin B_6, though. B_6 counteracts the effects of levodopa when the medicine is taken by itself. Medical experts say that B_6 does not have this effect if levodopa is taken in combination with carbidopa (in the drugs Sinemet and Atamet).

Pellagra

Decoding a Turn-of-the-Century Mystery

Offer someone sow bellies and cornmeal grits for dinner tonight, and you'll probably find yourself eating alone. But in the deep South less than 100 years ago, these foods were the staple diet that's thought to have caused an outbreak of a niacin-deficiency disease called pellagra.

Characterized by a progressive decline that often starts with itchy, red skin, moves on to diarrhea and depression and ends in death, pellagra afflicted more than 100,000 people in 1914.

"The incidence was of such alarming proportions that the U.S. Surgeon General called for a special investigation of 'one the knottiest and most urgent problems of the present time,' " says Marvin Davis, Ph.D., chairman of the Department of Pharmacology at the University of Mississippi at Oxford.

An experiment involving orphans in Jackson, Mississippi, who had pellagra soon provided clues to the mystery. Just a few days after doctors added milk, meats and eggs to the corn grit diet of the children, their pellagra disappeared, says Dr. Davis.

To confirm dietary deficiency as a cause, another study was conducted, this time involving convicts. When pellagra-free prisoners agreed to eat nothing but sow bellies, corn grits, gravy and fried mush for five months, nearly all developed pellagra.

To eliminate lingering doubts that pellagra might be an infectious disease, Dr. Davis says, still another study was launched involving convicts. The prisoners, and the experimenters themselves, were injected with blood from people with pellagra or were exposed to their nasal or throat excretions. When the subjects didn't come down with the disease, researchers realized that pellagra could not possibly be infectious.

True Grits Not Enough

Although researchers soon figured that poor diet was causing pellagra, it wasn't until 1937 that researchers pinpointed the exact source of the problem. Corn not only contains a form of niacin, a B vitamin, that the body cannot easily use but also can create an amino acid imbalance, says Dr.

Prescriptions for Healing

These days, pellagra is rare. Once this niacin-deficiency disease is diagnosed, doctors recommend niacinamide, a form of niacin that is known to have fewer side effects.

Nutrient	Daily Amount
Niacinamide	300–400 milligrams, taken as 3 or 4 divided doses

MEDICAL ALERT: *If you have symptoms of pellagra, you should see your doctor for proper diagnosis and treatment.*

This amount of niacinamide is prescribed for severe cases of pellagra and should be taken only under medical supervision.

Davis. Amino acids are the building blocks of protein, the stuff of which the body is made.

Eating corn as part of a well-balanced diet is not a problem, but a diet that consists almost exclusively of corn and corn products is devastating. In fact, the turn-of-the-century pellagra tragedy led to the fortification of flours and cereals with niacin. As a result, pellagra is now rare.

A few people still get pellagra, however, for reasons that have nothing to do with eating corn. Alcoholics and individuals with severe gastrointestinal problems often have difficulty getting enough niacin. Even then, diagnosing pellagra is not easy. The early symptoms, such as reddening of the skin, cracked lips, weight loss, tiredness, confusion and mild diarrhea, can be subtle, says William M. Hendricks, M.D., director of the Asheboro Dermatology Clinic in North Carolina.

Niacin to the Rescue

Fortunately, the effects of early-stage pellagra are easily reversed. "In general, the main therapy is to get patients back on a healthy diet and, in the case of alcoholics, to get them off of their alcohol and on to some kind of niacin supplementation," says Dr. Hendricks. (For the full story on the role of nutrients in treating alcoholism, see page 69.) He generally prescribes niacinamide, a form of niacin that's known not to produce undesirable side effects.

For severe cases, Dr. Hendricks recommends 100 milligrams of niacinamide three or four times daily for several weeks. Since high amounts of niacin can be toxic, he suggests that this amount be taken only under the supervision of a physician.

The amount of niacinamide a person with pellagra should take really depends on the condition of the individual and should be determined by a doctor, he says.

Some of the best food sources of niacin are chicken breast, tuna and veal. The Daily Value for niacin is 20 milligrams.

Phlebitis

Staying Out of Deep Trouble

You might think you've been kicked in the leg or you've pulled a muscle, but you can't for the life of you remember just when or where or how it happened. That's because it didn't happen. That painful knot you feel in your calf isn't a bruise or a muscle injury. It's phlebitis, a swollen, inflamed vein that can be caused by anything from staying put too long to birth control pills.

Phlebitis is not uncommon. And it's not necessarily serious when it occurs in a superficial vein, since these veins are numerous enough to permit your body to rechannel the flow of blood, bypassing the inflamed vein.

Phlebitis that occurs in deep veins, called thrombophlebitis, is a serious matter. It usually involves formation of a blood clot in the vein, and it can lead to life-threatening circulation problems. "If the clot breaks free, it can travel to the brain, lungs or heart and cause devastating damage," explains Robert Ginsburg, M.D., director of the cardiovascular intervention unit at the University of Colorado Health Sciences Center in Denver.

Thrombophlebitis doesn't always have clear symptoms, but it can be detected with ultrasound. It must be treated promptly with blood-thinning medication. Superficial phlebitis, which is most likely to occur in varicose veins, responds to a judicious combination of exercise and resting with your feet elevated. "Stopping smoking is also important, since chemicals in tobacco get into the bloodstream and promote clotting," Dr. Ginsburg says.

These nutritional approaches may also help prevent phlebitis and its worst consequences.

B Vitamins May Help Stop Clots

Several years ago researchers discovered that people with high blood levels of an amino acid called homocysteine had a high risk of developing damage to endothelial cells, the cells lining artery walls. Once these cells are damaged, cholesterol deposits can build up fast. These people frequently suffered from severe heart disease, experiencing heart attacks in their twenties and thirties.

Dutch researchers discovered a second problem connected with homocysteine. They found elevated blood levels of this substance in people who had recurring blood clots in their veins. As the blood levels of homocysteine increased, so did people's risk of forming clots. Even moderately elevated levels of homocysteine were linked to two to three times the normal risk of recurrent blood clots.

What do B vitamins have to do with all of this? Researchers now know that three B vitamins—folate (the naturally occurring form of folic acid), vitamin B_6 and vitamin B_{12}—help break down and clear homocysteine from the blood. "Deficiency of any one could lead to high levels of homocysteine," explains Jacques Genest, Jr., M.D., director of the cardiovascular genetics laboratory at the Clinical Research Institute of Montreal, a research center that has done pioneering work on homocysteine and heart disease.

Dr. Genest usually measures blood levels of folate and vitamin B_6 in people found to have high blood levels of homocysteine. (He has found that the people he studies, mostly middle-aged men with coronary heart disease, aren't usually low in vitamin B_{12}.) Then he provides supplements as necessary.

"We've found that 2.5 milligrams (2,500 micrograms) of folic acid or 25 milligrams of vitamin B_6 reduces homocysteine levels to normal in most people," he says. Some people may need to take both, he says, and people at risk for vitamin B_{12} deficiency (older people, strict vegetarians and those with absorption problems) also need to make sure their blood levels of B_{12} are adequate. Dr. Genest recommends taking 2 micrograms of B_{12} a day.

The high amounts of folic acid and vitamin B_6 that Dr. Genest recommends are available only through supplements and, in the case of folic acid, should be taken only under medical supervision. Folic acid can actually mask signs of a vitamin B_{12} deficiency. Even those eating a healthy diet, with two

Food Factors

If you're trying to prevent a recurrence of phlebitis, the research done by Daniel Mowrey, Ph.D., director of the American Phytotherapy Research Laboratory in Lehi, Utah, points to a few foods that might help.

Eat foods that go with the flow. Certain foods have anti-clotting properties, says Dr. Mowrey. "They may reduce the tendency for blood platelets to stick together or to the sides of blood vessels," he explains. These foods include garlic, onions, ginger and cayenne, a hot red pepper.

to three servings of fruits and three to four servings of vegetables a day, get only about 190 micrograms of folate a day. As for B_6, men get about 1.9 milligrams and women get about 1.2 milligrams a day through foods such as chicken, fish, pork and eggs.

Dietary vitamin B_{12} is less of a problem. Most people do get enough from meats, dairy products and eggs, with men getting almost eight micrograms and women getting about five micrograms a day. People with absorption problems, however, usually need to get injections of this vitamin.

Vitamin E May Improve the Flow

Evidence is mounting that vitamin E helps protect against cardiovascular disease by helping to block the chemical processes that lead to atherosclerosis, or hardening of the arteries.

Prescriptions for Healing

These nutrients won't cure a raging case of phlebitis. But some medical experts feel that they might help prevent a recurrence.

Nutrient	Daily Amount
Folic acid	2,500 micrograms
Vitamin B_6	25 milligrams
Vitamin B_{12}	2 micrograms
Vitamin E	200–600 international units

MEDICAL ALERT: *If you have phlebitis, you should be under a doctor's care.*

Consult your doctor before supplementing your diet with these B vitamins. Blood tests need to be done to determine your exact deficiencies before a doctor can prescribe the best combination and amounts. In addition, folic acid in doses exceeding 400 micrograms daily can mask symptoms of vitamin B_{12} deficiency.

If you are taking anticoagulant drugs, you should not take vitamin E supplements.

Vitamin E plays an additional role, one that's particularly important to people with phlebitis. Several studies indicate that vitamin E can help protect against potentially life-threatening blood clots. Specifically, vitamin E helps prevent platelets, components involved in blood clotting, from sticking to each other and to blood vessel walls.

"Sticky platelets can cause blood clots to build up fast," explains Joseph Pizzorno, Jr., N.D., a naturopathic physician and president of Bastyr University in Seattle. Studies suggest that reducing platelet stickiness with vitamin E could have a role in the treatment of "thromboembolic events," or traveling blood clots, especially in people with Type I (insulin-dependent) diabetes, who are at particularly high risk for blood-clotting problems.

If you're going to take vitamin E, Dr. Pizzorno suggests that 200 to 600 international units daily should do the trick. Some research suggests that 200 international units is enough to reduce platelet adhesion.

People taking anticoagulants (sometimes called blood thinners or heart medicine) should not take vitamin E supplements.

Premenstrual Syndrome

Putting an End to Monthly Discomfort

Ask ten women what premenstrual syndrome feels like, and you'll probably get ten different answers.

A few of those answers will be pretty predictable: bloated, sore, headachy. Other women feel okay physically but ride an emotional roller coaster of anxiety and depression.

And—something you probably don't want to hear if you have premenstrual syndrome—some women don't experience any premenstrual symptoms at all.

Experts estimate that as many as 50 percent of menstruating women in the United States have some degree of premenstrual syndrome, or PMS. Whether you're one of them depends on a variety of factors, including your genetic inheritance, how much stress you're under, whether you drink alcohol or caffeine and how much you exercise. Age is also a factor: Women in their thirties and forties are more likely to get PMS than younger women.

Food Factors

How you feel in the days before your period depends at least in part on what you eat and drink all month long.

Don't turn to the bottle. Resist the temptation to unwind with a cocktail. While it has been said that severe premenstrual syndrome (PMS) drives some women to drink, research suggests that drinking is more than a reaction to monthly discomfort. Studies show that women who drink moderately throughout the month (ten or more drinks per week) are more likely to have premenstrual symptoms than lighter drinkers or teetotalers.

Don't be so refined. If you experience PMS every month like clockwork, it's possible you're just too refined, at least as far as your diet is concerned. Some studies show that women who get PMS eat more refined sugar and carbohydrates, such as breads, cakes, pastas and other starchy foods made of white flour.

"These foods are generally poor in vitamins, minerals and fiber. So if a woman gets most of her calories from them, she's going to wind up deprived of essential nutrients," says PMS researcher Guy Abraham, M.D., founder of Optimox, a Torrance, California, company that manufactures nutritional supplements. Replacing these refined foods with their heartier cousins, whole-grain breads and cereals and naturally sweet fresh fruits, will result in a more nutrient-dense diet and possibly fewer premenstrual symptoms, he says.

And finally, some researchers believe that nutrition exerts a powerful influence on how a woman feels both before and during her period. PMS researcher Guy Abraham, M.D., became so convinced of the importance of nutrition that he left his teaching position at the University of California, Los Angeles, UCLA School of Medicine to found Optimox, a Torrance, California, company that manufactures nutritional supplements. "Nutrition is the single most important factor in whether or not a woman will have PMS," says Dr. Abraham. "This is why we see so much PMS among women in their thirties. Most of them have been pregnant, which has depleted their bodies of nutrients, so they're more likely to be deficient in the B vitamins and magnesium."

Here's what researchers have learned about the nutrition connection.

Kick the can. The cola can, that is. While the caffeine in your coffee, tea or soda doesn't cause PMS, it can aggravate symptoms in some women, says Dr. Abraham.

Go easy on sugar and salt. This can be difficult when you're craving chocolate and potato chips, but giving in to your cravings can create a vicious cycle, according to Dr. Abraham. Sugar and salt affect the way your body uses the hormone insulin, and excesses of either can create sharp fluctuations in your blood sugar levels. These fluctuations can lead to increased appetite, fatigue, dizziness and more cravings. And both sugary and salty foods can aggravate monthly water retention, according to Dr. Abraham.

Love those veggies. "In Asian countries, where the typical diet includes more vegetable protein such as tofu, PMS is much less common," says Dr. Abraham. "The ratio of vegetable protein to animal protein is directly related to PMS. Countries that have high ratios have a low incidence of PMS, and those that consume a lot of animal protein and fat, such as the United States, have the highest incidence."

But regardless of where you live, you can enjoy the benefits of an Asian diet by limiting the meats and other animal products that you eat or by eliminating these foods altogether. "Vegetarian women seem to have much milder premenstrual symptoms or none at all," says Dr. Abraham.

Calcium: Woman's Best Friend

If you've picked up a health book or magazine lately, you know all about calcium's role in preventing osteoporosis, the brittle-bone disease that incapacitates thousands of women (and men) each year. But if scientific studies are any indication, there may be another, more immediate reason to add a calcium supplement to your medicine chest.

A study conducted at Metropolitan Hospital in New York City found that a daily supplement of 1,000 milligrams of calcium reduced premenstrual symptoms in 73 percent of the women who took it. The women, who normally experienced premenstrual symptoms every month, reported less breast tenderness and swelling and fewer headaches and abdominal cramps when they took the calcium supplements every day during the preceding

Prescriptions for Healing

Getting the right nutrients can make a big difference in whether you suffer monthly symptoms of premenstrual syndrome. Here's what some experts recommend.

Nutrient	Daily Amount
Calcium	500–1,000 milligrams
Magnesium	300–400 milligrams
Manganese	2 milligrams
Vitamin B_6	150–200 milligrams
Vitamin E	400 international units (d-alpha-tocopherol)

MEDICAL ALERT: *If you have heart or kidney problems, you should talk to your doctor before taking magnesium supplements.*

High doses of vitamin B_6 can cause side effects and should be used only under the supervision of your doctor.

If you are taking anticoagulant drugs, you should not take vitamin E supplements.

month. They also reported less discomfort during their periods.

It isn't clear exactly why calcium relieves PMS, but the researchers suspect that it eases the muscular contractions that lead to cramping.

And this isn't the only study to find a connection between calcium and PMS. A small study at the U.S. Department of Agriculture Grand Forks Human Nutrition Research Center in North Dakota found an intriguing connection between a diet low in both calcium and the trace mineral manganese and PMS. Women who experienced PMS on a low-calcium, low-manganese diet had fewer symptoms when their diet was supplemented with the two minerals.

What's interesting, says James G. Penland, Ph.D., head researcher at the Grand Forks Human Nutrition Research Center and one of the authors of the study, is that the diet that produced the worst premenstrual symptoms is actually closest to the way most American women eat. Dr. Penland's studies show that most women get about 587 milligrams of calcium a day, nowhere near the 1,000 milligrams they're supposed to get to build healthy bones and prevent osteoporosis.

Manganese intake among American women is only about 2.2 milligrams a day. That's a little more than the Daily Value for this mineral.

While researchers continue studying the connection between calcium and manganese and PMS, a daily supplement that includes both minerals can't hurt and might help if you're prone to PMS, says Dr. Penland. Check to see if your multivitamin/mineral formula provides 2 to 5 milligrams of manganese. As for calcium, "I would recommend increasing your intake of low-fat, calcium-rich foods such as low-fat yogurt and milk. If that is difficult, then I suggest taking 500 to 1,000 milligrams of supplemental calcium a day," he says.

Mellow Out with Magnesium

Magnesium is another mineral that seems to have a beneficial effect on women with PMS. A few studies have found lower magnesium levels in women with PMS than in women without symptoms. Other studies suggest that increasing magnesium levels might reduce or eliminate premenstrual discomfort, especially emotional symptoms such as tension and anxiety.

Magnesium deficiency causes a shortage of dopamine, a chemical found in the brain that regulates mood, according to Dr. Abraham. This shortage may have something to do with the premenstrual tension and irritability that many women experience.

In one Italian study of 28 women with PMS, a magnesium supplement of 360 milligrams was associated with fewer cramps, less water retention and an overall improvement in premenstrual symptoms.

The Daily Value for magnesium is 400 milligrams. The best sources of magnesium are nuts, legumes, whole grains and green vegetables, all of the staples of a low-fat, high-fiber diet. But if your diet leans more toward white bread, white rice, meats and dairy products, your body is probably coming up short on magnesium.

To help even things up, Dr. Abraham recommends a magnesium supplement of 300 to 400 milligrams. "Your body will tell you exactly how much magnesium you need within that range. Too much will cause diarrhea, so I tell women to take magnesium to bowel tolerance." If you have heart or kidney problems, be sure to talk to your doctor before taking magnesium supplements.

Vitamin E Smooths Out Rough Edges

Vitamin E also seems to lessen the severity of premenstrual symptoms. In two separate studies, a team of Baltimore scientists examined the effect of vitamin E supplements on women prone to PMS. The women received vitamin E in the form of d-alpha-tocopherol every day for two consecutive menstrual cycles. The supplement made a substantial difference in premenstrual symptoms such as mood swings, cravings, bloating and depression.

The women in the study, like most women with PMS, had normal dietary intakes of vitamin E. But the amount of vitamin E in the typical diet apparently isn't enough to treat some PMS, according to Robert S. London, M.D., assistant professor of obstetrics and gynecology at Johns Hopkins University School of Medicine in Baltimore and one of the authors of the study.

"The average person consumes a small amount of vitamin E in foods such as vegetable oils, but this certainly isn't enough to have any effect on PMS," says Dr. London. "The effect was clearly dose-responsive: 400 international units was much more effective than 200 international units. It's impossible for a woman to get these levels of vitamin E through diet alone."

It isn't clear why vitamin E has an effect on PMS. Some experts have suggested that it works by slowing the production of prostaglandins, hormonelike substances thought to play a role in premenstrual symptoms.

If you'd like to try vitamin E for PMS, experts generally advise a dosage of 400 international units daily. Take it for at least six weeks to give it a chance to work, advises Dr. London. "It usually takes about that long," he says. The d-alpha-tocopherol form of vitamin E used in the study is readily available; just check the label before you buy. (Other forms of the vitamin haven't been studied for PMS.)

Beat PMS with B_6

Finally, if you're bothered by premenstrual weight gain and emotional symptoms, vitamin B_6 can help control them, says Dr. Abraham. In a study of 25 women with PMS, Dr. Abraham found that a high-dose supplement of B_6 reduced premenstrual weight gain and lessened the severity of other premenstrual symptoms.

The women in the study were given high doses of vitamin B_6: 500 milligrams a day for three months. (The Daily Value is only 2 milligrams.) B_6 at this level eases PMS by changing blood levels of two female hormones, estrogen and progesterone, according to Dr. Abraham. But high doses of the vitamin can be dangerous, so supplementation should be used only under the supervision of your doctor.

If you'd like to try vitamin B_6 for premenstrual symptoms, Dr. Abraham recommends taking it as part of a B-complex supplement. "B_6 taken by itself can cause deficiencies of other nutrients, so it's important to balance it with the other B vitamins," he says.

You should also make sure you're getting enough magnesium, he adds. "I generally recommend taking twice as much magnesium as vitamin B_6. So if you're taking 300 to 400 milligrams of magnesium, you need 150 to 200 milligrams of B_6."

Prostate Problems

Dealing with a Common Condition

For most men, it seems as inevitable as gray hair and wrinkles. At first you notice a little hesitancy when trying to start the flow of urine. Your urine stream may be weak or intermittent. You find yourself getting up at night to urinate, or you feel like your bladder is still partly full after you've gone. These are all signs of benign prostatic hyperplasia (BPH), an enlargement of the prostate gland.

Statistics suggest that BPH is hard to avoid. More than half of all men over age 50 have significant prostate enlargement, and the rest have at least some. Simply getting older seems to be the main risk factor.

Enlargement does not inevitably lead to drugs or surgery, however. Some doctors contend that it's possible to slow enlargement enough to avoid surgery and drugs, especially if you take the right steps at the first signs of problems. The steps they recommend include dietary changes, herbs and nutritional therapy.

"If a man wants to stay out of the operating room and avoid cancer of the prostate, he needs to go full blast—to avoid the high-fat junk foods and environmental toxins that contribute to prostate problems and to start a wise nutritional program that includes the basic supplements that affect the prostate," says James Balch, M.D., a urologist in Greenfield, Indiana, and author of *Prescription for Cooking and Dietary Wellness*.

Small Gland, Big Problems

While most men may think of the prostate as nothing but trouble, the truth is that this chestnut-size gland does serve a useful purpose. Located just below the bladder, the prostate encircles the urethra, the tube that passes urine from the bladder to outside the body. The prostate produces semen and secretes it into the urethra, providing the liquid medium that sperm cells need for nourishment as well as to exit the body.

Prostate enlargement problems occur when the cells in the inner core of the gland, surrounding the urethra, grow to form fibrous nodules, eventually squeezing in on the urethra and blocking the flow of urine. The cells apparently grow in response to hormones, especially testosterone, and the growth seen in older men may be related to alterations in hormone balance associated with aging, experts say.

Nutritional intervention for BPH includes a healthy low-fat, high-fiber diet, weight loss if necessary, vitamin and mineral supplements and, in some cases, essential fatty acids such as flaxseed oil, says Dr. Balch. Some doctors also consider two herbs, saw palmetto and pygeum (a tree bark used extensively in Europe for this problem), an essential part of treatment. One product, Prostata, from Gero Vita International, combines all of these herbs and nutrients, says Dr. Balch.

Research findings are disappointingly slim when it comes to nutrition and BPH, however. Here's what studies show.

Zinc May Shrink Enlarged Gland

Zinc is highly concentrated in the prostate gland, but many doctors think zinc deficiency has little, if anything, to do with prostate enlargement. Some doctors, however, do recommend zinc for BPH, and with some apparent success. "It's not something I'd prescribe as a sole therapy. But I do use it, and it does seem to have some beneficial effects," Dr. Balch says.

And there is a bit of scientific evidence supporting its use.

One doctor, Irving Bush, M.D., professor of urology at the University of

Food Factors

More than any vitamin or mineral, fat may influence prostate health, say the experts. Here are some dietary changes that they recommend.

Lose that gut. Men with 43-inch waists or greater are 50 percent more likely than normal-weight men to report symptoms of prostate enlargement or to have surgery for this condition, Harvard University researchers report. Losing about 7 inches of waistline, about 35 pounds in most cases, could be a method of treating and preventing prostate enlargement, they say.

The best way to shake this stubborn fat? Eliminate alcohol and cut way back on sugar and dietary fat. At the same time, burn calories by walking, biking, swimming or running.

Trim the fat. A lean diet may be the best way yet to slash your risk of prostate cancer, experts say. Avoid saturated and hydrogenated fats (hard at room temperature) and stick to monounsaturated fats (olive oil or canola oil) for cooking.

Flush it. Drinking plenty of fluids—two to three quarts of water every day—helps prevent the bladder infections, cystitis and kidney problems sometimes associated with an enlarged prostate, doctors say.

Fiber up. A high-fiber diet helps reduce your risk of prostate cancer by slightly lowering your body's levels of reproductive hormones. In population studies, men who eat the most fiber, from beans, whole grains, fruits and vegetables, are least likely to develop prostate cancer.

Health Sciences/Chicago Medical School, senior consultant at the Center for Study of Genitourinary Diseases in West Dundee, Illinois, and former chairman of the Food and Drug Administration panels on gastroenterology, urology and dialysis, did a small study of the use of zinc in treating BPH. The men in the study took 150 milligrams of zinc sulfate every day for two months, followed by 50 to 100 milligrams a day as a maintenance dose. Dr. Bush found that 14 of the 19 men experienced shrinkage of the prostate.

And researchers at the University of Edinburgh Medical School in Scotland found that in test tube experiments using prostate tissue, high doses of zinc inhibited the activity of 5-alpha-reductase, the enzyme that

Prescriptions for Healing

Some doctors recommend a veritable smorgasbord of nutrients to treat benign prostatic hyperplasia (BPH). Solid scientific evidence that these nutrients help is sadly lacking, but some doctors say that they see a difference in men who take them. Here's what is often recommended.

Nutrient	Daily Amount
Beta-carotene	15,000 international units
Magnesium	400 milligrams
Selenium	50–200 micrograms
Vitamin A	10,000 international units
Vitamin B_6	2 milligrams
Vitamin C	1,000–5,000 milligrams
Vitamin E	600 international units
Zinc	160 milligrams (Vicon-C), taken as 2 divided doses

MEDICAL ALERT: *If you have symptoms of BPH, you should see your doctor for proper diagnosis and treatment.*

If you have heart or kidney problems, you should talk to your doctor before starting magnesium supplements.

Doses of selenium that exceed 100 micrograms daily should be taken only under medical supervision.

Vitamin C in doses of more than 1,200 milligrams daily can cause diarrhea in some people.

If you are taking anticoagulant drugs, you should not take vitamin E supplements.

Zinc in doses exceeding 15 milligrams daily should be taken only under medical supervision.

converts testosterone to its more powerful cousin, dihydrotestosterone.

"Stimulation of the prostate gland by dihydrotestosterone contributes to its growth, so reducing levels of this hormone should lead to a reduction in prostate size," says Fouad Habib, Ph.D., a cell biologist at the University of Edinburgh Medical School.

Unfortunately, zinc hasn't been tested in men with BPH in any large scientific studies, and until it is, most doctors will remain skeptical.

Dr. Bush continues to prescribe zinc to his patients with BPH. He uses Vicon-C from Whitby Pharmaceuticals, a product that offers 80 milligrams of zinc sulfate per capsule, along with vitamin C, several B vitamins and magnesium. (This amount of zinc is well above the Daily Value of 15 milligrams.) He recommends two capsules a day, after meals, and says it may take about six months to begin to see results. "It's not going to work for everyone, since gastrointestinal absorption and the presence of binding proteins are different in everyone," he admits. "But I think it's worth a try."

It's important to work with a doctor knowledgeable in nutrition if you want to try zinc for prostate problems, experts say. Normal amounts of zinc, up to 20 milligrams a day, have no effect on prostate enlargement, Dr. Habib says.

On the other hand, too much zinc is just plain toxic, Dr. Balch says. "My opinion is that if you go above 80 to 100 milligrams a day, you're skating on thin ice," he says. And other experts suggest not taking more than 15 milligrams daily without medical supervision. Too much zinc can cause anemia and immunity problems.

Other Nutrients Round Out the Program

Zinc isn't the only nutrient that doctors use to treat BPH. Dr. Balch, for instance, adds a smorgasbord of supplements: 10,000 international units of vitamin A, 15,000 international units of beta-carotene (which converts to vitamin A in the body), 600 international units of vitamin E, 1,000 to 5,000 milligrams of vitamin C and 50 to 200 micrograms of selenium daily. All of these have been associated with reduced risk of cancer.

If you would like to try a nutritional program along these lines, you should discuss it with your doctor. The amounts of vitamins A, E and C that Dr. Balch recommends are significantly higher than the Daily Values of these nutrients. Vitamin C can cause diarrhea when taken in high doses, and high doses of selenium—more than 100 micrograms daily—can be toxic. (A Daily Value has not been established for beta-carotene.)

Dr. Balch also prescribes magnesium and vitamin B_6. The Daily Value for magnesium is 400 milligrams; for vitamin B_6, it's 2 milligrams. (If you have heart or kidney problems, be sure to talk to your doctor before taking magnesium supplements.)

"I'm well aware that there is nothing most doctors would call evidence that these nutrients help BPH," he says. "In my own experience, however, men who eat healthy diets and take these supplements have all-around better health and are less likely to require surgery."

Psoriasis

Prescription Vitamin D Delivers Hope

For years, experts and people with psoriasis scratched their heads (not to mention other body parts) in despair over medical science's inability to fight this troubling skin disease. Then groundbreaking research by Michael F. Holick, M.D., Ph.D., director of the General Clinical Research Center and chief of the Section of Endocrinology, Diabetes and Metabolism at Boston University Medical Center, unleashed the dramatic healing power of vitamin D and revealed just how to make it work against psoriasis.

A Plague Called Plaques

Vibrant, healthy skin seems to just happen for some people. Like clockwork, they shed skin cells in the form of minute, invisible flakes while new cells push to the surface in a 15-stage cycle that is as natural as it is uneventful. And every 28 to 30 days, they're clad in a completely new suit of skin.

Not so for people with psoriasis. It's as if parts of the skin-renewing cycle were put on fast-forward—really fast-forward. Within four to five days, the affected patches of skin, called plaques, undergo just five changes before they pile up like the Sunday paper. The result: red, itchy, scaly plaques that often cover the knees, elbows and scalp.

Nor does psoriasis stop at the surface. "It ranges from localized mild patches on the skin to a totally disabling total body disease," says Nicholas

Lowe, M.D., clinical professor of dermatology at the University of California, Los Angeles, UCLA School of Medicine. About 25 percent of the four to five million psoriasis cases in the United States are so bad that people are completely disabled, often with a crippling form of arthritis.

While experts say that such prolific skin shedding is caused by some as yet unknown genetic problem, things such as stress, infections, cuts, scrapes, certain medications (quinine, beta-blockers and lithium, among others) and alcohol can also spark flare-ups. "While psoriasis is an inherited disease, a whole series of other events can bring out the disease in a person who is ge-

Fishing for a Cure

Some experts think that there's something fishy about treating psoriasis with fish oil. But at least one study, done several years ago, showed that the fatty acids found in fish may be beneficial after all.

In a Finnish study, 80 people with psoriasis took two capsules containing fatty acids from fish three times a day for eight weeks. At the end of the study, 7 people were completely healed, and 13 reported 75 percent healing. Those who showed the best results in the study had the least severe cases, the researchers noted.

"It's neither the best treatment for psoriasis nor the only treatment that people should use, but it may be of some benefit," says Michael F. Holick, M.D., Ph.D., director of the General Clinical Research Center and chief of the Section of Endocrinology, Diabetes and Metabolism at Boston University Medical Center.

Thirty-four of the people included in this Finnish study also had psoriatic arthritis, a form of arthritis related to psoriasis. All 34 reported less severe joint pain after taking the capsules. Fatty acids from fish apparently act as an anti-inflammatory, and that action is particularly effective in some cases of psoriatic arthritis that involve considerable inflammation, says Dr. Holick.

Atlantic herring and pink salmon are among the fish highest in helpful fatty acids. Unfortunately, you'd have to eat between one and two pounds a day to get close to the dose of fish oil that the volunteers took during the study. So you might want to ask your doctor about taking fish oil capsules to help combat psoriasis.

Food Factors

These dietary tips may help you keep your psoriasis at bay.

Ban the booze. Alcohol and psoriasis apparently go together like martinis and olives. One study of 362 men between ages 19 and 50 found that many drank heavily before they developed psoriasis—twice as much as those who were psoriasis-free. Heavy drinking also increases the risk of infection, which is known to trigger psoriasis, according to the researchers.

Give acid the slip. One small study showed a reduction of psoriasis symptoms among people who avoided acidic foods such as coffee, tomatoes, soda and pineapple. If you discover that certain foods cause you problems, listen to your body and avoid them, says Michael F. Holick, M.D., Ph.D., director of the General Clinical Research Center and chief of the Section of Endocrinology, Diabetes and Metabolism at Boston University Medical Center.

Bring on the veggies. Could eating less protein help tame your psoriasis? Some reports have suggested improvement in symptoms when people with psoriasis ate a vegetarian diet low in protein for several weeks.

netically predisposed," says Dr. Lowe.

Defeating Psoriasis with Vitamin D

Added to milk and other dairy products, vitamin D has long been known as the cure for rickets, a disease that causes bone deformity and stunted growth in children.

Special receptors in your skin also make use of sunlight-produced vitamin D, a fact that has led some to try tanning in an attempt to end their psoriasis. In fact, nude sunbathing at the Dead Sea in Israel has become such a popular treatment for psoriasis that the *Wall Street Journal* suggested the influx (about 10,000 visitors a year and growing!) is creating a modern mecca for psoriasis treatment.

Why the Dead Sea? The location's low elevation prevents the sun's harshest rays from reaching sunbathers, allowing them to stay out longer without burning, experts say. The Dead Sea's mineral-rich water, so salty that plants and fish can't survive, is also thought to help psoriasis.

Researchers exploring the role of vitamin D receptors in the skin have found a way to help people with psoriasis. Dr. Holick discovered that skin cells have receptors for what is called activated vitamin D, essentially the hormone that prevents skin cells from growing and shedding too rapidly.

The next step was to develop a superpotent yet nontoxic form of activated vitamin D, strong enough to slow the growth of psoriatic skin cells. "We wanted to take advantage of the observation that we had made, using a high enough concentration to alter the growth of the skin cells without harm," Dr. Holick explains.

Applied to the skin as an ointment (Dovonex), activated vitamin D, available only by prescription, not only slows skin cell growth to levels much closer to normal but also reduces itching and inflammation, says Dr. Holick. "Among those who Dovonex use topically, upward of 50 to 60 percent have seen significant improvement," he says. Such improvement usually begins to appear in two to three weeks.

And all of this is accomplished without the common reaction to megadoses of vitamin D: raised calcium levels, which can cause kidney stones and high blood pressure. "It's purposely formulated as an ointment. That way, it stays in the skin and doesn't usually enter the blood," says Dr. Holick.

Wouldn't megadoses of over-the-counter vitamin D have the same positive effect on psoriasis? Not at all, says Dr. Holick. "The reason is that the body is very particular about the amount of vitamin D that it takes in. It will not make any more activated vitamin D (1,25-dihydroxy vitamin D_3), regardless of how much of the vitamin you take. You can become vitamin D–intoxicated, but you won't be able to treat your psoriasis," says Dr. Holick.

Virtues of Vitamin A

Although it's reserved for more severe cases, a superpotent form of vitamin A called etretinate (Tegison) is also available for psoriasis, but only by prescription.

Taken orally, activated vitamin A helps skin cells grow to maturity before shedding. Unfortunately, it also has a downside. "When used clinically to have an effect on psoriasis, almost all of the vitamin A derivatives create a series of unwanted side effects," says James G. Kreuger, M.D., Ph.D., assistant

Prescriptions for Healing

Ask your doctor about Dovonex, a prescription topical form of superpotent vitamin D, and etretinate (Tegison), a prescription oral form of superpotent vitamin A.

Many doctors also recommend a multivitamin/mineral supplement containing the Daily Values of folic acid and iron.

professor of medicine at Rockefeller University in New York City, who heads an investigative group in psoriasis research. Side effects include birth defects, dry mouth and hair loss.

In some cases, Dr. Lowe uses both etretinate and six grams of omega fatty acids, which are found in fish oil, to limit any side effects. "We take blood tests when we have people on these drugs, but it's usually okay to combine them," he says.

Unfortunately, taking a regular form of vitamin A won't help psoriasis at all, says Dr. Lowe.

The Case for a Multivitamin

Although no one suggests that any vitamin or mineral taken orally can cure psoriasis, there is some evidence that psoriasis itself can cause certain vitamin and mineral deficiencies.

In a study of 50 people hospitalized with psoriasis, researchers found that some were low in protein, iron and folate (the naturally occurring form of folic acid), according to Janet Prystowsky, M.D., Ph.D., assistant professor of dermatology at Columbia Presbyterian Hospital in New York City.

Rapid skin cell growth and shedding deplete stores of protein, iron and folate because psoriatic skin seems to take precedence over other parts of the body, she says. "While nutritional supplementation is not a remedy for psoriasis, it could improve the general health of a person with the disease," according to Dr. Prystowksy.

Raynaud's Disease

Defrosting Frigid Digits

Is it possible that Moses had Raynaud's disease?

The Bible tells of how the Hebrew leader, high on a mountaintop, watched his hand turn snow white after he touched a rod that God had commanded him to pick up. There's no doubt that Moses was a little anxious at the time. After all, God was asking him to do something pretty scary, since the rod he picked up had been a snake only moments earlier. God then ordered Moses to stick his hand inside his shirt, where it promptly regained its normal color.

People with Raynaud's don't need to be in such a chilly and frightening situation to experience this disease's finger-blanching symptoms. Just a bit of cold or nervousness can often set off symptoms, according to Jay D. Coffman, M.D., chief of peripheral vascular medicine at Boston University Medical Center.

Chilled to the Bone

Raynaud's is actually an extreme exaggeration of a normal response, says Dr. Coffman. When our hands are exposed to cold, the tiny arteries in our fingertips constrict, shunting blood to the interior of the body, where it can stay warm. When our hands sense warmth, the arteries relax, allowing normal blood flow to the fingers to resume.

In Raynaud's, however, arteries clamp down and stay clamped for the slightest reason. Taking a tray of ice cubes from the refrigerator or getting tense may bring on symptoms, explains Dr. Coffman. Fingers turn first white as blood drains out, then blue as poorly oxygenated blood pools in them. Then they flush red as oxygenated blood returns. An entire episode may take less than a minute or go on for hours.

Some people, mostly young women, develop Raynaud's for no apparent reason. "These women also tend to have more migraines and other conditions linked to overreactive blood vessels," says Dr. Coffman.

For some, Raynaud's is an early symptom of an autoimmune disease such as scleroderma or lupus. (An autoimmune disease results when the immune system attacks the body itself rather than going after viruses and bacteria.) "Both of these diseases cause scarring in blood vessels and changes in blood

Food Factors

You'd be hard-pressed to find an Eskimo with Raynaud's disease. But if you can't find whale blubber at your local supermarket, try this fishy alternative.

Have a sardine sandwich. A study by researchers at Albany Medical College in New York found that the omega-3 fatty acids concentrated in fatty fish such as salmon, mackerel, tuna and, yes, sardines seemed to help keep blood vessels open in some people with Raynaud's disease.

The same study found that symptoms stopped altogether in 5 of 11 people taking 12 fish oil capsules (a total of 3.96 grams in the form of eicosapentaenoic acid and 2.64 grams in the form of docosahexaenoic acid) daily for two consecutive six-week periods. The other 6 people extended the amount of time that they could keep their hands submerged in cold water before blood flow to their fingers shut down from 31 to 47 minutes, an increase of 50 percent.

In a comparison group of nine people with Raynaud's taking olive oil, only one person showed any significant improvement.

proteins that can impair circulation in small blood vessels," Dr. Coffman says.

Certain medications, including beta-blockers (used to treat high blood pressure) and ergot (used to treat migraines), can cause Raynaud's, Dr. Coffman says. So can carpal tunnel syndrome and certain blood-clotting abnormalities. So it's smart to see your doctor to figure out what is causing your symptoms, says Dr. Coffman.

In the United States, nutritional therapy generally isn't used much for this disorder, says Dr. Coffman. Two nutrients, niacin and vitamin E, are sometimes recommended to help relieve symptoms, however. Here's how they work.

Niacin Keeps Blood Vessels Open

One of the B-complex vitamins, niacin is well-known for its talents in dilating blood vessels. Take enough of this nutrient, and you'll experience the "niacin flush," a burning, itching, reddening, tingling sensation, usually in the face, neck, arms and upper chest, that may persist for a half-hour or even longer. In fact, a slow-release form of niacin called inositol nicotinate is available overseas as a drug called Hexopal and is prescribed precisely for Raynaud's disease.

Inositol nicotinate is available in this country in health food stores but can be obtained from some doctors who commonly use nutritional therapies in their practices. Look for inositol hexaniacinate, a form of inositol nicotinate that is less likely to cause flushing. (One brand name is Flush-Free HexaNiacin from Enzymatic Therapy.) In a number of studies, people who took this drug had fewer and shorter finger-freezing attacks.

"If you try inositol nicotinate, take 500 to 1,000 milligrams three or four times a day," suggests Mary Dan Eades, M.D., medical director of the Arkansas Center for Health and Weight Control in Little Rock. "The inositol combination slows the release of the niacin."

Or you can take nicotinic acid, although it also causes flushing. Depending on your sensitivity, flushing may occur at doses as low as 50 milligrams. Dr. Eades recommends taking the lowest dose that relieves your symptoms and taking no more than 100 milligrams a day without medical supervision.

Regardless of the form in which it's taken, niacin has been known to cause liver damage in high doses. If you have liver disease, Dr. Eades feels that it's best to take no more than the Daily Value of niacin, 20 milligrams, without medical supervision.

Niacin can thaw your icy fingers, Dr. Coffman agrees. "But I don't recommend it, because people don't like the side effects," he says. In addition to itching and flushing, niacin may cause nausea, headaches and intestinal cramps.

Vitamin E May Improve Blood Flow

Most doctors consider so-called case reports, in which a physician reports his observations of a patient who has a particular disease or is undergoing a particular treatment, a less reliable means of assessing a treatment than scientific studies. In fact, there are no studies to show the potential benefits of vitamin E for Raynaud's disease. But several case reports attest to its benefits, and one report in particular stands out because of the dramatic results obtained.

The report, by Samuel Ayres, Jr., M.D., a Los Angeles dermatologist, told of a 45-year-old man who for six months had had worsening ulcers and gangrene on the tips of his fingers. Dr. Ayres prescribed 400 international units of vitamin E twice a day, along with vitamin E applied to the fingertips. Within eight weeks, the man's fingers had completely healed, and they remained healed one year later on a maintenance dose of vitamin E. Dr. Ayres says that he has treated an additional 20 people in his practice who

Prescriptions for Healing

Nutrients that preserve circulation in the tiny capillaries of the fingers are most helpful for Raynaud's disease. Many doctors suggest these.

Nutrient	Daily Amount
Inositol nicotinate	1,500–4,000 milligrams, taken as 3 or 4 divided doses
or	
Nicotinic acid	Up to 200–300 milligrams
Vitamin E	800 international units, taken as 2 divided doses

MEDICAL ALERT: Both inositol nicotinate and nicotinic acid are forms of niacin. Niacin has been known to cause liver damage in high doses. If you have liver disease, it's best to take no more than the Daily Value of niacin, 20 milligrams, without medical supervision.

Depending on your sensitivity, nicotinic acid may cause flushing at doses as low as 50 to 75 milligrams. Doctors recommend staying at the lowest dose that relieves your symptoms and going no higher than 100 milligrams a day without medical supervision.

Check with your doctor before taking more than 600 international units of vitamin E daily, as high doses can cause side effects in some people. If you are taking anticoagulant drugs, you should not take vitamin E supplements.

had circulation problems in their hands, the majority of whom have benefited from taking vitamin E supplements.

"Vitamin E could be helpful for a number of reasons," Dr. Eades says. "It may improve blood flow through tiny capillaries by reducing the tendency for cells to stick to the sides of blood vessel walls and to each other. Plus it may speed the healing of and reduce the scarring from ulcers, which are sometimes associated with Raynaud's disease."

Check with your doctor before taking more than 600 international units of vitamin E daily, as high doses can cause side effects in some people.

Restless Legs Syndrome

When Your Legs Have a Life of Their Own

What happens when you want to sit still but your legs want to move?

"When I look back, I just don't know how I functioned. I walked the floor at night and dragged myself around during the day for so many years that it's a wonder I survived," recalls Carol Walker, a Holmdel, New Jersey, woman who has had restless legs syndrome since she was a teenager. Her words only begin to describe the problems associated with this strange but apparently not-so-uncommon neurological sleep disorder.

People who experience restless legs syndrome have sensations in their legs, usually at night, that make moving their legs irresistible. Some people even describe these sensations as feeling like painful electric shocks. "It feels like creeping, crawling sensations or pins and needles, like there are ants crawling around inside your legs," Walker says. "It's just the most horrible feeling in the world."

Like many, she would get up, walk around, massage her legs, rub them against the sheets—do anything but sleep for hours every night. "I would usually fall asleep around 5:00 in the morning," she recalls, "and sleep for a few hours before I'd have to get up and start my day."

But she also found it hard to sit much during the day. She remembers, as a teenager, trying to hold still in a movie or a car and thinking "If I don't move my legs, I am going to scream."

"I know that sounds strange, but that's the way it was," she says. Luckily, she enjoyed dancing, so she wasn't a complete social misfit.

Finding the Answers

Walker is also typical in that it took years until she was diagnosed. She endured a misdiagnosis of multiple sclerosis for eight years. "If you get a doctor who has never heard of this condition, you see a look of disbelief when you try to describe your symptoms," she says.

Restless legs syndrome was previously thought to affect only 2 to 5 percent of people, says Pickett Guthrie, director of the Restless Legs Syndrome Foundation in Raleigh, North Carolina. But estimates of its incidence are now as high as 10 percent. "After an article appeared in *Modern Maturity* magazine, we got 31,000 letters," Guthrie says. "This condition apparently is much more common in the elderly than was previously assumed. The medical world is just now acknowledging that this is an important medical condition."

No one really knows what causes restless legs. It does tend to run in families, however, and may appear as "growing pains" in children or as pregnancy-related "leg cramps." And it tends to get worse as people get older, experts say.

"One theory that restless legs is associated with a problem in the brain related to dopamine, a neurotransmitter involved in movement, has been proposed. That's because even small amounts of a drug containing dopamine (levodopa) improve symptoms in most people," says Arthur Walters, M.D., associate professor of neurology at the University of Medicine and Dentistry of New Jersey in New Brunswick. That drug is what seemed to help Walker most.

Walker also takes vitamins and minerals, particularly folic acid. And many doctors agree that nutrients can play roles, at least in some cases. Restless legs syndrome has been associated with at least two nutritional deficiencies: iron and folate (the naturally occurring form of folic acid).

"How deficiency of either of these nutrients might cause this problem isn't known," admits June Fry, M.D., Ph.D., professor of neurology and director of the Sleep Disorders Center at the Medical College of Pennsylvania in Philadelphia. "Both of these nutrients are required in the brain and peripheral nerve tissues, but we don't know the details or the actual mechanism behind a possible link. These deficiencies may be not actual causes of restless legs but exacerbating factors, something that makes the underlying disease worse. In my experience, even after a deficiency is corrected, other treatment may be necessary to control the condition."

Here's what research shows.

Iron Weighs In as a Factor

It was back in the 1960s that Swedish neurologist Karl Ekbom, M.D., noted that about one of four people with restless legs syndrome had iron-deficiency anemia and that when these people were treated with iron for their anemia, their legs calmed down, too.

Although case reports of iron's benefits continued in the intervening decades, little research was done that would confirm these findings until researchers at Royal Liverpool University Hospital in England delved into the matter again.

They gave 35 older people with restless legs 200 milligrams of iron (ferrous sulfate) three times a day for two months, without telling the people

Food Factors

Other than helping to offset iron or folate deficiency, foods don't seem to play much of a role in the development of restless legs syndrome. Pay heed, however, if you're a coffee fan.

Junk the java. In a study of 62 people with restless legs, researchers at St. Mary's Hospital in Passaic, New Jersey, found that the elimination of caffeine and other related compounds in tea, chocolate and cola caused improvement in restless legs symptoms.

Incidentally, caffeine and other components of coffee and tea as well as sugar can rob your body of iron, folate, magnesium and other nutrients that play roles in restless legs syndrome.

that it might help their restless legs. When the people were later quizzed on their symptoms, about one-third reported substantial reductions in severity, says Shaun O'Keeffe, M.D., the study's main researcher. "While their symptoms weren't entirely gone, many people got enough relief that they did not require medication for the problem," says Dr. O'Keeffe.

Those obtaining the most relief from iron supplements were people with low blood levels of ferritin, an iron-protein complex that is the main storage form of iron in the body. "None of these people had actual iron-deficiency anemia, and most even had normal blood levels of iron," Dr. O'Keeffe notes.

Experts suggest that if you have been diagnosed with restless legs syndrome, you should have your doctor check your blood level of ferritin. If it is low or borderline, you may benefit from iron supplements.

"How much iron you need depends on your iron level," Dr. Fry says. If you are so low that you have anemia, you may need to take several hundred milligrams a day for a few months.

Your doctor will monitor your dosage by periodically checking your blood ferritin level. Once your level is well within the normal range, a maintenance dosage can be established, or you may be able to get enough iron from iron-rich foods such as clams and fortified cereals.

Note that it's important to determine the cause of your iron deficiency and to correct it. Many of the people Dr. O'Keeffe and Dr. Fry saw were found to have stomach or intestinal bleeding.

The Daily Value for iron is 18 milligrams. Since daily intake of high amounts of iron can be harmful, don't take more than the Daily Value in supplements unless your doctor confirms the need with a blood test.

Prescriptions for Healing

Nutrients play roles in some cases of restless legs syndrome. Here's what experts say might help.

Nutrient	Daily Amount
Folic acid	5,000–20,000 micrograms
Iron	18 milligrams
Magnesium	400 milligrams
Vitamin E	100–400 international units

MEDICAL ALERT: The Daily Value for folic acid is 400 micrograms. Higher doses may hide important symptoms of pernicious anemia, a vitamin B_{12}–deficiency disease, so be sure to talk to your doctor before starting supplementation.

The amount of iron recommended here is the Daily Value. Your doctor, however, should prescribe your iron dosage based on the results of a blood test that measures your blood level of ferritin.

If you have heart or kidney problems, be sure to consult your doctor before starting magnesium supplementation.

If you are taking anticoagulant drugs, you should not take vitamin E supplements.

Folic Acid May Aid Some

While you're having your blood checked for iron deficiency, it might be worthwhile to have your doctor check your blood level of another nutrient: folate, a B vitamin that is essential for normal nerve function. Deficiency of this nutrient appears to be associated with restless legs problems in a small percentage of people.

Your doctor can determine if you're coming up short in this essential nutrient by measuring folate levels in your red blood cells, which is a more accurate way to determine your real status than simply measuring blood levels, Dr. O'Keeffe says.

There is no established dosage of folic acid to treat restless legs, so your doctor is likely to prescribe an amount that corrects your deficiency. Some doctors have given up to 20,000 micrograms a day, but most stick to 5,000 to 7,000 micrograms a day. If folic acid is going to help your problem, it should do so within a few weeks, Dr. O'Keeffe adds.

Since the Daily Value for folic acid is only 400 micrograms, you should talk to your doctor before taking a higher amount. High doses of folic acid can mask the symptoms of pernicious anemia, a condition caused by a deficiency of vitamin B_{12}. For this reason, your doctor should also check your blood for B_{12} deficiency and provide a supplement if necessary, notes Dr. O'Keeffe.

"Especially in the elderly people I see, folate deficiency often means that people are deficient in other B vitamins as well," Dr. O'Keeffe adds. So your doctor may add a supplement for more than one B vitamin.

Vitamin E: Popular but Unproven

Vitamin E is a popular supplement among many people with restless legs syndrome, reports Guthrie. "Lots of people say that they take it," she says. Whether or not it actually helps is another question. "Some think it does; others don't know," she says.

Although there are a few reports from doctors that vitamin E in doses of 100 to 400 international units daily has helped this condition, no studies have been done to confirm its effectiveness. Doctors who treat this condition don't tend to recommend vitamin E.

Vitamin E may help maintain blood circulation if you have peripheral vascular disease, or poor circulation in your legs, Dr. Fry says. "I am not convinced that circulation problems cause restless legs symptoms, however," she adds. If you decide to take vitamin E supplements, don't neglect other, possibly more helpful treatments for this condition.

A Case of Mistaken Identity

It's possible that what you and your doctor think is restless legs is instead severe leg cramps. This mistake is fairly common, says Dr. Walters. One way to tell: "If quinine (a drug used to treat malaria that also calms nerve firing in muscles) helps your problem, you probably have leg cramps, not restless legs syndrome," Dr. Walters says. If you are interested in trying quinine for your leg problems, talk to your doctor.

If you think you are experiencing leg cramps, it might be helpful for you to make sure that you are getting the Daily Values of calcium, magnesium and potassium (and sodium, too, if you've been on a very restrictive diet). These minerals all play roles in muscle contraction and relaxation. Deficiency of any one can lead to muscle cramps. (If you have heart or kidney problems or diabetes, be sure to check with your doctor before taking magnesium or potassium supplements.) For the full details on using nutrients to deal with leg cramps, see page 353.

One study, from Romania, suggests that magnesium supplements can also help bona fide restless legs. So it might be worth your while to make sure you're getting the Daily Value of this mineral, which is 400 milligrams. Most people fall short of that amount.

Rheumatoid Arthritis

Cooling Down the Inflammation

Even though there are doctors who specialize in the disease (they're called rheumatologists), rheumatoid arthritis remains something of a medical mystery. No one knows exactly what causes it, and no one knows why the disease seems to come and go. No one knows why some people get it so badly that they are permanently crippled or why a few lucky people have a single flare-up and never again have symptoms.

"There's a lot we still have to learn about this disease," admits Robert McLean, M.D., clinical assistant professor of medicine at Yale University School of Medicine and an internist in New Haven, Connecticut.

In a person with rheumatoid arthritis, the body's own infection-fighting immune cells attack joint tissue and cause inflammation, with pain, redness, heat and swelling. The inflammation doesn't always confine itself to joints; sometimes other organs, such as the skin, heart and lungs, can be affected.

Rheumatoid arthritis is usually treated by simply suppressing symptoms. Doctors prescribe anti-inflammatory drugs such as aspirin or ibuprofen. For severe cases, they may recommend steroid drugs, which dampen the body's immune response and so reduce inflammation. They may recommend other medications that modulate the immune system in different ways, including cancer chemotherapy drugs such as methotrexate (Folex), azathioprine (Imuran) and cyclophosphamide (Cytoxan).

These drugs do reduce pain and swelling, but at a price. Most have side effects, from stomach upset to bone loss and reduced resistance to infection.

Traditional medicine tends to discount any possible benefit of nutritional therapy for rheumatoid arthritis. The Arthritis Foundation, for instance, holds firm to its position that except for a slight benefit from fish oil, no nutritional therapy has been proven to help any kind of arthritis. And indeed, the kind of large clinical trials that might confirm that nutrition does help have yet to be done.

Nutritional Backup for Treatment

Doctors who prescribe nutritional therapy take these tactics: They eliminate foods from the diet that may aggravate rheumatoid arthritis; they add anti-inflammatory fats such as fish oil; and they provide optimum amounts of nutrients, including those nutrients thought to help reduce inflammation and other vitamins and minerals needed for general good health.

"It's a simple premise," says Robert Cathcart, M.D., a physician in private practice in Los Altos, California, who specializes in nutritional therapy. "People who have a chronic disease such as this need extra amounts of certain nutrients to help their bodies fight the disease."

People with rheumatoid arthritis have been found to be low in a number of nutrients. One study by Finnish researchers, for instance, found that people with low blood levels of vitamin E, beta-carotene and selenium (a mineral with anti-inflammatory properties) had more than eight times the risk of developing rheumatoid arthritis compared with people with high levels of these nutrients.

Doctors who specialize in nutritional therapy use an array of nutrients to fight rheumatoid arthritis. "I find that a broad approach is best," says Joseph Pizzorno, Jr., N.D., a naturopathic physician and president of Bastyr University in Seattle. "People won't necessarily be cured of their arthritis, but they will get enough relief to be able to cut back on their medications, and they are often willing to put up with a bit of discomfort in exchange for fewer side effects from drugs."

Here, then, is what doctors who practice nutritional therapy recommend.

(continued on page 488)

Food Factors

The strongest evidence to date that diet has anything to do with rheumatoid arthritis comes from studies of omega-3 fatty acids.

Make fish your dish. Mackerel, salmon and tuna all contain omega-3 fatty acids, which are known to be anti-inflammatory. At least six studies have shown that diets rich in these fatty acids help reduce the pain and stiffness of rheumatoid arthritis and the biochemical signs of inflammation.

Evidence so far suggests that about six grams of these fatty acids a day seems to have an anti-inflammatory effect. If you're not taking fish oil capsules, try eating two or three meals of fatty fish each week. It might be up to four months before you notice any improvement in your condition.

Some doctors recommend plain old cod liver oil, in doses of up to three tablespoons (nine teaspoons) a day. In fact, there's some evidence that it reduces pain and swelling.

Even though cod liver oil has been used over the years with apparent safety, it is possible to get too much of a good thing. That's because unlike omega-3 fatty acids, cod liver oil contains hefty amounts of vitamins A and D. Although it's important to get the Daily Values of both of these nutrients, more than 15,000 international units of vitamin A (3 times the Daily Value) or 600 international units of vitamin D (1½ times the Daily Value) can be toxic if taken over a long period of time, even if taken in foods. In addition, research has found that vitamin A can cause birth defects when taken in doses of 10,000 international units during early pregnancy.

So don't mix cod liver oil with supplements, even in modest doses, without knowledgeable medical supervision, especially if you are a woman who is pregnant or of childbearing age. And stop your regimen if you develop headaches, nausea or vomiting.

Cut back on other fats. Doctors who prescribe fish oil say that this oil works better to relieve pain and stiffness when it's used along with a diet low in animal fats.

That makes sense, since fats compete with each other for use in the body's production of biochemicals called prostaglandins. When the body selects fish oil, as it does when fish oil molecules are abundant, the prostaglandins produced are anti-inflammatory. When the body chooses arachidonic acid from animal fats, the prostaglandins produced are pro-inflammatory.

Cut back on fats by going easy on meats (especially lunchmeats), whole-fat dairy products (such as ice cream, cheeses and butter), mayonnaise, baked goods and salad dressings.

Pinpoint possible trouble foods. Most doctors believe that only a small percentage of people with inflammatory arthritis have symptoms that are aggravated by foods. But many nutrition-oriented doctors believe that more people than previously suspected have food-related arthritis symptoms and that everyone with arthritis should at least try an elimination diet to detect trouble foods.

"Research is looking at the possibility that some people develop antibodies (a normally protective immune system reaction to invasion) against proteins they eat and that those antibodies then go on to attack similar proteins in the body," says Robert McLean, M.D., clinical assistant professor of medicine at Yale University School of Medicine and an internist in New Haven, Connecticut. "So the idea of food-related arthritis is not so far out as it once seemed."

You may want to keep a food diary for a few weeks to see if certain foods seem to be contributing to your symptoms. "One quick way to figure out if foods are part of your problem is to put yourself on a week-long program of eating foods that you don't normally eat or to go on a juice fast," says Jonathan Wright, M.D., a doctor in Kent, Washington, who specializes in nutritional therapy and is author of *Dr. Wright's Guide to Healing with Nutrition*. If you improve during this time, then you'll need to slowly reintroduce foods to see if your symptoms flare.

Almost any food may cause problems, but milk, wheat, sugar, corn and soy appear to be common triggers. Some people also seem to have trouble with tomatoes, potatoes, eggplant, paprika, green and red bell peppers and chili peppers, all members of the nightshade family.

Quench the Flames with Vitamin C

When it comes to rheumatoid arthritis or other conditions that involve inflammation, nutrition-oriented doctors almost always include vitamin C in their prescriptions.

"The theory is that all inflammation is mediated by free radicals, and if you can get rid of the free radicals, you get rid of the inflammation," Dr. Cathcart says. "This is easier said than done."

Free radicals are molecular bad guys that grab electrons from your body's healthy molecules. This electron stealing harms cells. Free radicals congregate in gangs in rheumatic joints because immune cells generate free radicals in their attack on joint tissue. Vitamin C and other antioxidants disarm free radicals by offering their own electrons and so spare cells.

Doctors recommend different amounts of vitamin C, but most call for at least 600 milligrams a day. Dr. Cathcart usually recommends as much ascorbic acid (another name for vitamin C) as an individual can tolerate without developing diarrhea and gas. That may be up to 60,000 milligrams a day, which is well above the Daily Value of 60 milligrams.

He suggests taking powdered ascorbic acid, which can be mixed with water. This mixture should be drunk through a straw to keep it away from teeth, he warns, because ascorbic acid can erode tooth enamel. Powdered ascorbic acid is available in health food stores and through vitamin supply houses.

Although there's good reason to think that vitamin C could be helpful in treating inflammation, and studies with laboratory animals indicate potential benefits, there are no studies with humans to show that large amounts of this nutrient help people with rheumatoid arthritis. Vitamin C is considered safe, even in large amounts, because any extra is eliminated in the urine. If you want to take large amounts of vitamin C—more than 1,200 milligrams a day—it's still a good idea to discuss it with your doctor.

Selenium May Help Stop Inflammation

Selenium is essential to the body in small amounts. It is thought to be helpful for rheumatoid arthritis because it, too, fights inflammation. Selenium is used in the body for the production of glutathione peroxidase, an enzyme that works inside joints to round up free radicals.

In one study done in Belgium, 15 women with rheumatoid arthritis who took 160 micrograms of selenium or 200 micrograms of selenium-enriched yeast every day for four months experienced significant improvement in joint movement and strength compared with women receiving placebos (blank pills).

Doctors who recommend selenium for people with rheumatoid arthritis prescribe 200 to 300 micrograms a day. In large amounts, selenium can be toxic, so experts say that it's probably best not to take more than 100 micrograms a day without medical supervision.

Studies show that people generally get about 108 micrograms of selenium a day in their diets. Top food sources include seafood, meats and whole grains.

Vitamin E Adds Anti-inflammatory Power

Doctors add vitamin E to their rheumatoid arthritis prescriptions because it, too, cleans up free radicals and may fight joint inflammation.

In one study, Japanese researchers looked at laboratory animals deficient in vitamin E as well as at those given large doses of vitamin E. When both groups were given toxins that cause joint damage similar to that caused by rheumatoid arthritis, those deficient in vitamin E had many more of the biochemical markers of inflammation in their blood.

Doctors who recommend vitamin E generally call for amounts far beyond the Daily Value of 30 international units. "I recommend 400 international units a day," Dr. Pizzorno says. Since foods contain relatively little vitamin E, that amount is available only in supplements.

Beta-Carotene May Reduce Swelling

People with rheumatoid arthritis who become vegetarians often report that their symptoms of pain and swelling are relieved.

Such a diet may be helpful in several ways. In particular, a veggie-dense diet is likely to include more than the normal slim pickin's of foods that contain beta-carotene, the yellow pigment found in carrots, winter squash, cantaloupe and other orange and yellow fruits and vegetables.

Like vitamins C and E and selenium, beta-carotene rounds up free radicals. In one study done in Switzerland using laboratory animals, beta-carotene helped stop symptoms of a type of experimentally induced arthritis similar to rheumatoid arthritis.

Doctors who include beta-carotene in their anti-arthritis formulas recommend about 25,000 international units a day. That amount is considered safe, says Dr. Cathcart.

Prescriptions for Healing

Most doctors who treat rheumatoid arthritis do not make dietary recommendations beyond that of eating a balanced diet.

Those who do provide nutritional therapy make sure that a person is getting at least the Daily Value of every essential vitamin and mineral. They might recommend larger doses initially, if necessary, to restore normal blood levels of these nutrients. These doctors also recommend continuing to take large doses of some of the nutrients known to play roles in regulating inflammation in the body. Here's their daily prescription.

Nutrient	Daily Amount
Beta-carotene	25,000 international units
Copper	2 milligrams (Daily Value) or 3 milligrams (1 milligram for every 10 milligrams of zinc)
Selenium	200–300 micrograms
Vitamin C	600–60,000 milligrams
Vitamin E	400 international units
Zinc	30 milligrams (zinc picolinate or zinc citrate)

MEDICAL ALERT: *Anyone with rheumatoid arthritis should be using vitamin and mineral supplementation only after discussing it with his physician.*

Doses of selenium that exceed 100 micrograms daily should be taken only under medical supervision.

If you want to take more than 1,200 milligrams of vitamin C daily, discuss it with your doctor, as large doses can cause diarrhea in some people. If you're taking vitamin C in the form of powdered ascorbic acid, be sure to drink the mixture through a straw, since ascorbic acid can erode tooth enamel.

If you are taking anticoagulant drugs, you should not take vitamin E supplements.

Doses of zinc that exceed 15 milligrams daily should be taken only under medical supervision.

Zinc Zeros In on Pain

Think zinc belongs only on your galvanized trash can? Think again.

Another mineral that fights inflammation, zinc is an important component of the nutritional package for rheumatoid arthritis. Several studies have shown that people who have rheumatoid arthritis have low blood levels of zinc, often associated with high levels of inflammatory biochemicals in the blood.

"Our bodies use zinc, along with copper, to make an inflammation-fighting enzyme called superoxide dismutase. This enzyme is found in inflamed joints, where it neutralizes free radicals," says Jonathan Wright, M.D., a doctor in Kent, Washington, who specializes in nutritional therapy and is the author of *Dr. Wright's Guide to Healing with Nutrition*. Zinc also functions as a building block for 200 or so other enzymes that play essential roles throughout the body, including repairing joints and helping the immune system to do its job.

In one study by researchers at the University of Washington in Seattle, people with rheumatoid arthritis who took 50 milligrams of zinc three times a day for three months experienced significant improvement in joint swelling, morning stiffness and walking time compared with when they were not taking zinc.

In another study, people with psoriatic arthritis, an inflammatory condition that is a combination of arthritis and the skin disease psoriasis, improved while taking 250 milligrams of zinc three times a day. In this study, relief of symptoms reached its peak after about four months of zinc supplementation and continued for several months after participants stopped taking zinc supplements.

"I recommend taking no more than 30 milligrams of zinc picolinate or zinc citrate without medical supervision," says Dr. Wright. Some doctors start their patients at amounts of up to 150 milligrams a day, then cut back as blood levels of zinc rise to normal. But prolonged high doses of zinc can cause problems, Dr. Wright warns. That's why most experts feel that it's a good idea not to take more than 15 milligrams (the Daily Value) of zinc daily without medical supervision.

Most people get 10 to 15 milligrams of zinc a day through foods, although older people may get only half of that amount. Whole grains, wheat bran, wheat germ, beef, lamb, oysters, eggs, nuts and yogurt all contain good amounts of zinc. (*Note:* Because bacteria in raw oysters can cause serious illness in people with certain health conditions, make sure oysters are fully cooked before you eat them.)

The Copper Connection

For years, doctors have been fascinated—and stumped—by copper's possible link to rheumatoid arthritis. Blood levels of copper are often elevated in people with rheumatoid arthritis, which leads some researchers to believe that copper is being drawn out of body tissue stores and transported by the blood to fight inflamed joints.

What is known is that copper, like zinc and selenium, is used to form anti-inflammatory compounds in the body, including superoxide dismutase and ceruloplasmin, a protein found in the blood. Both of these biochemicals are known to help counteract the inflammation that occurs with rheumatoid arthritis.

Copper is also essential for the body's manufacture of connective tissue, the ligaments, tendons and such that wrap around a joint like rubber bands and keep it stable.

And in the body, copper combines with salicylate, a compound found in aspirin, and improves the drug's pain-relieving ability, Dr. Wright says. "People who take copper supplements often find that they can get by with less aspirin or other nonsteroidal anti-inflammatories," he says.

Doctors who recommend copper supplements say that people should make sure they are getting either the Daily Value of two milligrams or one milligram of copper for every ten milligrams of zinc that they take. The body works on a delicate balance of zinc and copper; too much zinc interferes with copper absorption and can lead to copper deficiency. Higher amounts of copper should be used only under medical supervision. Even in small amounts, copper can be toxic.

Studies show that generally, women get about 1 milligram a day and men get 1.6 milligrams a day in their diets. For food sources, try shellfish, nuts, seeds, fruits, cooked oysters and beans.

Copper bracelets have commonly been promoted as a remedy for the aches and pains of arthritis. The Arthritis Foundation states that "there is no scientific evidence" that copper bracelets have any benefit for arthritis. If you want to get copper into your system, you'll have to take it orally.

Rickets

Building Strong Bones

Was Tiny Tim, the lovable crippled child in Charles Dickens's classic *A Christmas Carol*, suffering from the vitamin D–deficiency bone disease called rickets?

One expert argues that it's likely, since nineteenth-century London was, as he puts it, "miserable." Any sunlight capable of piercing the English gloom was almost certainly trapped by industrial smog back then.

Sunlight is not the only potential source of rickets-preventing vitamin D, of course. But the Cratchit family's meager diet was hardly healthful enough to prevent a case of the infamous disease that crippled so many nineteenth-century children.

Bah, humbug, retort other experts. The Cratchit child clearly had some other crippling disease.

That the experts amuse themselves by debating Tiny Tim's condition says a lot about the frequency of rickets today. Aside from cases in which people avoid certain foods or the sun for dietary or religious reasons, this condition, called common rickets in children and osteomalacia in adults, is more a medical curiosity than an ongoing concern.

Almost Gone, but Not Forgotten

Still, doctors have to be prepared to diagnose either. Not too long ago, at Children's Hospital of New Jersey in Newark, doctors were looking at the x-rays of a 15-month-old girl suffering from respiratory problems when they discovered that bones in her shoulder were frayed. This is a common sign of rickets, says Robert Rapaport, M.D., director of the Division of Pediatric Endocrinology and Metabolism at the University of Medicine and Dentistry of New Jersey/New Jersey Medical School in Newark.

Further investigation revealed that the child came from a strict religious home where she wore clothing that covered all but her nose and forehead. The combination of her manner of dress and the absence of dairy products in her diet contributed to her condition, reports Dr. Rapaport.

An unusual case, perhaps, but "these kinds of cases demonstrate that vitamin D–deficiency rickets is still around," says Dr. Rapaport. "Both health care professionals and parents need to be educated about factors that predispose to rickets and about measures that can prevent its development."

Without sunlight (vitamin D is synthesized in the skin by the action of ultraviolet light) or dairy products, both sources of vitamin D, young, growing bones are unable to perform a task known as mineralization, which is the process that adds minerals needed for bone development, says Binita R. Shah, M.D., professor of clinical pediatrics and director of pediatric emergency medicine at the State University of New York Health Science Center at Brooklyn. Dark skin, colder climates, abundant clothing and industrial pollution are all potential barriers to vitamin D production by the skin, says Dr. Shah.

Boning Up on Vitamin D

Bone is a dynamic organ that is constantly being formed and re-formed, says Dr. Shah. Vitamin D is essential for bone formation and mineralization. It also ensures that there are proper amounts of calcium and phosphorus on hand for bone growth. It does this in three ways: first, by making certain that these minerals are absorbed in the intestines; second, by bringing calcium from bones into the blood; and third, by aiding the reabsorption of calcium and phosphorus by the kidneys, says Dr. Shah.

"When you see a case of rickets, the body is desperately trying to make bone, but adequate calcium and phosphorus aren't available. It's a poor effort, resulting in unmineralized bone accumulation," says Dr. Shah.

As a result, a child with rickets will have ankles and wrists that flare, with noticeable knobby bumps, and weakened leg bones that bow under the child's own weight. Other symptoms include a lack of muscle tone, a disproportionately large head and forehead and delayed infant milestones such as sitting up, standing and the appearance of teeth.

Prevention of rickets and osteomalacia is as simple as including good sources of vitamin D, such as fish (especially sardines and salmon) and fortified milk, in the diet. Dr. Shah recommends human milk for infants, but in this case, she stresses the importance of vitamin D supplementation, since human milk contains little vitamin D. For infants who are not given human milk, infant formula contains all of the necessary nutrients. Also, fortified whole milk is a very important part of an infant's diet, notes Dr. Shah. Since fortified milk is important for adults as well, she adds, skim milk may be a wise choice for them.

Because of fortification, an eight-ounce glass of milk provides about 100 international units of vitamin D. The Daily Value is 400 international units. Experts say that taking more than 600 international units of vitamin D a day can be toxic, with symptoms that may include high blood pressure, kidney failure and coma. For this reason, daily doses exceeding 600 international units should be taken only under medical supervision.

For confirmed rickets cases, Dr. Shah prescribes something called stosstherapy, a form of treatment that provides a total of 600,000 international units of vitamin D, given in a single day in six divided doses. This amount of vitamin D is highly toxic and should be taken only under the supervision of a physician. Used more often in Europe, stosstherapy is preferred when there's doubt whether a child will continue to get appropriate amounts of vitamin D to treat rickets. "This kind of therapy not only heals the rickets but also maintains vitamin D levels for three months," says Dr. Shah. Another benefit: Doctors know in four to seven days whether the rickets is caused by diet or another factor, such as heredity.

Prescriptions for Healing

Because vitamin D is so readily available from sunshine and fortified milk products, rickets, a vitamin D–deficiency disease, is relatively rare in this country. Here's what doctors recommend for both prevention and treatment.

Nutrient	Daily Amount
Prevention	
Vitamin D	400 international units
Treatment	
Vitamin D	600,000 international units, taken as 6 divided doses (administered in 1 day under the supervision of a doctor)

MEDICAL ALERT: *Doses of more than 600 international units of vitamin D a day can be toxic. Symptoms may include high blood pressure, kidney failure and coma. Vitamin D in such high daily doses should be taken only under the supervision of your doctor.*

Scleroderma

Softening Rock-Hard Skin

Talk about being a prisoner in your own body. People with scleroderma—literally, hard skin—can become encased in thick scar tissue. The disease can turn a formerly animated face into an expressionless mask and stiffen hands into claws. About one in three people with the disease may also have problems with the intestines, kidneys, heart or lungs.

Scleroderma, like lupus and rheumatoid arthritis, is an autoimmune disease. This means that the immune system, the white blood cells that normally protect against bacteria, viruses and other foreign invaders, turns renegade and attacks the body's own tissues. In this case, the attack is on connective tissue called collagen. Collagen is found throughout the body, including in the skin, the muscles and the organs.

The immune system attack first produces inflammation that can make the joints hurt and cause the hands to become puffy. Ultimately, scar tissue forms and makes the skin thick, hard and shiny. Muscles can become weak. And almost everyone with scleroderma also has Raynaud's disease, an extreme sensitivity to cold in the hands and feet. Raynaud's disease causes blood vessels to constrict and fingers and toes to turn white, resulting in stinging pain and discomfort.

Battling Toxic Exposure

Just what causes most cases of this relatively rare disease is not known, says David Pisetsky, M.D., medical adviser to the Arthritis Foundation and author of *The Duke University Medical Center Book of Arthritis*. A clue to the cause is provided by the occurrence of similar problems in people who have been exposed to environmental chemicals such as polyvinyl chloride (found in soft plastics) and trichlorethylene (a grease dissolver used in manufacturing and dry cleaning). Coal miners may develop scleroderma after years of work, and outbreaks of similar connective tissue diseases have been associated, in Spain, with contaminated cooking oil and, in the United States, with contaminated tryptophan, an amino acid supplement used to treat insomnia.

Doctors treat scleroderma with drugs that suppress the immune system and reduce inflammation. They may also recommend medications that help the heart and kidneys function better. Antibiotics and drugs that stimulate gut motility, or the movement of food from one end of the digestive tract to the other, can combat the bacterial overgrowth and absorption problems that sometimes accompany scleroderma.

Nutrition isn't thought to play much of a role in the development or progression of scleroderma. "But nutrition does play an important role in maintaining the best possible health despite the disease," says Sheldon Paul Blau, M.D., clinical professor of medicine at the State University of New York at Stony Brook and co-author of *Living with Lupus*.

Most doctors who offer nutritional therapy to their patients with scleroderma are helping them to absorb nutrients more easily by recommending liquid or intravenous feedings and supplements, says Dr. Blau. Some doctors, he says, further suggest dietary changes and add nutrients that are thought to help reduce inflammation and stress on organs such as the heart and kidneys. Here's what they recommend.

Inflammation Fighters

Doctors agree: Scleroderma starts with inflammation, and its progress depends on how much inflammation continues to occur in the body. That's one reason some doctors recommend that patients with any sort of inflammatory disease—rheumatoid arthritis, lupus or scleroderma—make sure they are getting optimum amounts of vitamin E, selenium and beta-carotene, a yellow pigment found in dark green, leafy vegetables and in orange and yellow fruits and vegetables. These nutrients, known as antioxidants, are thought to help to dampen inflammation by neutralizing some of the biochemicals associated with the process.

Inflammation produces unstable molecules called free radicals, which damage a cell by grabbing electrons from healthy molecules in the cell's outer membrane. Antioxidants offer free radicals their own electrons, disarming the free radicals and saving cells from harm.

As yet there hasn't been much in the way of actual scientific study of the use of antioxidants to treat scleroderma. In one study using laboratory animals, supplemental vitamin E helped prevent calcium deposits in soft tissues, which can be a problem for people with scleroderma. In another study, three people with scleroderma who took 800 to 1,200 international units of vitamin E daily had reductions in the stiffness and hardness of their hands, re-

Food Factors

Doctors agree: If you have scleroderma, healthy eating habits can help you function better. Here's what they recommend.

Subtract fat. Chances are you've heard this advice a few times before, as prevention for heart disease and cancer. In the case of a chronic inflammatory condition such as scleroderma, you'll want to cut back on the fat in your diet, especially saturated fat, because fat helps fuel the fire of inflammation. High-fat meals are also harder to absorb than low-fat meals.

To do this, stick to low-fat dairy products, lean meats and reduced-fat salad dressings. "I tell people to eat mostly vegetarian," says Sheldon Paul Blau, M.D., clinical professor of medicine at the State University of New York at Stony Brook and co-author of *Living with Lupus*.

Fill in with fish. The oil in fatty fish such as mackerel, salmon and tuna actually has a mild anti-inflammatory effect, Dr. Blau says. Some people take fish oil capsules, but since you want to stay low-fat, a better tactic may be to replace high-fat dishes such as macaroni and cheese with broiled fish, he says.

Use yogurt to your advantage. Although antibiotics may be essential to knock out harmful bacteria in your digestive system, these powerful medications also destroy helpful bacteria. Eating plenty of yogurt or taking acidophilus tablets restores these friendly bacteria to the bowel, which helps protect it from a new bout of harmful overgrowth, says Dr. Blau.

ductions in calcium deposits in soft tissues and, in two of these people, healing of ulcerated fingertips.

And studies of animals with another, more common inflammatory disease, lupus, do show that these nutrients can help stop damage from inflammation, says Dr. Blau.

He recommends daily intake of 1,000 international units of vitamin E, 25,000 international units of beta-carotene and a multivitamin/mineral supplement that includes 50 micrograms of selenium and 15 milligrams of zinc. (Zinc is used by the body to produce a free radical–quenching enzyme.) Vitamin E in doses exceeding 600 international units daily can cause side effects, so it's a good idea to talk to your doctor about supplementing in this high amount.

Dr. Blau does not recommend supplemental vitamin C for people with scleroderma, however. (Vitamin C is also an antioxidant.) That's because vitamin C promotes the body's production of collagen, and scleroderma involves the overproduction of collagen. In fact, one study attempted to treat

Prescriptions for Healing

Although most doctors do not recommend supplements to people with scleroderma, some doctors say they've found that certain supplements may help the two biggest problems that people with scleroderma face: malabsorption and inflammation. Here's what they recommend.

Nutrient	Daily Amount
Beta-carotene	25,000 international units
Selenium	50 micrograms
Vitamin B_{12}	1,000 micrograms
Vitamin E	1,000 international units
Zinc	15 milligrams

Plus a multivitamin/mineral supplement containing the Daily Values of all essential vitamins and minerals

MEDICAL ALERT: *If you have scleroderma and wish to take these nutrients, you should discuss it with your doctor, especially if you have kidney damage or high blood pressure.*

Vitamin E in doses exceeding 600 international units daily can cause side effects, so it's a good idea to talk to your doctor about supplementing in this high amount. If you are taking anticoagulant drugs, you should not take vitamin E supplements.

scleroderma by putting people on a very low vitamin C diet. "We never found out whether a vitamin C–deficient diet helped," Dr. Blau explains. "Vitamin C is found in so many foods that it was impossible to keep people on a C-deficient diet." He does not tell his patients with scleroderma to avoid eating vitamin C–rich foods.

Vitamin E and beta-carotene are considered safe, even in fairly large amounts. But if you have scleroderma, check with your doctor before you take supplements of these or any other nutrients, especially if you have kidney damage or high blood pressure, Dr. Blau cautions.

Fighting Absorption Problems

Perhaps the biggest nutritional problem that people with scleroderma face is malabsorption. Their intestines absorb less than normal amounts of nutrients from foods because of scarring and bacterial overgrowth. Doctors often recommend treatment with antibiotics to knock out the bad bugs and help restore some absorption. But some people also require liquid nutritional supplements or, in some cases, intravenous nutrition.

But even people who don't require special feeding formulas can benefit from taking a multivitamin/mineral supplement, says Dr. Blau. "These people have an especially hard time absorbing the fat-soluble vitamins A, D, E and K, and they can develop an array of symptoms associated with deficiencies of these nutrients if they do not get adequate amounts," he says.

Dr. Blau says he has seen people with scleroderma develop softened bones from a lack of vitamin D and hemorrhaging from a lack of vitamin K. That's one reason he urges people with scleroderma to see a rheumatologist (a doctor who specializes in these sorts of diseases) for their care.

"These symptoms are not a normal course of scleroderma, and you need to see a doctor who knows what symptoms can be prevented with proper nutrition," he says.

In addition to deficiencies of fat-soluble vitamins, people with scleroderma are at particular risk for vitamin B_{12} deficiency, says Dr. Blau. Fatigue, memory loss and abnormal gait can be signs of low B_{12} levels. Most people with absorption problems require injections of B_{12} to restore blood levels to normal. Oral doses of 1,000 micrograms a day (well above the Daily Value of 6 micrograms) may maintain normal blood levels in people with only minor absorption problems, he says.

Scurvy

Solved with Vitamin C

Chances are the last time you heard someone mention scurvy, an Errol Flynn type was being forced to walk the plank at swordpoint in a bad old pirate movie: "We'll make shark bait outta ya, ya scurvy dog!"

The name given to a set of symptoms that develop during a severe long-term shortage of vitamin C, scurvy is rare these days. But make no mistake: At one time, scurvy was a plague of epic proportions. In fact, one expert maintains that after famine, scurvy is "probably the nutritional deficiency disease that has caused the most suffering in recorded history."

Source of Sailors' Suffering

Once called the scourge of the navy, scurvy killed or incapacitated countless sailors during the age of naval exploration. Often long sea voyages, even aboard grand sailing ships led by legendary explorers such as Ferdinand Magellan and Vasco da Gama, literally became death trips for the crew. In fact, da Gama lost 100 of 160 men to scurvy during one ten-month voyage.

Soldiers bogged down on long winter campaigns often suffered the same fate: wounds that wouldn't heal, muscle pain, bleeding gums, lost teeth, fatigue, kidney failure, pneumonia and, finally, death.

Between 1556 and 1857, more than 100 scurvy epidemics occurred throughout Europe, including Ireland's infamous Great Potato Famine (potatoes were that country's main source of vitamin C).

Many early medical experts thought that scurvy was contagious, and no one had any idea what caused the disease. Finally, James Lind, a young Scottish physician in the British navy, theorized that sailors' diets, which often consisted of nothing more than biscuits and salted meats such as beef and pork, lacked "acidic principles."

To test his theory, Dr. Lind divided some sick sailors into groups. A few sailors ate oranges in addition to the ship's rations; others ate lemons. Still others were given vinegar. One group even drank seawater!

Within six days, the sailors who ate the oranges and lemons were healthy enough to be reassigned to active duty. And for his part, Dr. Lind had shown that this devastating illness could be cured with the right nutrients. In 1753, Dr. Lind published *A Treatise on Scurvy*, describing the study and his recommendations for treatment.

Dr. Lind's observations weren't implemented for another 50 years. But they had impact, and not just on health. Soon British sailors were known as limeys, a nickname that poked fun at the lime juice they drank while at sea.

Scurvy Still Exists

Healthier diets featuring lots of vitamin C–containing foods have come close to ending scurvy in America in this century. And yet several factors raise the possibility of a future increase in cases. Among these factors is changing demographics. "Although scurvy is considered uncommon in the United States, the two populations at greatest risk, the institutionalized elderly and alcoholics, are increasing," says Kevin C. Oeffinger, M.D., associate professor of family medicine at the University of Texas Southwestern Medical Center at Dallas.

Prescriptions for Healing

Although scurvy is extremely rare, doctors still see an occasional case. What's more common is a condition known as sub scurvy. Here's how the experts treat both.

Nutrient	Daily Amount
For Scurvy	
Vitamin C	500–1,000 milligrams for 1 week; then 100 milligrams for 1 month; then 60 milligrams thereafter
For Sub Scurvy	
Vitamin C	200 milligrams

MEDICAL ALERT: Anyone with scurvy should be under medical care and should receive a vitamin prescription from a doctor.

Dr. Oeffinger had read about scurvy when he was in medical school, but it wasn't until just a few years ago that he came face-to-face with his first case. A 59-year-old man arrived at a Waco, Texas, emergency room accompanied by his sister and complaining of sore, bleeding gums, an outbreak of small purplish red spots on his legs and arms (actually hemorrhaging blood vessels), fatigue and weakness. The man later told Dr. Oeffinger that he had eaten nothing but crackers and eight to ten beers a day for six months.

What's wrong with this dietary picture? Virtually everything. But the man's obvious lack of fruits and vegetables, the best sources of vitamin C, gave him scurvy.

Once a person starts to get scurvy, the disease itself makes it hard to make the kinds of dietary changes needed to overcome it, explains Dr. Oeffinger. That puts people in a real medical emergency.

"It becomes a snowball effect, so to speak," says Dr. Oeffinger. "Because they lose their appetites as a symptom of the disease, their chances of eating something with vitamin C are lowered. In addition, they start getting painful gum changes that make it uncomfortable for them to eat, and that's a further impediment to them eating a normal diet."

Who's at Risk

While few doctors ever see full-blown cases of scurvy, nutrition experts warn that a potentially large number of older folks teeter on the brink of a condition known as sub scurvy. Living alone or in nursing homes, they might eat just enough fruits and vegetables to get the Daily Value of vitamin C, which is 60 milligrams.

But the Daily Value of vitamin C might not be enough for some older people, according to Tapan K. Basu, Ph.D., co-author of *Vitamin C in Health and Disease* and professor of nutrition at the University of Alberta in Edmonton. Many older folks take aspirin or other analgesics daily to manage arthritis pain, and that can reduce the amount of vitamin C in the body by as much as 50 percent, he explains. "You get a combination effect of aspirin impeding vitamin C absorption in the gastrointestinal tract as well as damaging the vitamin C itself," he says.

People with ulcers are also at risk for sub scurvy. Avoiding acidic foods to help keep pain at bay often means cutting back on solid sources of vitamin C such as oranges and lemons, says Dr. Basu.

Smoking a pack of cigarettes a day has also been found to cut the amount of vitamin C in your body by 50 percent. As a result, the Food and Nutrition

Board of the National Research Council recommends that smokers get 100 milligrams of vitamin C daily.

Combine all three—prolonged low vitamin C intake, smoking and daily aspirin use—and you're well on your way to sub scurvy. Symptoms include delayed wound healing, small red spots that show up particularly when pressure is applied to the arms, severe fatigue and bleeding gums.

Treating Deficiency

How much vitamin C does it take to overcome the symptoms of scurvy and sub scurvy? The amount pretty much depends on how severe the deficiency is in the first place, says Dr. Basu.

To begin with, a person with full-blown scurvy should be under a doctor's care. During the first week of treatment, between 500 and 1,000 milligrams of vitamin C a day is usually enough to replenish depleted reserves and help end symptoms such as bleeding gums and those purplish red spots, says Dr. Basu. During the second week, he reduces the daily dose to 100 milligrams and then prescribes that level for the next month. After that, the Daily Value (60 milligrams) is usually enough to avoid a recurrence, he says.

But how much vitamin C should you take if you think you're at risk for sub scurvy? Generally, 200 milligrams a day, says Dr. Basu.

For those who use aspirin frequently, Dr. Basu suggests waiting three hours after taking your aspirin to take vitamin C, giving your body enough time to absorb the aspirin without harming the vitamin C. Taking vitamin C soon after a meal and not on an empty stomach is the answer for people with ulcers. You could also try ester-C, a calcium-based version of vitamin C, to prevent acid-related pain, he advises. This form of vitamin C is available in health food stores, he says.

Shingles

Chickenpox Revisited

Childhood chickenpox is usually no big deal. A rash of itchy blisters, a touch of fever, a couple of days in bed and a few bowls of ice cream, and you're better. You might not even remember having had it.

But the virus that causes chickenpox remains in your body in nerves at the base of your spine, and it may reactivate years later as a searing case of shingles, or herpes zoster, its medical name.

When the virus flares, it moves out along the pathway of whatever nerve is involved, usually on the trunk, neck or face. The nerve becomes inflamed and extremely sensitive to touch. The area where the nerve reaches the skin burns and stings, then erupts in a splay of painful blisters that may last for up to a week or longer.

Shingles isn't something that you can just shrug off. And you shouldn't ignore it, even if you could. Doctors consider it a "pain emergency" and can offer some relief. Some studies also suggest that post-herpetic neuralgia, the lingering pain that sometimes follows an attack of shingles, is less likely to occur if you are treated within 72 hours of the onset of blisters with high doses of drugs that stop the virus from multiplying.

People with infections such as HIV and those taking chemotherapy drugs for cancer or immunity-suppressing drugs to protect organ transplants are at highest risk for a shingles episode. And your risk goes up simply as you get older.

"Most doctors use drugs to treat shingles, and a few drugs now in the pipeline may provide more help than ever," says Stephen Tyring, M.D., Ph.D., professor of dermatology, of microbiology and immunology, and of internal medicine at the University of Texas Medical Branch at Galveston.

Still, some doctors add nutritional therapy to their treatments, hoping to reduce inflammation, protect nerves and restore strong immunity, says Richard Huemer, M.D., a doctor in private practice in Vancouver, Washington, with a special interest in nutrition. Here's what they recommend.

Vitamin B_{12} May Aid Recovering Nerves

It's considered an old-fashioned remedy, and it apparently doesn't work for everyone. But some doctors give their patients with shingles injections of vitamin B_{12}.

"It's true that this treatment has been around for a while, and it's one of the things we do where we can be pretty sure that we are going to get beneficial results," Dr. Huemer says. "Usually, it helps relieve the pain, probably more than anything else we offer, and it seems to shorten the course of the illness."

A study by Indian researchers reported that 21 people with shingles showed "dramatic response," as judged by relief of pain and the speed with which blisters disappeared, starting the second or third day of treatment with vitamin B_{12} injections. What's more, none developed the lingering pain of post-herpetic neuralgia.

Vitamin B_{12} is known to play an important role in nerve function, Dr. Huemer says. "It's needed by nerves to maintain the protective myelin sheath, a thick layer of fatty membranes that wraps around nerves and insulates them," he explains.

Injections of vitamin B_{12} are absorbed more efficiently by the body than supplements. If you're interested in B_{12} injections, you'll need to enlist the aid of your doctor. Doses vary. Dr. Huemer gives up to 2,000 micrograms once or twice a week until symptoms improve, then tapers off the dose. Other doctors may give 500 micrograms daily for six days, then weekly for six weeks.

It's impossible to get this large amount of vitamin B_{12} from foods. Supplements can be helpful at 1,000 to 2,000 micrograms a day, according to Dr. Huemer. Absorption from supplements isn't as beneficial as injections, he explains. This amount of B_{12} is extremely high (the Daily Value is only 6 micrograms) and should be taken only under a doctor's supervision.

Along with vitamin B_{12}, some doctors give injections of folic acid and the rest of the B-complex: thiamin, riboflavin, niacin, vitamin B_6 and the like. "Many of these vitamins work together, and restoring all of them helps people get better faster," says Robert Cathcart, M.D., a doctor in private practice in Los Altos, California.

Vitamin C May Dry Up Blisters

It's not exactly what you would call recent research. But two studies, one from 1949 and another from 1950, suggest that people having shingles outbreaks get substantial relief from intravenous doses of large amounts of vitamin C.

In one of the studies, by researchers in North Carolina, seven of eight people with shingles reported relief from pain within two hours of the first dose, drying of blisters within one day and complete clearing in three days. In the other study, French researchers reported that they were able to cure all 327 people with shingles with three days of intravenous vitamin C.

Vitamin C may help bolster immunity in several different ways, explains Raxit Jariwalla, Ph.D., head of the virology and immunodeficiency programs at the Linus Pauling Institute of Science and Medicine in Palo Alto, California. Additionally, studies show that in large doses, vitamin C can inhibit

Food Factors

The shingles virus, herpes zoster, responds to the same dietary changes used for herpes simplex, the virus that causes cold sores and genital herpes. Here are the details.

Pay attention to amino acids. Research indicates that large doses of lysine, an essential amino acid, inhibit replication of the virus responsible for shingles.

"I recommend 2,000 to 3,000 milligrams of lysine a day during a shingles outbreak, more in stubborn cases," says Robert Cathcart, M.D., a doctor in private practice in Los Altos, California. Although lysine is commonly found in foods such as beef, pork, eggs and tofu, it may be necessary to take a supplement in order to get this high amount. The amino acid appears to have no side effects, since it's taken in high doses for only a short period of time, Dr. Cathcart adds. Lysine supplements are available in health food stores.

Ax arginine-rich foods. These include chocolate, nuts and seeds. Lysine seems to work best when people cut back on arginine, another amino acid, says Dr. Cathcart. That's because lysine may work by blocking the virus's ability to absorb arginine.

replication of certain types of viruses, including those in the herpes family, Dr. Jariwalla says. It can also impair the ability of certain viruses to cause infection, he adds.

How vitamin C exerts its antiviral action isn't known, Dr. Jariwalla says. "It's probably by a multi-targeted effect rather than a single effect," he says.

By virtue of its antioxidant ability, vitamin C can also neutralize inflammation-causing biochemicals that are produced by immune cells as they do battle, Dr. Jariwalla says. That talent may help spare nearby cells that would otherwise be damaged by the battle between immune cells and viruses.

Many of the doctors who prescribe vitamin C for viral infections use it both intravenously, as neutralized sodium ascorbate, and in the largest oral dose that can be tolerated without causing diarrhea, Dr. Cathcart says. "We literally flood the body with vitamin C," he says. This large amount helps keep both blood levels and levels inside cells high enough to dampen inflammation, he explains. He usually gives daily intravenous doses for three to five days, by which time the blisters are gone. "I've never had a case that

Prescriptions for Healing

The main treatment for shingles consists of drug therapy. There are, however, a few nutrients that some doctors recommend.

Nutrient	Daily Amount
Vitamin B_{12}	1,000–2,000 micrograms
Vitamin C	Largest dose tolerated without diarrhea, as prescribed by your doctor
Vitamin E	400–600 international units

MEDICAL ALERT: *If you have shingles, you should be under a doctor's care.*

The amount of vitamin B_{12} recommended here is many times the Daily Value and should be taken only under medical supervision. Depending on the severity of your condition, your doctor may choose to administer B_{12} by injection.

Before prescribing a high dose of vitamin C, your doctor should determine how much of this nutrient you can tolerate. Some people experience diarrhea with amounts of more than 1,200 milligrams daily. For this reason, it's important that you discuss this therapy with your doctor.

If you are taking anticoagulant drugs, you should not take vitamin E supplements.

goes on to post-herpetic neuralgia or neuritis," he says. "This handles it very nicely."

Large amounts of vitamin C can cause diarrhea. For this reason, Dr. Cathcart explains, a doctor should determine how much vitamin C can be tolerated without diarrhea before a high dose is prescribed. In addition, notes Dr. Jariwalla, the amount of vitamin C that a person can tolerate before a laxative effect is experienced increases with the severity of illness or infection. If you'd like to try this therapy for shingles, you should discuss it with your doctor.

While it's impossible to get a high-enough dosage of vitamin C from foods, many doctors suggest that you'd still do well to include citrus fruits in your daily diet. That's because the white rinds and membranes of citrus fruits contain bioflavonoids, chemical compounds related to vitamin C that are also potential immunity boosters and inflammation fighters.

Vitamin E May Ease Long-Irritated Nerves

One of the worst potential consequences of a shingles attack is pain that just won't quit, caused by chronic nerve inflammation. Although it hasn't been studied recently, several older research reports suggest that high doses of vitamin E can help resolve this persistent pain.

One report, published in 1973 by Los Angeles dermatologists Samuel Ayres, M.D., and Richard Mihan, M.D., found "highly gratifying results" with vitamin E used orally and topically. Of 13 people treated, 9 experienced complete or almost complete relief from pain, 2 were moderately improved, and 2 were slightly improved. Two of those who experienced complete or almost complete relief from pain had had post-shingles pain the longest: one for 13 years, the other for 19 years.

Vitamin E is incorporated into the fatty membranes of all cells, including nerve cells, which are protected by the myelin sheath, the thick wrapping of fatty membranes mentioned earlier, explains Dr. Huemer. There, vitamin E helps shield cells from the damage that occurs during a viral attack. Vitamin E can neutralize harmful biochemicals that are produced by immune cells as they ward off viruses. It may help stop the damage that can lead to lingering inflammation, Dr. Huemer says.

Dr. Ayres and Dr. Mihan used high doses of vitamin E in their study: 1,200 to 1,600 international units daily. Dr. Huemer simply recommends 400 international units a day. Consider medical supervision for doses of more than 600 international units daily.

Order the Complete Package

Vitamin E, along with other nutrients, stimulates immunity in other ways that may be helpful to people with shingles, especially those who seem to have weakened immunity, says Dr. Cathcart. "Many of my patients with herpes zoster have low immunity, so I work with an array of nutrients to rebuild their systems," he explains. These nutrients include vitamin A, the B-complex vitamins, zinc, selenium and others. For the full story on boosting your immune system, see page 320.

Smog Exposure

Protection from Pollution

From campfires to jet engine exhaust, where there's civilization, there's smog, a combination of noxious chemicals, light-as-air particles and moisture that hangs in a yellowish gray haze over cities. Smog not only makes your eyes sting and lungs twitch but can even nibble the nose off a marble statue of Ulysses S. Grant.

Smog contains a long lineup of chemical nasties, including ozone, nitrogen dioxide, sulfur dioxide and tiny particles of everything from asbestos to soot, that can settle deep in the lungs and cause general havoc. "Smog is a soup that contains a lot of stuff, and people inhale everything that's in it, a whole bunch of toxic chemicals," says Daniel Menzel, M.D., Ph.D., professor in the Department of Community and Environmental Medicine at the University of California, Irvine. "They're a significant threat to people's health."

A high concentration of or long exposure to any one of these chemicals can cause shortness of breath, wheezing, coughing, bronchitis, pneumonia, headaches, inability to concentrate, chest pain and, in some cases, lung cancer.

Smog Hurts

Breathing smog changes the way that lung cells do business, Dr. Menzel explains. In some people, the lungs become supersensitive, reacting to smog exposure with inflammation, bronchial spasms, coughing, asthma attacks or increased production of mucus.

Smog can also make lung cells vulnerable to attack by bacteria and viruses that are always in the air. Smog can kill cells, making the lungs less efficient at doing their job of gas exchange (absorbing oxygen and releasing carbon dioxide). And some of the chemicals in smog can cause genetic mutations in cells that lead to cancer in the lungs or nasal passages.

Many of the harmful interactions between the noxious substances in smog and lung cells happen during a chemical process known as oxidation. This is the same process that causes butter to turn rancid and iron to rust. Oxidation, as you might guess, is a chemical reaction that requires oxygen in

Food Factors

Antioxidant nutrients are your surest protection against damage from chemical exposure. But these additional dietary adjustments may help, experts say.

Scratch the saturated fat. Researchers at the National Cancer Institute in Rockville, Maryland, reported a strong association between saturated fat intake and adenocarcinoma, a type of lung cancer that is most common in nonsmokers. They found that women who consumed the greatest amounts of fat, typically from hamburgers, cheeseburgers, meat loaf, cheeses and cheese spreads, hot dogs, ice cream and sausage, had six times the risk of lung cancer of those who ate the least fat.

Think raw. Researchers at Yale University found that the risk of lung cancer among men and women eating lots of salad greens and other raw vegetables, along with fresh fruits, was almost half of the risk seen among people not putting these foods on their plates.

order to take place, and there's plenty of oxygen in the lungs. During oxidation, free radicals, which are unstable molecules of harmful chemicals, snatch electrons from the healthy molecules that compose the cells in order to balance themselves. This starts a chain reaction of electron stealing. The end result: serious damage to cells.

The best way to deal with smog, of course, is to avoid it as much as possible. Don't run along heavily trafficked roads. Aerobic exercise makes you breathe deeply, so you draw pollutants deep into your lungs. And don't smoke cigarettes. Smoking exposes your lungs to some of the same toxins found in smog, plus it makes your lungs more sensitive to smog's effects.

If you can't avoid smog entirely, you may want to protect yourself by taking nutrients that provide a measure of internal pollution protection: vitamins A, C and E, beta-carotene and selenium.

Vitamin E Equals Protection

Vitamin E, found in wheat germ, certain vegetables, nuts, seeds and vegetable oils, is well-known both for its ability to enhance the immune system and as an antioxidant. Antioxidants offer their own electrons to free radicals, disarming those renegade molecules and protecting healthy molecules from damage.

"Vitamin E is the strongest antioxidant found in the body," Dr. Menzel explains. "It gets incorporated into cell membranes, where it shields cells from harm. It helps stop the chain reaction that starts with exposure to smog and so is very effective at limiting the amount of damage done to cells."

Researchers at Yale University School of Medicine have shown just how well vitamin E does its job in the lungs. They found that nonsmokers had only half of the normal risk of developing lung cancer if they took vitamin E supplements.

"In our study, we weren't able to determine the amounts of vitamin E that people took, but the protective effect was apparent, and it was almost as strong as the protection offered by eating lots of fruits and vegetables," says Susan Taylor Mayne, Ph.D., a research scientist in the Department of Epidemiology and Public Health at Yale University School of Medicine and the study's main researcher.

Prescriptions for Healing

For healthy lungs, avoid smog-filled areas and supplement your diet with these nutrients, which some doctors recommend as protection against air pollution.

Nutrient	Daily Amount
Beta-carotene	25,000 international units
Selenium	50–200 micrograms
Vitamin A	5,000 international units
Vitamin C	1,200 milligrams
Vitamin E	600 international units

MEDICAL ALERT: *Selenium in doses exceeding 100 micrograms daily can be toxic and should be taken only under medical supervision.*

If you are taking anticoagulant drugs, you should not take vitamin E supplements.

Doctors who recommend vitamin E suggest that you take 600 international units a day. This amount is considered safe, but it's more than you can get from even the best food sources. Research indicates that the Daily Value of vitamin E, 30 international units, is not enough to offer optimum smog protection, Dr. Menzel says.

Orange Aid for Air Pollution

Vitamin C is another well-known antioxidant. Like vitamin E, it helps stop free radical chain reactions.

Vitamin C helps maintain healthy lung function both in the general population and in people with asthma, say researchers at Harvard Medical School. They found that people who were getting at least 200 milligrams of vitamin C (about three oranges' worth) a day did best on tests that measured their lungs' capacity to expand and draw in oxygen.

"This study demonstrates, for the first time, that high dietary intake of vitamin C–rich foods is associated with improved levels of pulmonary function," says study co-author Scott Weiss, M.D., associate professor of medicine and associate physician in the Channing Laboratory at Brigham and Women's Hospital in Boston. "Getting enough vitamin C may prove to play an important role in reducing your risk of chronic lung disease."

Here again, usual dietary amounts may not be adequate protection, Dr. Menzel says. Researchers who recommend nutritional therapy to offset the effects of smog exposure suggest that you get about 1,200 milligrams of vitamin C a day. That amount is considered to be within the safe range, but it does require taking supplements.

Vitamins C and E work together in the lungs, and Yale University researchers have shown that a combination of the two helps keep lung tissue healthy. In one study, people who took daily supplements of 1,500 milligrams of vitamin C and 1,200 international units of vitamin E built up levels of a protective protein that prevents enzymes released during inflammation from destroying the lung's elastic properties. People with emphysema, for instance, who've lost lung elasticity from years of cigarette smoking, struggle for every breath.

Treat Your Lungs to a Carrot

The research evidence that's piling up about the protective effects of beta-carotene looks more and more like a cornucopia of fruits and vegetables.

Those that contain beta-carotene, the yellow pigment found in carrots, cantalope and other orange and yellow fruits and vegetables, apparently help shield lungs from air pollution. "In population studies, foods rich in beta-carotene seem to offer strong protection against lung cancer, even among nonsmokers," says Dr. Mayne.

Unfortunately, a highly publicized 1994 study of male Finnish smokers found that 20 milligrams (about 33,000 international units) of supplemental beta-carotene a day did not reduce the incidence of lung cancer. Does that mean you shouldn't take beta-carotene to help protect your lungs from smog?

Some researchers feel that this study tested amounts of beta-carotene that were too little and given too late. They believe that there are still plenty of good reasons to get enough of this nutrient, Dr. Menzel says. Both beta-carotene and vitamin A (beta-carotene is converted to vitamin A in the body) help keep cells on track as they grow and divide and so help prevent genetic mutations that can lead to cancer, he explains.

Most experts recommend getting beta-carotene from foods rather than supplements, as foods contain many other substances that may also be important for cancer prevention. Dr. Menzel suggests that people get about 25,000 international units of beta-carotene a day from foods or supplements. That's roughly the amount found in one cup of chopped, cooked spinach, 1¼ large carrots or 2½ large sweet potatoes. Some doctors also recommend taking the Daily Value of vitamin A, which is 5,000 international units.

Selenium Shields Cells

Medical researchers round out their antipollution prescriptions with the mineral selenium. "Selenium is needed in the body to activate glutathione peroxidase, an important antioxidant enzyme that helps keep lung tissue elastic," Dr. Menzel explains.

Doctors recommend getting from 50 to 200 micrograms of selenium daily from foods and supplements. Studies show that most people get about 108 micrograms a day from foods. (Rich sources of selenium include grains, seeds and fish.) So it's probably not necessary to take a supplement. If you do take a supplement, don't exceed 100 micrograms daily without medical supervision. In high amounts, selenium can be toxic.

Smoking

Damage Control while Kicking the Habit

Unless you live on another planet, you know the evils of smoking. And if you're a smoker, you've likely tried to quit more than once. And you plan to try again. That's good.

While kicking the habit is your number one priority, there are measures you can take nutritionally to block smoking's path of destruction while you work on "butting out" once and for all. For a little motivation, it helps to first understand how cigarette smoke damages your body.

A Radical Habit

Though all of the harmful reactions caused by smoking are not completely understood, researchers agree that the lion's share of smokers' ailments are the result of free radicals. Free radicals are unstable molecules that are missing electrons. They pillage your body's healthy molecules for replacement electrons, leaving more free radicals and damaged cells and tissues in their wake. This process is called oxidation, and it's what makes iron rust and fruit turn brown. And scientists are beginning to believe that oxidation is what makes people age.

Though free radicals are formed during everyday functions such as breathing, environmental stress factors such as smoking dramatically accelerate their production. In fact, each puff on a cigarette generates millions of free radicals, making smokers much more susceptible than nonsmokers to the ravages of oxidative tissue damage.

To fight this free radical onslaught, you need a strong defense. And according to research, one of the best defenses consists of nutrients known as antioxidants, most notably vitamins C and E and beta-carotene. Antioxidants act as your body's kamikaze fighters, protecting your body's healthy molecules by sacrificing their own electrons to neutralize hostile free radical invaders.

Though antioxidants aren't miracle cures and certainly shouldn't lure you into a false sense of security about smoking, these nutrients can help stave off smoking-related damage while you're kicking the habit. Here's what experts recommend.

Food Factors

When it comes to smoking, the health advice is clear: Don't do it. But if you're still lighting up, one of the best ways to help protect yourself is by improving your diet. Here's how.

Eat fruits and veggies. "The evidence overwhelmingly shows that people who eat high levels of fruits and vegetables have lower rates of cancer," says Eric Rimm, Sc.D., assistant professor in the Department of Epidemiology at Harvard School of Public Health.

In fact, in a study in Japan, where cigarette consumption per capita is among the highest in the world and the incidence of lung cancer is among the lowest, researchers evaluated the effects of eating raw vegetables, green vegetables (especially lettuce and cabbage) and fruits in 282 smokers. They found that the relative risk of lung cancer was markedly decreased in those who included fruits and raw vegetables in their daily fare.

Experts recommend that for optimum protection, smokers eat seven half-cup servings of fruits and vegetables every day.

Go easy on acids. If you're trying to quit via a nicotine replacement product such as nicotine gum or a nicotine patch, then steer clear of orange juice, grapefruit juice and other acidic beverages, says Thomas M. Cooper, D.D.S., professor of oral health sciences at the University of Kentucky in Lexington and co-author of *The Cooper/Clayton Method to Stop Smoking*. "By making your urine more acidic, you clear your body of nicotine faster, which is what you don't want if you're trying to minimize withdrawal with a nicotine replacement product," he explains.

E Is Essential for Smokers

When it comes to protecting your body from smoking's nasty side effects, vitamin E, an antioxidant found in sunflower seeds, sweet potatoes and kale, is a top performer.

One of vitamin E's most important functions for smokers is slowing the progression of atherosclerosis, a condition in which the coronary arteries harden from deposits of cholesterol, calcium and scar tissue, gradually restricting blood flow and leading to heart disease. Studies show that before atherosclerosis can occur, LDL cholesterol, the "bad" kind, has to undergo oxidation-related changes that allow it to deposit on artery walls. Vitamin E helps prevent those changes.

"Our data from two separate studies of men and women suggest that both smokers and nonsmokers taking vitamin E supplements reduce their risk of heart disease by 30 to 40 percent," says Eric Rimm, Sc.D., assistant professor in the Department of Epidemiology at Harvard School of Public Health.

Additionally, investigators believe that vitamin E's ability to scavenge free radicals can protect tissues from smoke irritation and discourage the cell mutation that marks cancer and other tobacco-associated chronic diseases.

For optimum effects, experts recommend getting 100 to 200 international units of vitamin E a day. Since you would have to eat between 10 and 20 cups of foods such as chopped kale and diced sweet potatoes to reach that amount, supplements are generally called for.

Beta-Carotene Protection

Ever notice how Popeye is able to puff away on that pipe, yet never suffer from the smoking-related ailments typically seen in a man his age? That may be the result of his penchant for spinach, a vegetable rich in beta-carotene, which appears to have protective, immunity-building effects against cancer.

But before you start popping beta-carotene, you should know that although supplementation is considered okay by most experts, doctors say it's even better to eat beta-carotene-rich foods such as spinach and other dark green, leafy vegetables as well as cantaloupe, carrots and other orange and yellow fruits and vegetables. Why? Because studies show that beta-carotene is good, but it's probably not the whole story.

On the one hand, myriad small studies have found positive results from beta-carotene supplementation in smokers. Canadian researchers, for example, found that 25 smokers experienced significant reductions in oxidation-related damage after receiving 20 milligrams (about 33,000 international units) of beta-carotene daily for just four weeks.

But in one large study from Finland of 29,133 male heavy smokers between 50 and 69 years of age, those who received 20 milligrams (about 33,000 international units) of beta-carotene for five to eight years not only didn't reap any benefits but actually experienced a higher incidence of lung cancer.

Which study should we believe? Both, says Jeffrey Blumberg, Ph.D., associate director and chief of the antioxidants research laboratory at the Jean Mayer USDA Human Nutrition Research Center on Aging at Tufts University in Boston. Dr. Blumberg contends that the Finnish study represents what we already know: "You can't undo a lifetime of damage by taking a vitamin pill for five years.

"That population was at extraordinarily high risk," says Dr. Blumberg. "They smoked an average of a pack a day for 35 years. Most of them were overweight. They had high cholesterol. They had moderate to high alcohol consumption. It would have been a public health nightmare if the study had worked, because it would have said 'Smoke and drink and eat all you want. This pill can turn around all of the damage.' "

Actually, the group in the Finnish study that did not receive supplements also taught us something, says Dr. Blumberg. "Among the people who weren't supplemented, those who had the highest blood levels of beta-carotene had the lower risk of lung cancer," he says.

The bottom line? Dr. Blumberg recommends that everyone, smokers and nonsmokers, get between 16,500 and 50,000 international units of beta-carotene daily.

Finally, it's important to remember that beta-carotene is just one of many related substances called carotenoids that protect the body from cell damage, says Dr. Rimm. "All of the carotenoids function a little differently, so getting beta-carotene from fruits and vegetables covers a lot more bases than just taking a supplement." It's best to strive for getting as much of your 16,500 to 50,000 international units a day as possible from foods. If you're having trouble meeting your needs in this way, then talk to your doctor about supplementation.

Vitamin C for Healthy Cells and Sperm

It's a joke among male smokers that they don't feel as bad about smoking when they buy packs with the "Do not smoke while pregnant" warning on the side panel. Well, according to researchers, it may be time for male smokers to get a warning of their own.

Studies have found a connection linking smoking, low levels of ascorbic acid (vitamin C) and sperm abnormalities. These abnormalities could play roles not only in infertility in men but also in birth defects and childhood cancer in their offspring, the studies show.

"We've known that many gene mutations come through the male line, but since women carry the babies, most of the birth defect studies are done on women," says Bruce Ames, Ph.D., professor of biochemistry and molecular biology and director of the National Institute of Environmental Health Sciences Center at the University of California, Berkeley. "We're looking

Prescriptions for Healing

Let's say it again: If you smoke, the only way to truly prevent smoking-related diseases is to quit. In the meantime, however, some doctors recommend these nutrients to help preserve your health.

Nutrient	Daily Amount
Beta-carotene	16,500–50,000 international units
B-complex supplement containing . . .	
Biotin	300 micrograms
Folic acid	400 micrograms
Niacin	20 milligrams
Pantothenic acid	10 milligrams
Riboflavin	1.7 milligrams
Thiamin	1.5 milligrams
Vitamin B_6	2 milligrams
Vitamin B_{12}	6 micrograms
Calcium	1,500 milligrams
Vitamin C	180–2,000 milligrams
Vitamin E	100–200 international units

Plus a multivitamin/mineral supplement containing the Daily Values of all essential vitamins and minerals

MEDICAL ALERT: *Some people may experience diarrhea when taking vitamin C in doses that exceed 1,200 milligrams daily.*

If you are taking anticoagulant drugs, you should not take vitamin E supplements.

into the effects of paternal smoking on sperm damage, and the effects of antioxidant depletion are significant."

Smokers must ingest two to three times the daily intake of vitamin C recommended for nonsmokers, or about 180 milligrams, just to maintain comparable levels of ascorbic acid, says Dr. Ames. He has also found that as a group, smokers tend to make their deficiencies worse by not eating enough vitamin C–rich foods.

While studying the vitamin C consumption of 22 smokers and 27 nonsmokers, Dr. Ames and his colleagues found that the smokers consumed less vitamin C than the nonsmokers. In addition, the level of oxidative damage in the sperm was 52 percent higher in the smokers than in the nonsmokers.

Of course, sperm are not alone in their need for vitamin C. The rest of your body, whether you're male or female, needs it, too. And because smokers have too little vitamin C in their bodies and need more vitamin C to fight free radical damage, experts suggest that they take much more than nonsmokers: up to 2,000 milligrams a day, if they are older and smoke heavily. Just keep in mind that the Daily Value for vitamin C is only 60 milligrams. Higher amounts are considered safe but may cause diarrhea in some people.

Calcium May Help Prevent Bone Loss

Research shows that people, especially women, who smoke accelerate the bone loss that occurs naturally with age, putting them at greater risk for osteoporosis, a condition of brittle, easily fractured bones.

In fact, a study done at the University of Melbourne in Australia looked at 41 pairs of female twins between 27 and 73 years of age in which one of the twins smoked and the other did not. The researchers reported that by the time women reach menopause, those who smoke a pack a day throughout adulthood have an average bone density deficit of 5 to 10 percent compared with those who are smoke-free.

Though the only surefire way to stem this bone deterioration is to snuff your cigarette habit, some doctors recommend stepping up your calcium intake in the meantime to nourish your bones. And while it will help to increase your intake of calcium-filled foods, including low-fat dairy products and certain vegetables such as broccoli, the best way to get the 1,500 milligrams that experts recommend is through supplements.

Better Body Function with B-Complex

Because the B vitamins are essential for maintaining physical and mental fitness and healthy skin, eyes, nerves and tissues—things that are deteriorated by smoking—many experts also recommend taking supplements of the B-complex vitamins.

Especially important, say researchers, is folic acid, a nutrient that is often deficient in smokers and one that your lungs love. Studies have shown that increased folic acid intake can lessen symptoms of bronchitis as well as reduce the number of abnormal or precancerous bronchial cells in smokers. Plus inadequate folic acid intake has been linked to increased susceptibility to cancerous changes in the lungs of smokers.

"Not only does smoking deplete the B vitamins, but smokers' diets often aren't as good as those of nonsmokers, so smokers don't get enough of these nutrients to begin with," says nutritionist James Scala, Ph.D., author of *If You Can't/Won't Stop Smoking*. Dr. Scala recommends that smokers take a B-complex supplement that contains the Daily Values of all of the B vitamins.

Finish Off with a Multivitamin

"Because smoking depletes the body of all vitamins, smokers absolutely need to take a multivitamin/mineral supplement on top of their specific nutritional supplements," says Dr. Scala.

He also stresses the importance of smokers' adding more fruits and vegetables to their diets. "Smokers generally eat poor diets, which contributes to their nutritional deficiencies," he says.

Sunburn

Protecting Yourself from Harmful Rays

You're all ready for a day at the beach. You have a blanket, a radio and a big bottle of baby oil . . . oops. Nix the oil. You've heard the warnings about ultraviolet rays and skin cancer, so it's on with the sunscreen instead, right?

Right. But somehow, whether it's from snoozing too long in the midday warmth or forgetting to reapply your lotion after a dip in the ocean, you, like most people, probably still manage an occasional burn. Maybe not one of the Maine lobster scorches that you got as a kid, but a fairly vivid shade of pink nonetheless. Worse yet, studies show that even if you never forget your sunscreen, unless you block out 100 percent of the ultraviolet rays, lolling in the sun will damage your skin whether you burn or not.

What's a sun worshiper to do—carry a parasol? That certainly helps, say the experts. Limiting your time in the sun, especially during midday hours, is absolutely essential. And if you want some extra protection, take your vitamins and minerals. According to research, oral supplements of vitamin E and selenium, as well as topical applications of vitamins C and E, can give your sunscreen a boost by partially preventing the skin damage that occurs once you've been exposed.

How Sunburn Does Damage

To understand how vitamins and minerals can help shield you from sun damage, it helps to know how that damage comes about in the first place.

Sunlight exposes skin to two types of ultraviolet rays: UVA and UVB. UVB rays are high-intensity rays absorbed by the surface of the skin. They are the primary cause of sunburn and immediate skin damage. UVA rays are of lower intensity, but they penetrate below the skin's surface, causing long-term damage such as premature wrinkles.

Both types do significant damage by forming free radicals, unstable molecules that steal electrons from your body's healthy molecules to stabilize themselves. Though some free radicals are formed during everyday functions such as breathing, environmental stress factors such as sun exposure create additional droves of them.

Although you have natural defenses against free radicals generated by sun exposure, they often aren't enough. Sunscreen does a good job of protecting you, but many brands still block predominantly UVB rays. Even those that block both UVB and UVA rays generally allow some exposure. Look for a sunscreen labeled "broad-spectrum coverage," suggests Douglas Darr, Ph.D., director of technology development at the North Carolina Biotechnology Center in Research Triangle Park. And look for the ingredients oxybenzone and methoxycinnamate, which absorb some UVA rays. Remember that only clothing and zinc oxide totally block UVB and UVA rays.

Fortunately for your skin and your body, there are chemical substances that mop up free radicals by offering them electrons, sparing healthy molecules from harm. These substances, known as antioxidants, include vitamins C and E and the mineral selenium. Sun exposure, however, quickly depletes your skin's supply of these antioxidants.

Although you can get some protection through oral supplementation of these nutrients, researchers agree that the best protection generally comes from topical application. Currently, you have to apply a separate cream along with your sunscreen, but some researchers hope that future sunscreens will have the nutrients built right in.

"No one is proposing that vitamins will ever replace sunscreen, but they

Food Factors

Although there are no foods that you can eat to protect your skin from the sun, there are a few that can add fuel to the fire. Here's what you might want to avoid before a day at the shore.

Don't be a silly rabbit. While you certainly shouldn't stop eating carrots, these vegetables, along with celery, parsley, parsnips and limes, contain psoralens, chemicals that may make you unusually sensitive to the sun.

"Though most people would have to eat huge amounts of these foods before they would have problems, some people are really sensitive to these chemicals. For them, the effects can be quite nasty," says Douglas Darr, Ph.D., director of technology development at the North Carolina Biotechnology Center in Research Triangle Park.

And even if you're not psoralen-sensitive, you should wash your hands after handling these fruits and vegetables, because anyone's skin can be more susceptible to burning after direct contact with the chemical.

can make sunsreen better. It would also be nice to replace some of the chemicals in sunscreen with vitamins," says Dr. Darr. "Right now we're soaking in all of these chemicals that are photodecomposing into unknown compounds. And because there are no lifetime studies, we can't make the blanket statement that they are completely safe."

Here's what the research says about adding vitamins and minerals to your sun protection regimen.

The Vitamin C Solution

Vitamin C is well-known for its role as a collagen (skin tissue) builder when used topically. It's also a pretty impressive sun protectant, say the experts. But don't get it confused with sunscreen, says John C. Murray, M.D., assistant professor of medicine at Duke University Medical Center in Durham, North Carolina. Vitamin C creams can't absorb ultraviolet rays.

"Sunscreen is a chemical that acts as a shield and absorbs ultraviolet light, so you're not as red," he explains. "Vitamin C is a photoprotectant. It possibly works by scavenging the free radicals caused by sun exposure."

Also, unlike sunscreen, you can't wash off vitamin C, says Dr. Murray.

"Once you put it on, it's soaked into your skin," he says. "You can't rub it off."

To measure vitamin C's effectiveness, researchers at Duke University Medical Center studied ten fair-skinned individuals. They found that when the volunteers applied a 10 percent vitamin C solution, the amount of ultraviolet light needed for them to burn increased by an average of 22 percent for nine of them. And once they did burn, half of the volunteers experienced much less severe burns than they would have without the solution.

So can you get the same protection from eating a lot of oranges?

No, because you just can't eat enough oranges, says Sheldon Pinnell, M.D., chief of dermatology at Duke University Medical Center. Dr. Pinnell helped develop a 10 percent vitamin C lotion called Cellex-C. The preparation provides far more—20 to 40 times more—vitamin C to the skin than you could achieve by ingesting the vitamin, he says.

Don't try spraying your skin with orange juice, either; you'll just make yourself sticky, says Dr. Murray. "Vitamin C is very unstable," he says. "It needs to be in a special preparation to stay effective."

Cellex-C is available without a prescription from dermatologists, plastic surgeons and licensed aestheticians (full-service beauty salon operators) and by mail order from Cellex-C Distribution, 2631 Commerce Street, Suite C, Dallas, TX 75226 (1-800-423-5592). For best results, apply the lotion daily and after a sunburn. For sunbathing, apply along with sunscreen 15 to 30 minutes before sun exposure. Used alone, Cellex-C is not an appropriate beach product.

Extra Protection with Vitamin E

Like vitamin C, vitamin E is a free radical scavenger. But unlike vitamin C, vitamin E is being recommended by researchers for after-sun use, rather than pre-sun use, to soothe your skin and prevent a burn after exposure.

In fact, it's even effective if you apply it a half-day later, say researchers at the University of Western Ontario in London, Ontario, but it's better to do it as soon as possible. In studies using laboratory animals, the researchers found that vitamin E acetate, which converts to vitamin E in the body, prevented inflammation, skin sensitivity and skin damage when applied up to eight hours following UVB exposure.

"At this time, I wouldn't recommend that people apply vitamin E before sun exposure, because when vitamin E is exposed to ultraviolet light it produces a free radical, which in itself can be damaging," says John R. Trevithick, Ph.D., professor in the Department of Biochemistry at the University of Western Ontario. "But if you fall asleep in the sun and start to get a sunburn that you want to prevent from getting worse, vitamin E oil is a good idea."

Vitamin E can also work from the inside out. As an oral supplement, it can significantly reduce the inflammation and skin damage caused by sun exposure, says Karen E. Burke, M.D., Ph.D., a dermatologic surgeon and dermatologist in private practice in New York City. If you are inadvertently

Prescriptions for Healing

Unlike the usual prescriptions, wearing your nutrients is often better than taking them when it comes to sunburn. Here are the doses that some doctors say work best against sun damage.

Nutrient	Daily Amount/Application
Oral	
Selenium	50–200 micrograms (l-selenomethionine)
Vitamin E	400 international units (d-alpha-tocopherol), taken before sun exposure
	2,000 international units, taken as 5 divided doses for 1 or 2 days after sun exposure
Topical	
Vitamin C	10% lotion (Cellex-C)
Vitamin E	5%–100% cream or oil, applied after sun exposure
Zinc oxide	As an ointment

MEDICAL ALERT: Selenium can be toxic in high amounts. For this reason, doctors recommend that doses exceeding 100 micrograms daily be taken only under medical supervision.

If you are taking anticoagulant drugs, you should not take oral vitamin E supplements.

Vitamin E creams and oils contain the ester form of the nutrient, which can cause allergic reactions in some people.

exposed to sun, take a lot of vitamin E: five capsules of 400 international units each for one to two days, says Dr. Burke. For optimum protection, Dr. Burke recommends taking daily supplements of 400 international units of vitamin E in the form of d-alpha-tocopherol. (It's okay to take oral vitamin E before you go out in the sun.)

To boost your intake of vitamin E, try cooking with sunflower oil or safflower oil and adding more nuts, whole grains and wheat germ to your daily fare. Vitamin E oil and vitamin E–fortified creams can be bought over the counter in drugstores. These products contain the ester form of vitamin E, which can cause allergies, and they're not very effective in reducing sun damage, says Dr. Burke.

Selenium Also Shines

Like vitamins C and E, the mineral selenium can quench free radicals at the cellular level, says Dr. Burke, thereby reducing the inflammation and skin damage associated with too much sun.

Although she's hoping that a cream will soon be available that can be used as an adjunct to sunscreen, Dr. Burke says that in the meantime, you can get some of the benefits by taking selenium supplements.

For best results, she suggests that people take 50 to 200 micrograms of selenium in the form of l-selenomethionine, depending on where you live and your family history of cancer. Superior food sources of selenium include fish such as tuna and salmon as well as cabbage. Selenium can be toxic in doses exceeding 100 micrograms daily; such high amounts should be taken only under medical supervision.

Zinc Oxide: The Lifeguard's Standby

You know the white stuff that lifeguards wear on their noses? It's zinc oxide, and it may look funny, but it's a great skin protectant.

"In this case, the zinc is acting not as a micronutrient but as a physical blocker of ultraviolet light," explains Norman Levine, M.D., chief of dermatology and professor at the University of Arizona College of Medicine in Tucson. "And it does a terrific job."

If you don't like the white, zinc oxide is now being broken down into nearly invisible particles and put into sunblocks. It's also available in designer colors, for those who like their zinc on the wild side.

And remember, since zinc works as a topical barrier, upping your dietary zinc may make you healthier, but it won't protect your skin.

Surgery

Minding Your Mending

No doubt about it: Surgery is a major insult to your body. Even though it's done with the best of intentions and in a clean environment, your body needs to put out extra effort to mend from even minor surgery. And while you're recuperating, you're more vulnerable than usual to pneumonia, bedsores, urinary tract infections and other kinds of infections.

That's why good nutrition is vital both before and after surgery. "It gives your body the building blocks to fight off infection, replenish lost blood and mend tissues, all things that can help you heal as quickly as possible with the least pain and discomfort," explains Ray C. Wunderlich, Jr., M.D., author of *Natural Alternatives to Antibiotics* and a doctor in St. Petersburg, Florida, who practices nutritional/preventive medicine and health promotion.

Medical experts are well aware that every single nutrient your body normally needs is also needed when you're facing surgery, including everything from calories and protein to copper and vitamin B_6. "Keep in mind that every person's condition when undergoing surgery is different, so the types of vitamins and minerals that your doctor prescribes for you, if any, will depend on your own particular case," says Joanne Curran-Celentano, R.D., Ph.D., professor of nutritional sciences at the University of New Hampshire in Durham. "Because of the wide range of problems and conditions surrounding surgery, it is recommended that anyone who is about to undergo surgery check with his doctor before taking any kind of supplementation."

Not all doctors have the same approach to nutritional therapy and surgery. If you are facing surgery and want to pay special attention to nutrients that might be helpful, you'll have to find a doctor who uses methods that you feel most comfortable with.

Here are a few key nutrients that some doctors believe are important for getting your body on the high road to healing.

Vitamin C Speeds Healing

Doctors know that any kind of trauma, including surgery, can pull the plug on your vitamin C stores. After surgery, blood levels of vitamin C drop

Taking Your Supplements to the Hospital

You do everything possible to stay healthy, including taking supplements. So when you have to go into the hospital for surgery, you take your supplements with you. But the next thing you know, someone is telling you not to take them, and you're left wondering why.

The deal is this: "You just can't take whatever pills you were taking outside the hospital, even if they are vitamins," explains Alexandra Gekas, executive director of the National Society for Patient Representation and Consumer Affairs of the National Hospital Association. "Vitamins are considered medications, and in the hospital, you need your doctor's approval for every medication you take."

So how do you operate in this environment? "It's in your best interest to keep your doctor and other caregivers as informed as possible about what you're taking, in order to avoid any possible complications," says Gekas. Before your surgery, she suggests, get your doctor's approval for whatever supplements you want to take. Ask him to write his approval on your hospital chart. Then if anyone questions your taking them, refer that person to your chart.

Do note, though, that orders for "nothing by mouth" prior to surgery apply to everything—including supplements.

rapidly. And it's no secret that a vitamin C deficiency makes wounds heal slower. Delayed healing was noted hundreds of years ago in sailors with scurvy, a mystery disease at the time that turned out to be nothing more than severe vitamin C deficiency. "Today, it's more likely that people simply won't be getting enough vitamin C for optimum healing," Dr. Wunderlich says.

Many studies have shown that vitamin C is essential for the body to produce wound-healing collagen, which provides the basic structure for many tissues, including skin, bone and blood vessels. Vitamin C is also needed for the skin to produce elastin, a tissue that lets wounds stretch without breaking.

Vitamin C also helps maintain a healthy immune system, vital for anyone who's undergoing surgery, Dr. Wunderlich says.

One study, by Russian researchers, found that people who had gallbladder surgery who received 200 to 250 milligrams of supplemental vitamin C a

Finding Healthy Hospital Fare

Is hospital food really so bad? The answer you get depends on whom you ask. "It's not as bad as it used to be, but at most hospitals, there's still room for improvement," says Don Miller, R.D., a San Diego dietitian and chef who helps hospital kitchen staffs make their foods tasty and attractive.

These days, any hospital can come up with a low-fat, low-sodium, diabetic or vegetarian meal without having to order out, Miller says. The problem is, sometimes it just doesn't taste good. Miller reports that new trends in the hospital industry are changing the way that foods look and taste.

Instead of finding mushy string beans, wilted lettuce or processed meats, you might find steamed vegetables, a hearty romaine lettuce salad or brown rice, Miller says. And you can select from items on your menu to come up with the most nutrient-packed choices.

Look for these staples, offered in most hospitals: yogurt, whole-wheat bread, spinach, carrots, broccoli, orange or grapefruit juice, V-8 or vegetable juice, oatmeal, bran cereal, fruits, beans, skim milk, stewed prunes, baked potatoes, baked or broiled fish and chicken.

If you're concerned that a family member or friend who's in the hospital isn't eating, visit at mealtime to help, suggests Melanie Roberts Afrikian, a nutrition consultant in private practice in Wakefield, Massachusetts. "If you can't do that, ask the nursing staff to make that sure they help," she says.

day were able to leave the hospital one or two days earlier compared with people who simply got their vitamin C from foods.

At most hospitals, you're expected to get your vitamin C from foods such as citrus juices and fruits. Eight ounces of orange juice, for instance, offers about 124 milligrams, while one orange has about 70 milligrams.

Some doctors, however, recommend amounts of vitamin C that are much higher than you normally obtain from foods alone. Dr Wunderlich believes this to be especially important when you're recovering from surgery.

He tells his patients that "if you can take 1,000 milligrams of buffered or esterified vitamin C every eight hours for two weeks before and several weeks after surgery, you'll most likely be able to keep the vitamin C in your blood at a level that promotes optimum healing." Some people experience diarrhea and other digestive discomforts from such high levels of vitamin C. Buffered vitamin C and esterified vitamin C (a slow-release form) are easier on the stomach, says Dr. Wunderlich. Vitamin C can interfere with the results of certain diagnostic blood and urine tests, however, so it's important that you discuss supplementation with your doctor.

He also recommends 1,000 milligrams of bioflavonoids a day to some of his patients. These chemical compounds are related to vitamin C and are often found in the same foods as the vitamin, especially citrus fruits. Dr. Wunderlich maintains that bioflavonoids can help maintain blood vessel strength and control inflammation.

Food Factors

Protein, fiber and other components of foods are just as important to recuperation as vitamins and minerals. Here's what the doctor orders.

Find a friend in fiber. As people recovering from surgery know, moving the bowels is a much-anticipated event, and it's one that has to be initiated if it doesn't happen on its own. "That's why fiber is so important," says Joanne Driver, R.D., a dietitian in the critical care and surgical units of Marquette General Hospital in Michigan.

"I suggest prunes, prune juice, fruits, vegetables, legumes, whole grains—the kind of fiber that is beneficial in preventing constipation," she says. If your bowels need more help, try psyllium, another kind of fiber (found in Metamucil and similar bulk laxatives).

Keep on sippin'. Some experts recommend drinking the equivalent of six to eight eight-ounce glasses of fluids a day unless your doctor tells you that you need to restrict fluids. It helps prevent dehydration, helps the fiber work better and flushes out the bladder, which is prone to infection if you've had a urinary catheter.

Eat light and eat often. People recovering from surgery naturally prefer small, light meals, and that's what patients should be served, Driver says. "Don't try to coax someone to fill up on a regular-size meal; it will just make him uncomfortable."

Serve five or six mini-meals a day, she suggests. Old favorites include whole-wheat toast, custard, pudding, yogurt, fruits, sherbet, soup, half-sandwiches and fortified shakes.

Vitamin A Mends Skin

Vitamin A has been called the skin vitamin, and with good reason. At burn centers such as Shriners Burns Institute in Cincinnati, large amounts of vitamin A are added to liquid formulas designed to help prevent infection and promote the growth of new skin.

In studies with laboratory animals, vitamin A enhances healing that has been retarded by steroid drugs, immune suppression, diabetes or radiation, reports Thomas K. Hunt, M.D., professor of surgery at the University of California, San Francisco.

"Vitamin A works in many different ways," Dr. Hunt says. "It's required for cell growth and differentiation, or the ability of a cell to mature into its final form. This is important for the generation of new tissues." Vitamin A also seems to activate the production of connective tissue, including collagen, and to promote the growth of new blood vessels, he explains. That's important for nourishing newly forming tissues.

"Adequate vitamin A really is essential for anyone undergoing surgery," Dr. Wunderlich agrees. He recommends up to 25,000 international units of water-soluble vitamin A (available in health food stores) for certain patients undergoing surgery. Vitamin A can be toxic in doses exceeding 15,000 international units daily and has been found to cause birth defects in doses of 10,000 international units daily when taken during early pregnancy. For this reason, the dosage of vitamin A recommended here should be taken only under medical supervision, especially if you are a woman of childbearing age. And you should not use this therapy if you are pregnant.

Studies show that most people get about 5,000 international units a day from foods such as carrots, eggs and vitamin A–fortified milk.

Zinc Zeros In on Tissue Repair

Medical research shows that in people who are low in zinc, supplements can dramatically speed up the healing of surgical incisions. In a study by researchers at Wright-Patterson Air Force Base in Ohio, people taking 220 milligrams of zinc sulfate three times a day were completely healed in roughly 46 days, while a group taking no zinc required about 80 days to heal.

Zinc, like vitamins A and C, is needed in the body for many things, Dr. Wunderlich says. It's necessary for the production of collagen, the connective tissue that allows scars to form. It interacts with vitamin A, making the vitamin available for use. And it plays a vital role in immune function.

The people most likely to be short on zinc include those who've lost lots of fluid, those who've lost weight because of loss of appetite, those who've experienced loss of taste and those who've been getting lots of colds and infections, says Keith Watson, D.O., professor of surgery and associate dean for clinical affairs at the University of Osteopathic Medicine and Health Sciences in Des Moines, Iowa. "In addition to slow healing," he says, "bedsores, skin changes and depression can also be signs of zinc deficiency."

It's hard to determine if someone is actually short on zinc, Dr. Watson says. "So we may give a patient zinc and other nutrients, since an isolated deficiency is rare," he says. "Then if he doesn't soon start improving, we'll check his zinc status to see if the amount we are giving is bringing the patient's blood level back to normal."

Dr. Wunderlich recommends 15 milligrams of zinc citrate (an easily absorbed form) twice daily to a number of his patients undergoing surgery. It's best to take this much zinc only under your doctor's care, as amounts exceeding 15 milligrams daily can be toxic.

Vitamin E: For Healing Hearts

Some doctors add vitamin E to their on-the-mend menus, especially for people who've had heart surgery. There's some evidence that vitamin E helps stop the process of atherosclerosis, or the buildup of fatty deposits in arteries. And one study, by researchers at the University of Toronto, suggests that it can also help limit tissue damage during coronary bypass surgery.

In this study, half of a group of people undergoing bypass surgery took vitamin E before their operations. The other half took placebos (blank pills). After the surgery, the people taking 300 international units of vitamin E for two weeks prior to surgery had "small but significant" improvement in heart function compared with the people taking the placebos.

"Heart cells can be damaged when their blood supply is cut off and then restarted, a condition called reperfusion injury," says Donald Mickle, M.D., professor of clinical biochemistry at the University of Toronto and one of the study's authors. When oxygenated blood circulates through the oxygen-deprived heart, free radicals can form and can injure the heart cells, he says. (Free radicals are unstable molecules that steal electrons from your body's healthy molecules to balance themselves.)

Vitamin E is known as an antioxidant. In the right place at the right time, it neutralizes harmful free radicals by giving up its own electrons, sparing healthy molecules from harm.

"Our study suggests that for people at high risk—those with unstable

Prescriptions for Healing

Every nutrient is important when it comes to bouncing back from surgery. The problem is that nutrient needs vary widely depending upon your current nutritional status and the kind of procedure that you'll be having. Your best bet is to have a frank discussion about nutrition with your doctor well before your surgery. Many doctors recommend that their patients take multivitamin/mineral supplements both before and after surgery. Some suggest additional supplements as well. You should let your doctor know what you are currently taking and ask whether any changes are in order.

angina, for instance—treatment with vitamin E prior to bypass surgery may be of benefit," Dr. Mickle says. (For people who require immediate surgery, a water-soluble form of vitamin E that can be given intravenously just prior to or during surgery is being developed, he says.)

Doctors who recommend vitamin E to their surgery patients often prescribe about 400 international units of vitamin E daily. Don't take more than 600 international units without your doctor's okay, especially if you've had a stroke or bleeding problems in the past. "In large amounts, I'd say more than 800 international units, vitamin E can enhance bleeding problems," Dr. Wunderlich says. If you're taking anticoagulants, it's best not to take vitamin E supplements.

In fact, when you're going into surgery, it's a good idea to be aware of any and all nutritional therapy you are taking that might interfere with blood clotting, Dr. Wunderlich advises. "Some of my heart patients take garlic for their conditions, and since garlic can cause bleeding problems, I recommend stopping the garlic for a few weeks prior to surgery," he says.

"Remember, taking any kind of supplementation may interfere with your surgical procedure and recovery," says Dr. Curran-Celentano. "To be safe, take supplements only under medical supervision." A few weeks prior to surgery, you might want to discuss any supplements you've been taking with your doctor.

The most commonly offered bit of advice, from doctors and dietitians alike? Ask your doctor about taking a multivitamin/mineral supplement that provides the Daily Value of every essential nutrient. And if necessary, get enough protein and calories by adding nutritional liquids to your menu.

Taste and Smell Problems

Sense-sational Nutrition

Imagine being unable to smell a bank of honeysuckle blooming along a country road or to savor the sweetness of a freshly picked raspberry. Most of us would feel seriously deprived if we were denied these simple pleasures.

Unfortunately, that's what happens to people with taste and smell problems. (The two senses are so closely linked that people who can't smell often complain that they can't taste anything, either.)

For some people, these two vital senses may tend to decrease with age, for no apparent reason. For others, taste and smell drop off quickly, the result of a viral infection, a head injury or cancer therapy or as a side effect of certain prescription drugs.

People may also develop disturbing sensory changes, such as a metallic, bitter or salty taste that can occur by itself or be triggered by foods (citrus is a common culprit). In some cases, senses recover after a time, although they may never be as sharp as they once were.

Although most physicians are unfamiliar with these problems, it's still best to seek medical attention if something seems to be wrong with your sense of taste or smell. See your family doctor or an ear, nose and throat specialist, or call the nearest university hospital to find out if there's a taste and smell clinic nearby. Such centers draw on a variety of specialists to troubleshoot your problem.

While there are any number of treatments that your doctor may consider, you should be aware that one nutrient has definitely been linked to taste and smell disorders: zinc, an essential mineral, according to researcher Robert Henkin, M.D., Ph.D., director of the Taste and Smell Clinic of the Center for Molecular Nutrition and Sensory Disorders in Washington, D.C. Here's the latest thinking—and controversy—on this connection.

Zinc May Account for Good Taste

There's no doubt that people with severe zinc deficiencies, which are rare in the United States, often lose their sense of taste. But there's one thing that many of the doctors who treat taste and smell disorders apparently do not

Prescriptions for Healing

Doctors who recognize the role that nutrition can play agree that most taste and smell disorders are not caused by zinc deficiency alone but that deficiency may be a factor. Here's what these doctors recommend.

Nutrient	Daily Amount
Zinc	30 milligrams (zinc acetate or zinc gluconate)

MEDICAL ALERT: *Doses of zinc exceeding 15 milligrams daily should be taken only under medical supervision, as high amounts of this mineral can be toxic.*

know (or believe, for some reason): Even a relatively mild zinc deficiency can cause problems, says leading zinc researcher Ananda Prasad, M.D., Ph.D., professor of medicine at Wayne State University School of Medicine in Detroit.

"Years ago in Iran, we found aberrations in taste in young boys who were zinc-deficient. Their growth and sexual maturity were retarded, and they ate clay," he explains. "More recently, we found that volunteers made mildly zinc-deficient also lost some of their taste acuity." (Eating clay is a strange deficiency symptom known as geophagia.)

The volunteers, all healthy young men, weren't being seriously deprived of zinc, Dr. Prasad says. They ate what might be considered a fairly typical vegetarian diet, getting about five milligrams of zinc a day, one-third of the Daily Value. And they ate soy as their main source of protein. "Soy and grains contain phytates, compounds that interfere with the absorption of a variety of nutrients, including zinc," Dr. Prasad explains. The volunteers' sense of taste diminished after six months on the diet. (They also developed problems adapting their eyes to darkness.)

When these people were supplemented with 30 milligrams of zinc a day, their ability to taste returned in about two to three months.

Both taste buds and olfactory (smell) cells, which are found high in the nose, are specialized cells. They depend on zinc, along with other nutrients, for their growth and maintenance, Dr. Prasad explains.

Taste buds are especially dependent on zinc, says Dr. Henkin. He found that cells in the salivary glands make gustin, a zinc-dependent protein that is secreted in saliva. "Gustin is important in maintaining the sensation of taste," Dr. Henkin says. "It acts on the stem cells that are in the taste buds, causing these cells to differentiate, or to divide and develop into new taste bud cells."

Dr. Henkin believes that about 20 to 25 percent of taste and smell problems are zinc-related, not necessarily because people are zinc-deficient but because their bodies are unable to use zinc properly. "About half of these people benefit from additional zinc, but others don't improve no matter how much zinc they get," he says. He believes that these people have problems making gustin.

If you believe that your taste or smell problem may be linked to low zinc intake, discuss it with your doctor. And if your doctor recommends blood tests, keep in mind that the most commonly done tests, blood plasma and serum zinc levels, detect only severe deficiency, not mild to moderate deficiency, Dr. Prasad says. He measures the zinc content of lymphocytes (white blood cells), a much more sensitive test performed in only a few laboratories nationwide. Dr. Henkin, on the other hand, uses a measurement of zinc in saliva, which reflects the activity of the zinc-dependent enzyme that stimulates taste bud cells to grow and develop. This test, however, is not readily available.

Dr. Prasad believes most people can safely get up to 30 milligrams of zinc a day from foods and supplements. "More than that amount of zinc may interfere with copper absorption and so requires supplementation of 1 to 2 milligrams of copper daily, along with regular blood tests to check for anemia," he cautions. In addition, it's best to consult your doctor before taking zinc in doses of more than 15 milligrams daily, since large amounts of the mineral can be toxic.

Seafood and meats provide the most easily absorbed form of zinc. Eastern oysters are far and away the best source, with six cooked medium-size oysters providing about 76 milligrams of zinc. Three ounces of beef, veal, lamb, crab or pork provides about 7 milligrams of zinc. If you're taking supplements, zinc acetate and zinc gluconate deliver the goods with less stomach upset than zinc sulfate, Dr. Prasad says.

If zinc is going to improve your taste, it should begin to do so within three months, Dr. Prasad says. If you don't notice an improvement by then, it's likely that zinc is not going to help you. You should then cut back to the Daily Value, 15 milligrams, and consider some other cause of your problem, he advises.

Zinc-related sensory abnormalities, including decreased taste and smell acuity and problems adjusting your eyes in the dark, have been associated with a number of conditions, Dr. Prasad reports: liver disease, kidney disease, Crohn's disease, cystic fibrosis, Parkinson's disease, thyroid problems, multiple sclerosis, serious burns, Type II (non-insulin-dependent) diabetes, flulike infections, sickle-cell anemia and anorexia. These abnormalities have also been noted in people taking penicillamine, a rheumatoid arthritis drug. Dr. Prasad also believes that vegetarians and older people who don't eat much food, including meats, are often shortchanged on zinc. "Mild deficiency is much more common than most people realize," he says.

Tinnitus

Silencing the Ring

Susan J. Seidel, an otologist (hearing specialist) at the Greater Baltimore Medical Center, knows exactly how she developed the cicada-like chirp in her left ear.

"I was standing outside an airport, waiting to get on a plane, when a jet taxied toward our line," she recalls. "When it got close, it revved one of its engines to make a turn. The sound was so intense, I remember, that I clenched my teeth and thought 'Good grief, that's loud.' "

The blast lasted only a few seconds, but it set off the buzz that has pretty much stayed with her for more than 20 years. "I've gotten used to it, and lucky for me, it's in only one ear. But it has made me more interested in helping other people who have the same problem," she says.

Like Seidel, most of us have noticed that our ears can play their own tune for a time after being blasted by loud music or machinery, firecrackers or gunshots. Usually, the sound is barely noticeable, lasting anywhere from a few minutes to a couple of days.

For people with a condition called tinnitus, though, the ringing, hissing or buzzing becomes a persistent presence. Tinnitus, which in Latin means "tinkling like a bell," has been reported to reach volumes as high as 70 decibels. That's equivalent to having a vacuum cleaner in your head.

Tinnitus occurs when nerve cells in the cochlea, the tiny, snail shell–shaped inner ear, are damaged, explains Michael Seidman, M.D., director of the Tinnitus Center at the Henry Ford Hospital in Detroit. These nerves project hairlike endings into the cochlea, which is filled with fluid that moves in waves in response to sounds traveling through the ear. When a sound sends waves through the cochlea, the hairlike endings send a signal to the brain that gets interpreted as sound. When the sounds are too loud and the waves through the cochlea are too intense, the tiny nerve endings become damaged and may send abnormal signals that can cause hissing or buzzing.

Noise-induced spasms of the tiny arteries feeding the inner ears can also damage the tiny hairlike cells by cutting off their blood supply. The nerve cells can also be damaged by viruses, high blood pressure, high blood cholesterol and high insulin levels as well as by drugs, particularly aspirin and the *-mycin* antibiotics. Aminoglycosides such as gentamicin, which are often used to treat pneumonia, are probably the number one offenders, says Dr. Seidman. Tinnitus is often one symptom of Ménière's disease, a condition that is caused by excess fluid pressure in the inner ear.

Finally, degeneration of the aging ear, usually because of poor circulation, accounts for a large percentage of cases.

If you develop tinnitus, it's important to see a doctor to make sure that you don't have a tumor on an ear nerve or a damaged ear membrane, Dr. Seidman says. Both are treatable conditions.

While most doctors don't yet use nutrition to treat tinnitus, there is some intriguing new research, mostly from Israel, that holds promise for some people with this condition. Here's what doctors say may help.

Vitamin B_{12} Sheathes Ear Nerves

When it comes to nerves, vitamin B_{12} plays a special role. The body needs this nutrient to manufacture myelin, the fatty sheath that wraps around nerve fibers, insulating them and allowing them to conduct their electrical impulses normally.

A vitamin B_{12} deficiency can raise blood levels of homocysteine, an amino acid that is thought to be toxic to nerves. Low levels of B_{12} have been linked to a number of nervous system disorders, including memory loss, decreased reflexes, impaired touch or pain perception—and, apparently, tinnitus and noise-induced hearing loss.

Researchers from the Institute for Noise Hazards Research and Evoked Potentials Laboratory at Chaim-Sheba Medical Center in Ramat Gan and from Tel Aviv University, both in Israel, looked at a group of 385 people with tinnitus and found that 36 to 47 percent suffered from vitamin B_{12} deficiency. All of the people low in B_{12} received injections of 1,000 micrograms weekly for four to six months. At the end of that time, their hearing and tinnitus

Prescriptions for Healing

Tinnitus is one of those conditions that often resist treatment. Most ear specialists do not recommend nutrients to prevent or treat this condition. Some doctors, however, feel that certain nutrients can be helpful for some people. Here's what they recommend trying.

Nutrient	Daily Amount
Beta-carotene	100,000 international units, taken as 2 divided doses
Copper	1.5 milligrams (1 milligram for every 10 milligrams of zinc)
Magnesium	400 milligrams
Selenium	50–200 micrograms
Vitamin B_{12}	1,000 micrograms
Vitamin C	500 milligrams, taken as 2 divided doses
Vitamin E	400 international units
Zinc	15 milligrams

Plus a multivitamin/mineral supplement containing the Daily Values of all essential vitamins and minerals

MEDICAL ALERT: *If you have heart or kidney problems, be sure to talk to your doctor before beginning magnesium supplementation.*

Doses of selenium exceeding 100 micrograms daily can be toxic and should be taken only under medical supervision.

If you are taking anticoagulant drugs, you should not take vitamin E supplements.

were evaluated. Fifty-four percent reported improvement in their tinnitus, and approximately one-fourth reported reductions in the measured loudness of their tinnitus, according to Joseph Attias, D.Sc., head of the institute and one of the study's main researchers.

"Vitamin B_{12} deficiency is somehow associated with chronic tinnitus," says Dr. Attias. "Long-term exposure to noise may deplete body levels of B_{12} and so make the ears more vulnerable to noise-induced damage."

Most of the people in this study had tinnitus for six years or longer. "It's possible that people who are treated earlier for vitamin B_{12} deficiency may have more improvement in their tinnitus than occurred in this study," says Dr. Attias.

If you have tinnitus, and especially if you also have memory problems, ask your doctor to check your blood level of vitamin B_{12}, he suggests.

Although most people get enough vitamin B_{12} from foods, absorption problems can cause shortages, especially in older people. Strict vegetarians, who eat no meats, dairy products or eggs, are also at risk for deficiency, since B_{12} comes only from animal foods.

If your doctor determines that you have absorption problems, you'll need vitamin B_{12} shots for the rest of your life. If you don't have absorption problems, experts say that it's safe to take about 1,000 micrograms of B_{12} a day.

Magnesium May Shield Sensitive Ears

It's true that you won't find laboratory animals handling heavy artillery or using chain saws. But you can thank these creatures for another dietary recommendation for protecting ears: magnesium.

Magnesium-deficient lab animals exposed to noise have much more damage to the nerve cells in their cochleas than animals fed a diet adequate in magnesium, Dr. Attias says. What happens to these cells when the noise level gets too high? "The tiny hairs on these cells fuse or disappear, and they and their supporting cells eventually disintegrate, along with the nerve fibers going to these cells," explains Dr. Attias. Low levels of magnesium combined with noise exposure eventually deplete the cells' energy stores, leading to exhaustion, damage and death of the inner ear cells, he explains.

Low magnesium levels can also cause blood vessels, including the tiny arteries going to the inner ears, to constrict. (Remember, noise-induced vasospasm is thought to play a role in tinnitus.)

Human ears, even young, healthy, normal-hearing ones, can benefit from extra magnesium, Dr. Attias says. He found that Israeli soldiers who got an additional 167 milligrams of supplemental magnesium daily had less inner ear damage than soldiers getting placebos (blank look-alike pills). According to Dr. Attias, a more recent study showed that supplemental intake has this same protective effect against long-term noise exposure.

If you're faced with a noisy environment, you'll want to make sure that you're getting the Daily Value of magnesium, which is 400 milligrams, Dr. Attias says. Most people fall short in that regard, with men getting about 329 milligrams a day and women averaging 207 milligrams a day. Green vegetables, whole grains, nuts and beans are packed with magnesium. (If you're considering taking magnesium supplements, be sure to talk to your doctor first if you have heart or kidney problems.)

If your tinnitus includes a sensation of fullness in your ear and balance problems, experts recommend that you get adequate amounts of calcium and potassium as well. These additional symptoms could be a sign of Ménière's disease. (For the full details on treating Ménière's with nutrients, see page 381.)

Antioxidants May Help Spare Ears

Tinnitus is sometimes caused by impaired blood flow to the ears, which can happen in two ways, Dr. Seidman says. First, the tiny artery leading to the inner ear can get clogged with cholesterol, causing a kind of stroke in the ear, he explains. Second, loud noises can send this artery into spasm, reducing blood supply to the cochlea. In either case, an interrupted blood supply can lead to hearing problems.

That's where the antioxidant nutrients—vitamin C, vitamin E, beta-carotene and others—come in. "Antioxidants work by helping to prevent oxygen-caused damage to cell membranes," Dr. Seidman explains. Antioxidants also help keep arteries open and free of plaque buildup, experts say.

Dr. Seidman and some other ear doctors suggest that you consider a smorgasbord of antioxidant nutrients: 400 international units of vitamin E daily, 250 milligrams of vitamin C twice daily, 50 to 200 micrograms of the mineral selenium daily and about 50,000 international units of beta-carotene twice daily. Doses of selenium exceeding 100 micrograms daily can be toxic and should be taken only under medical supervision.

Zinc Can Make a Difference

Some parts of the body have much higher concentrations of certain vitamins and minerals than other parts. That's the case with the inner ear, which, like the retina of the eye, has a high concentration of zinc. That finding has led some doctors to speculate that zinc deficiency may play a role in inner ear problems such as tinnitus.

"We don't know much about how zinc works in the inner ear, but it's evident that the cochlea needs zinc to function properly," explains George E. Shambaugh, Jr., M.D., professor emeritus of otolaryngology and head and neck surgery at Northwestern University Medical School in Chicago. "Animals fed a diet low in zinc partially lose the ability to hear, and apparently, even the kind of marginal zinc deficiency often seen in older people worsens the hearing loss associated with ear damage from noise or aging." Zinc is involved in a wide array of functions, including helping to maintain healthy cell membranes and protecting cells from oxygen-related damage.

Dr. Shambaugh estimates that about 25 percent of the people he sees with severe tinnitus are zinc-deficient. Sometimes they also have poor appetite, hair loss, diminished taste or smell or skin problems. All of these symptoms are related to zinc deficiency. For these people, he recommends supplemental zinc, along with a potent multivitamin/mineral that supplies other nutrients.

Although Dr. Shambaugh and other ear, nose and throat specialists may initially give large doses of zinc, up to 150 milligrams a day, it's important to take no more than about 15 milligrams a day without medical supervision. Doctors monitor blood levels of zinc when they prescribe higher amounts. That's because zinc can be toxic in large doses. Zinc also interferes with copper absorption, so if you're taking high doses of zinc, you may need to take supplemental copper (the ratio that's generally recommended is 1 milligram of copper for every 10 milligrams of zinc). Copper, too, can be toxic, so follow your doctor's advice on this.

The Daily Value for zinc is 15 milligrams. According to Dr. Shambaugh, few people get 10 to 15 milligrams a day in their diets, while people over age 75 rarely get as much as 7 milligrams a day. Look to meats and shellfish for zinc; cooked oysters, beef, crab and lamb all offer good amounts.

Vitamin A May Aid Hearing

Like zinc, vitamin A is found in high concentrations in the cochlea. "All special sensory receptor cells, including the retina of the eye and the hair cells of the inner ear, depend upon vitamin A and zinc to function properly," Dr. Shambaugh says.

In one study, low blood levels of vitamin A were associated with decreased ability to hear. And in several studies, from 24 to 74 percent of people with tinnitus reported at least partial relief with vitamin A supplements.

"I recommend beta-carotene, which you can take without worrying about toxicity," Dr. Shambaugh says. (The body can use beta-carotene to make vitamin A.) He recommends taking 30 milligrams (about 50,000 international units) of beta-carotene twice a day.

Varicose Veins

Winning an Uphill Battle

That marbled look might work well on a fireplace mantel or a coffee table, but when it's on your legs—no way! You'd prefer them without those blue squiggles, thank you very much.

Why is it that some people have those squiggles and others don't?

To understand that, it helps to look at how the veins function. The heart pumps blood to the lungs to pick up oxygen. Then the blood travels back to the heart to be pumped out through arteries, thus delivering oxygen throughout the body. The heart pushes blood out through the arteries with a great deal of force. And when blood is making its return trip to the heart from various parts of the body, it moves through veins.

"Veins can't rely on the same forceful pressure that arteries have to move blood," explains Robert Ginsburg, M.D., director of the cardiovascular intervention unit at the University of Colorado Health Sciences Center in Denver. "Instead they use valves that open in one direction only, toward the heart, to keep blood from flowing backward. And they rely on muscle contractions to squeeze blood in the right direction." Inefficient? Well, send your complaints to Mother Nature.

Varicose veins, those blue bulges, develop when veins can't return blood to the heart efficiently. Blood pools in the veins, making them dilate. That hinders the valves' ability to close tightly and stop backward blood flow. Eventually, veins may become permanently dilated and scarred and take on a torturous configuration similar to a road map of West Virginia.

Varicose veins are not just a cosmetic problem. They can contribute to swollen, tired legs and muscle cramps.

Some people develop varicose veins because they have inherited structural problems with the valves in the upper parts of their legs, says Joseph Pizzorno, Jr., N.D., a naturopathic physician and president of Bastyr University in Seattle. "Even if just one or two valves fail, that can put enough pressure on the lower part of a vein so that it, too, has problems," Dr. Pizzorno says.

Other people have leaky valves because their veins are simply too weak to withstand the pressure of backflowing blood.

Most doctors' nutritional advice for varicose veins is limited to "Lose weight, eat more fiber." Both of these dietary measures help reduce pressure in veins. The few doctors who go beyond this advice to recommend nutritional supplements say they're focusing on nutrients that help maintain the structural integrity of the vein wall and help reduce the possibility of blood clots in veins. Here's what these doctors recommend.

Vitamin C Helps Fragile Veins

Keeping vein walls strong is important when it comes to preventing varicose veins or keeping them from getting worse, according to medical experts. Strong vein walls can resist more pressure without dilating, which allows the veins' valves to work better.

That's where vitamin C comes in. The body needs it to manufacture two important connective tissues: collagen and elastin. Both of these fibers are used to repair and maintain veins to keep them strong and flexible, explains Dr. Pizzorno. Vitamin C, he says, may be especially important for you if you bruise easily or have broken capillaries, which may show up on your skin as tiny "spider veins."

Even more important to keeping veins and capillaries in tip-top shape may be vitamin C's first cousin, bioflavonoids. Bioflavonoids are chemical compounds often found in the same foods as vitamin C.

Dr. Pizzorno recommends 500 to 3,000 milligrams of vitamin C and 100 to 1,000 milligrams of bioflavonoids daily. These high amounts are easily obtained only with supplements. Some people experience diarrhea with as little as 1,200 milligrams of vitamin C a day, so you should discuss taking this much with your doctor.

Vitamin E Keeps Blood Flowing

While there are no studies to show that vitamin E heals varicose veins, people with varicose veins apparently do use it, hoping that it will help prevent the biggest potential complication: blood clots.

"Vitamin E helps keep platelets, blood components involved in clotting, from sticking together and from adhering to the sides of blood vessel walls," Dr. Pizzorno explains. Research shows that reducing platelet stickiness with vitamin E could help people at particularly high risk for blood-clotting problems, such as those with diabetes.

If you're going to take vitamin E, aim for 200 to 600 international units

Food Factors

Certain foods can help minimize clotting, reduce pressure and strengthen vein walls. Spice up your menu with these suggestions.

Beef up on bioflavonoids. Deep-colored berries, such as cherries, blueberries and blackberries, contain these chemical compounds, as do the white membranes of citrus fruits. They're also found in wine and grape juice.

"Bioflavonoids are thought to reduce capillary fragility," says Joseph Pizzorno, Jr., N.D., a naturopathic physician and president of Bastyr University in Seattle. When fragile capillaries distend or break down, they can appear on the skin as red or blue "spider veins."

Reach for fiber foods. If you strain hard to move your bowels, you create pressure in your abdomen that can block the flow of blood back up your legs. Over time, the increased pressure may weaken vein walls, explains Robert Ginsburg, M.D., director of the cardiovascular intervention unit at the University of Colorado Health Sciences Center in Denver.

So avoid constipation by eating plenty of fiber-containing foods. Besides those berries, try other fruits as well as vegetables, beans and whole grains.

Pare down. Added body fat, especially around your middle, also creates pressure in your abdomen, making it harder for blood to return to your heart, explains Dr. Ginsburg. Keep your weight down, and chances are you'll have fewer problems with bulging veins.

Lick the salt habit. Too much salt can make your legs swell and stress already damaged veins. Dr. Ginsburg suggests cutting back by loading your diet with fresh fruits and vegetables as well as whole grains. You'll also be upping your intake of other minerals that help reduce fluid retention: potassium, magnesium and calcium.

daily, suggests Dr. Pizzorno. Some research suggests that 200 international units a day is enough to reduce platelet adhesion. If you've had bleeding problems or a stroke, it's important that you talk to your doctor before starting vitamin E supplementation. If you are taking anticoagulants, you should not take vitamin E supplements.

A Trace Mineral Helps Keep Veins Strong

We all know that minerals help keep bones strong. Studies show that some minerals do the same for blood vessels, helping to build and maintain the layers of tissues that form blood vessel walls.

Copper, which we all need in small amounts, is used in the body to knit together collagen and elastin, the same connective tissues that require vitamin C.

"Copper is involved in the cross-linking between the molecules that make up these tissues," explains Leslie Klevay, M.D., Sc.D., of the U.S. Department of Agriculture Grand Forks Human Nutrition Research Center in North Dakota. Research has shown that copper-deficient animals have weakened arteries and capillaries, two of the three types of blood vessels in our bodies (the third is veins), that can bulge out under pressure.

According to Dr. Klevay, little research has been done on copper's effect on veins. But because arteries and veins have similar structures, it is quite possible that the strength of veins depends on adequate copper levels, too. This is why everyone, including people with varicose veins, should make sure that they're getting adequate amounts of this trace mineral, Dr. Klevay says.

Copper is also needed to build and repair endothelial cells, the smooth protective cells lining the insides of blood vessels, Dr. Klevay explains. Getting adequate copper appears to help protect blood vessels against microscopic tears and rough spots, caused by high blood pressure and smoking, that can lead to the buildup of cholesterol-laden plaque and to blood clots.

The Daily Value for copper is two milligrams. Your best bet for getting enough? Include whole grains, nuts and seeds, along with shellfish (especially cooked oysters) and lean red meat, in your diet, recommends Dr. Klevay.

B Vitamins May Help Stop Clots

Endothelial cells are also damaged by high blood levels of an amino acid called homocysteine. The damage has been linked to early heart disease and, more recently, to increased risk of recurrent blood clots in veins.

That's where the three Bs come in. Researchers now know that folate (the naturally occurring form of folic acid) and vitamins B_6 and B_{12} help break down and clear homocysteine from the blood. "Deficiency of any one could lead to a high level of homocysteine," explains Jacques Genest, Jr., M.D., director of the cardiovascular genetics laboratory at the Clinical Research Institute of Montreal, a research center that has done pioneering work

Prescriptions for Healing

Using supplements to treat varicose veins is not standard medical practice, but some doctors feel that certain nutrients are helpful. Here's what they recommend.

Nutrient	Daily Amount
Copper	2 milligrams
Folic acid	2,500 micrograms
Vitamin B_6	25 milligrams
Vitamin B_{12}	2 micrograms
Vitamin C	500–3,000 milligrams
Vitamin E	200–600 international units

MEDICAL ALERT: Folic acid in doses exceeding 400 micrograms daily can mask symptoms of pernicious anemia, a vitamin B_{12}–deficiency disease, and should be taken only under medical supervision.

Some people may experience diarrhea when taking vitamin C in doses of more than 1,200 milligrams daily.

If you've had bleeding problems or a stroke, it's important that you talk to your doctor before starting vitamin E supplementation. If you are taking anticoagulants, you should not take vitamin E supplements.

on homocysteine and heart disease. "We've found that 2.5 milligrams (2,500 micrograms) of folic acid or 25 milligrams of vitamin B_6 reduces homocysteine levels to normal in most people," he says.

These high amounts of folic acid and vitamin B_6 are well above the Daily Values (400 micrograms and two milligrams, respectively) and are available only through supplements. This much folic acid should be taken only under medical supervision, as amounts exceeding the Daily Value can mask symptoms of pernicious anemia, a vitamin B_{12}–deficiency disease.

Even those eating healthy diets, with two or three servings of fruits and three or four servings of vegetables a day, get only about 190 micrograms of folate daily. As for vitamin B_6, men get about 1.9 milligrams a day and women average 1.2 milligrams a day through foods such as chicken, fish, pork and eggs. Some people may need to take both, and older people and strict vegetarians may also need extra vitamin B_{12}, Dr. Genest adds. He recommends taking 2 micrograms of B_{12} a day.

Water Retention

Beating the Bloat

Forget that "ashes to ashes, dust to dust" stuff. Water to water is more like it. Our aquatic ancestors brought the sea with them when they crawled on land, and human beings remain mostly fluid. We're 56 percent fluid, to be exact—but sometimes more, sometimes less, depending on the degree of bloat.

People who retain fluid know just how easy it is to swell up like a sponge. "Weight fluctuations of as much as four to five pounds in a single day are not uncommon in women with fluid retention problems," says Marilynn Pratt, M.D., a physician in private practice in Playa del Rey, California, who specializes in women's health.

Bloating occurs when fluid that normally flows through the body in blood vessels, lymph ducts and tissues gets trapped in tissues in the interstitial spaces, the tiny channels between cells. The fluid flows through the membranes of tiny blood capillaries into the tissue cells because of osmotic pressure (cell wall pressure), which is controlled by electrolytes such as sodium. A high sodium level attracts more fluid from the blood into the cells, where the fluid gets trapped and the cells become overhydrated. This occurs more readily in women, because their tissues are designed to fluctuate or expand for pregnancy.

Lots of things can cause waterlogged tissues: allergic reactions to foods, heart and kidney problems and prescription drugs such as hormones. In women, hormonal changes often cause bloating beginning seven to ten days prior to menstruation, as higher levels of estrogen and progesterone during that part of the cycle cause the body to retain salt (sodium) and therefore to retain fluid in tissues. "Replacement hormones (especially estrogen alone) can also cause substantial bloating and weight gain," says Dr. Pratt.

Food Factors

If you know that bag of salty chips is going to lead to water retention, then you pretty much know what you have to do to avoid the problem. Other dietary choices are not quite so obvious. Here's what many experts recommend.

Drink more water. If your fluid retention is caused by excess salt intake, cut back immediately and drink plenty of water, at least eight glasses a day, to help flush out the salt, says Marilynn Pratt, M.D., a physician in private practice in Playa del Rey, California, who specializes in women's health.

Watch out for MSG. MSG, or monosodium glutamate, also contains sodium. MSG is found in lots more than Chinese food; it's a common ingredient in processed foods. Read your labels for "MSG" or "hydrolyzed vegetable protein," which contains MSG, and avoid these foods as much as possible.

Avoid alcohol. Alcohol does act as a diuretic at first, making you lose excess water. But this loss of fluid can progress to the point of dehydration. And medical experts have another good reason for giving this advice: Alcohol depletes your body of important vitamins and minerals.

Try a natural diuretic. Several herbal teas have a mildly diuretic effect. Parsley tea is the best-known type. Brew two teaspoons of dried leaves per cup of boiling water and steep for ten minutes. Drink up to three cups a day.

Lose weight if you need to. Overweight women have more estrogen in their systems because fat tissue produces estrogen, Dr. Pratt says. This puts them at higher than normal risk for retaining fluid in their tissues and for adding to their overall weight. Overweight women need lots of water and must drastically reduce salt intake.

Ferret out food allergies. If you wake up in the morning congested, with puffy eyes and a headache, suspect a food allergy, says Joseph Pizzorno, Jr., N.D., a naturopathic physician and president of Bastyr University in Seattle. "In my opinion, wheat is by far the most common allergy-causing food, but it could be any food. So it's best to get tested," he says.

Usually, fluid retention is uncomfortable but not health-threatening. People who retain fluid because of heart or kidney problems, however, or who are taking diuretics (water pills) need to be under a doctor's care for their problems, says Dr. Pratt.

Nutritional changes for fluid retention are meant to counteract hormonal changes, balance the minerals that influence body fluid and eliminate foods that trigger bloating in some people. Here's what doctors say helps.

The Salt Connection

Most of us know that too much salt in our bodies can lead to temporary swelling. An evening's overload on movie popcorn or ballpark franks can leave us puffy-eyed and headachy, with stiff, swollen hands and feet, the next morning. "That's because our kidneys retain fluid in our bodies so that the excess salt can be diluted," explains David McCarron, M.D., professor of medicine and head of the Division of Nephrology, Hypertension and Clinical Pharmacology at Oregon Health Sciences University in Portland. And, contrary to what you might think, drinking more water will not worsen fluid retention and may even help.

And some researchers believe that too little salt in the diet can also cause fluid retention, Dr. McCarron says. "We speculate that too little salt may trigger the kidneys to secrete more of a hormone that conserves salt, in part by reducing urinary output," Dr. McCarron says. He recommends keeping salt intake at 2,400 milligrams (a little more than one teaspoon) a day, an amount thought to maintain optimum blood pressure.

For most people, this still means cutting back by about 1,000 milligrams (about a half-teaspoon) a day. Since most of our salt comes from processed foods, not from the shaker, the best way to cut back is to look for sodium-free or low-sodium versions of cheeses, nuts, crackers, lunchmeats, canned soups and vegetables.

"And women who are dieting may be eating a lot of celery, which has a higher level of sodium than any other vegetable," Dr. Pratt says. Munch on carrot sticks instead, she suggests.

Mix-and-Match Minerals

Getting too little potassium, calcium or magnesium in your diet can also contribute to fluid retention, Dr. McCarron says. "These minerals all play important roles in the fluid balance in your body—your body's ability to move

Prescriptions for Healing

There are a number of nutrients that can help relieve some cases of water retention. Here's what some experts recommend.

Nutrient	Daily Amount
Calcium	1,000–1,500 milligrams
Magnesium	400 milligrams
Potassium	3,500 milligrams
Vitamin B_6	200 milligrams, taken as 4 divided doses for 5 days before the start of menstruation
Plus a B-complex supplement	

MEDICAL ALERT: Doctors recommend limiting your sodium intake to no more than 2,400 milligrams a day.

Some doctors advise against supplementing calcium, magnesium or potassium without medical supervision if you have diabetes or heart, kidney or liver problems or if you are taking diuretics.

People who are taking nonsteroidal anti-inflammatory drugs, potassium-sparing diuretics, ACE inhibitors or heart medications such as heparin should also check with their doctors before supplementing potassium.

Vitamin B_6 can be toxic in large amounts. Do not take more than 100 milligrams a day without medical supervision. The higher dose suggested here may safely be consumed for the number of days noted to relieve premenstrual bloating.

fluid into and out of cells and from the bloodstream or lymphatic system into tissues and back again," he says.

He recommends getting about 3,500 milligrams of potassium a day (the Daily Value), an amount you can obtain by eating at least five servings of fruits and vegetables. (Potassium is lost in cooking water, though, so don't count on boiled potatoes or greens for this mineral unless you consume the water that they're cooked in.)

For magnesium, aim for the Daily Value of 400 milligrams, Dr. McCarron suggests. Most people fall short of this amount, with men getting about 329 milligrams a day and women averaging 207 milligrams a day. Nuts, legumes and whole grains supply the most magnesium; other good food sources are green vegetables and bananas.

And for calcium, doctors recommend striving for 1,000 to 1,500 milligrams a day. One quart of skim milk contains about 1,400 milligrams of calcium. On average, men between ages 30 and 70 get close to 1,000 milligrams a day, while women in the same age group consume only about 700 milligrams daily, at least 300 milligrams less than they need.

If you have heart, kidney or liver problems or diabetes, or if you're taking a diuretic to relieve fluid retention or high blood pressure, you should supplement these minerals only under medical supervision to make sure you don't develop dangerously high blood levels, says Dr. McCarron. People who are taking nonsteroidal anti-inflammatory drugs, potassium-sparing diuretics, ACE inhibitors or heart medications such as heparin should also check with their doctors before supplementing potassium.

Vitamin B_6 May Aid Hormone-Related Bloating

Most women don't need a calendar to tell them when that time of the month is imminent. Their tender breasts, swollen hands and feet and tightening blue jeans from abdominal swelling—all signs of fluid retention—mark time as well as any calendar.

In addition to the changes in mineral intake outlined above, some doctors recommend increases in the B vitamins, B_6 in particular. "Vitamin B_6 plays a role in the body's use of several hormones associated with fluid retention, including estrogen and progesterone," says Dr. Pratt. "By helping the body to metabolize these hormones, B_6 may help the liver metabolize excess amounts, which may be present during the premenstrual period."

In one study, in fact, 500 milligrams of vitamin B_6 daily relieved the breast tenderness, headaches and weight gain associated with water retention in 215 women.

If you'd like to try vitamin B_6 for hormone-related fluid retention, Dr. Pratt recommends taking 200 milligrams a day (50 milligrams four times a day) for the five days before your period begins. Take a B_6 supplement along with a supplement containing the rest of the B-complex vitamins. "These nutrients interact, so they work better when adequate amounts of all are available," Dr. Pratt says.

Vitamin B_6 can be toxic and can cause serious nerve damage in excessive amounts. For these reasons, it's best not to take more than 100 milligrams a day without checking with your doctor. You may, however, safely take up to 200 milligrams daily for five days to relieve premenstrual bloating, Dr. Pratt says. If your hands or feet start to feel numb or clumsy, stop taking B_6 and tell your doctor.

Wilson's Disease

Neutralized by Zinc

At age 22, the woman weighed 69½ pounds, consumed 700 calories a day, appeared depressed, didn't menstruate, chattered incessantly and worried constantly about everything and anything.

Her doctors suspected an eating disorder, so they admitted her to a hospital at the National Institutes of Health in Bethesda, Maryland, and began to run some tests.

Everything checked out normally until they looked at her liver. There the doctors found that the woman had almost 15 times the normal amount of copper tucked away, a sure sign that she had Wilson's disease, a condition in which various body tissues are slowly poisoned by copper.

Sunflower Eyes and Shaking Limbs

Copper is a nutrient that is required by all cells, most notably for the development of healthy nerves, connective tissue and the dark pigment in hair and skin. Everyone needs a little copper. In someone with Wilson's disease, however, a genetic error allows the metal to build up to toxic levels in the brain, liver, kidneys and eyes. The astronomical amounts that accumulate can result in impaired mental ability, dementia and liver failure.

Fortunately, the disease is rare, preventable and treatable. It occurs in about 30 of every 1,000,000 people, generally somewhere between the ages of 10 and 40 and most often among Eastern European Jews and their descendants.

Depending on where toxic levels of copper are accumulating, symptoms can range from malaise, fatigue, tenderness over the liver and perhaps low-grade fever—which together may seem to indicate a viral infection or acute hepatitis—all the way to eating disorders, the cessation of menstruation, shaking limbs and "sunflower cataracts," which are green, yellow or brown rings around the corneas.

"The biggest problem is recognition of the disease," says pioneering researcher George Brewer, M.D., professor of human genetics and internal medicine at the University of Michigan Medical School in Ann Arbor. "Many cases go unrecognized because the disease masquerades as, say, hepatitis or cirrhosis of the liver caused by alcohol."

Complicating recognition is the fact that symptoms frequently evolve over time rather than appearing all at once. "Instead of developing obvious neurological complications, for example, many people will have behavioral abnormalities for several years," explains Dr. Brewer. "They can become depressed, and they usually lose the ability to focus mentally. So if they're in school, their grades will drop. Or if they have jobs, they'll start to not perform as well. They'll become temperamental. They may become suicidal, and they can become exhibitionists.

"Often these behaviors are attributed to drug abuse, because you have people who have been normal and they sort of go off the deep end. Their spouses often leave during this period," he says.

The Blessing of Zinc

Fortunately, Wilson's disease is both preventable and treatable with zinc, according to Dr. Brewer.

In a series of studies at the University of Michigan, Dr. Brewer and his colleagues found that zinc induces formation of metallothionein, a substance that grabs on to any copper it can find and holds the copper in intestinal cells until they are sloughed off and excreted with other intestinal waste.

"The intestinal cells, like cells on the surface of your skin, turn over fairly rapidly," explains Dr. Brewer. "They have about a six-day life span. So when they slough into the intestines, they take the copper with them. It then goes out into the stool."

But zinc is not the first thing that doctors reach for when Wilson's disease is diagnosed. "Zinc is kind of leisurely acting for somebody who is symptomatic," says Dr. Brewer. "So we've developed a new drug called tetrathiomolybdate, a compound that works very nicely in the initial treatment of people with brain symptoms. We use it for eight weeks, and then we transition to zinc.

"For people with liver disease," he continues, "we use a combination of

Prescriptions for Healing

Zinc counteracts the toxic accumulation of copper that occurs in the brain, liver, kidneys and eyes of a person with Wilson's disease. Here's the amount recommended by George Brewer, M.D., professor of human genetics and internal medicine at the University of Michigan Medical School in Ann Arbor.

Nutrient	Daily Amount
Zinc	150 milligrams, taken as 3 doses spaced evenly throughout the day, each at least 1 hour before or after a meal

MEDICAL ALERT: Anyone with Wilson's disease should be under a doctor's care, especially since the amount of zinc recommended here can be toxic. Likewise, people who do not have Wilson's disease should not take this much zinc without the knowledge and consent of their doctors. Zinc can deplete copper in your body.

another drug, trientine hydrochloride (Syprine), and zinc. The trientine helps flush out the copper fairly rapidly."

Once on zinc-only therapy, a person with Wilson's disease is home free. "You're not trying to get rid of all of the copper in your body," says Dr. Brewer. "Copper is an essential nutrient, and without copper, people die. So what you're doing with zinc therapy is reducing the excessive load of copper and preventing it from reaccumulating."

That's why you can eat a normal diet. "The only two foods we ask people not to eat are liver, which is loaded with copper, and shellfish, which have intermediately high amounts," adds Dr. Brewer.

Sopping Up Copper

How much zinc does it take to sop up the extra copper in your body?

A study conducted by Dr. Brewer at the University of Michigan indicated that 150 milligrams of zinc a day, taken as three separate 50-milligram doses, each at least an hour before or after a meal, provides optimum copper removal. Because zinc can be toxic in such a high amount, it's important that you be under medical supervision while using this therapy.

Taking zinc with meals negates the mineral's effect. "If zinc is taken with a food, it's almost like not taking it, because it gets bound with material in the food and doesn't do much," says Dr. Brewer. "But if you split it away from food, as little as 25 milligrams will have a detectable effect on copper balance."

And that's also why people who do not have Wilson's disease should not take large amounts of zinc, adds Dr. Brewer. Since it takes a fairly small amount of zinc to have an effect on copper levels in the body, taking more than the Daily Value of zinc (15 milligrams) could easily make you copper-deficient within two to three weeks.

Preventing the Problem

Zinc also has the ability to prevent the onset of symptoms in people who have inherited the aberrant gene but have not yet developed any symptoms. Unfortunately, the only way to detect the possibility that you might have Wilson's disease before symptoms appear is to have it hit a brother or sister.

That's why siblings of those with Wilson's disease should have their urine monitored by their family physicians on a regular basis for elevated levels of copper, says Dr. Brewer. The odds are one in four that they will develop the disease at some time in their lives.

"Wilson's disease is an autosomal recessive disease," Dr. Brewer says. "That means the affected person has two doses of the abnormal gene that triggers the disease. The parents are obligatory carriers, but since each parent has only one dose, they will be completely normal."

Fortunately, even children who have inherited the disease will be completely normal, too—once they're put on zinc, says Dr. Brewer.

Wrinkles

Smoothing Out the Lines

Skin is like brand-new underwear. In the beginning, the elastic is snug and resilient, stretching and snapping right back into place. But after years of wear and tear, pulling and tugging and exposure to the elements, that elastic gradually gives, until one day . . . well, it's time to get new underwear.

Would that we could get new skin, too. Because after years of our laughing, crying, rubbing and, worst of all, sunning, our skin begins to give as well.

In fact, if it weren't for sun exposure, say the experts, our skin would stay relatively smooth into our eighties. That's why a dermatologist's first recommendation for wrinkle prevention is "Get out of the sun."

Sun exposure damages skin inside and out. First it attacks the epidermis, the thin, outermost tier of skin, forming a layer of dead cells that give skin a leathery appearance. Then it progressively damages the upper layers of the dermis, or the bulk of the skin, leaving them thinner, less resilient and more susceptible to wrinkling. Over time, the collagen and elastin fibers that form the dermis also break down, causing gradual drooping and sagging.

Fortunately, dermatologists say, the appearance of a few crow's-feet and laugh lines doesn't mean that you're on a slippery slope to Wrinkle City. By protecting yourself from the sun, shunning cigarettes and eating right, you can prevent many new wrinkles from occurring. You can also do some wrinkle erasing as well. Star players in getting rid of wrinkles once they've formed are some vitamin-derived compounds that are applied topically.

An A-Plus for Retin-A

Aside from plastic surgery, the best thing for getting rid of wrinkles is tretinoin, a vitamin A compound better known as Retin-A. No, it can't iron out deep lines, lift droops or undo severe damage, but Retin-A can erase the crow's-feet, fine lines and crinkling left by aging and the sun.

Retin-A, originally developed as an acne medication to unplug clogged pores, works against wrinkles by stimulating cell turnover, explains Retin-A creator Albert Kligman, M.D., Ph.D., professor of dermatology at the University of Pennsylvania School of Medicine and an attending physician at the Hospital of the University of Pennsylvania, both in Philadelphia. "Retin-A stimulates collagen production and blood flow into the dermis," says Dr. Kligman. "It creates tissue and makes the dermis thicker. In short, it returns skin to a more youthful condition and prevents many wrinkles from occurring."

But having heard that promise a thousand times before, you may wonder: Are the results noticeable?

Investigators at the University of Michigan Medical Center in Ann Arbor say they are. After studying 29 people who had sun-damaged skin, they reported that those who were treated for 10 to 12 months with Retin-A experienced an 80 percent increase in collagen formation compared with a

Food Factors

Ask most dermatologists about the best foods for healthy skin, and their answer will likely be "just eat a good, nutritious diet." But here are two specific dietary measures that they recommend to help avoid wrinkles.

Go easy on the spirits. Making too much merry can make your skin . . . well, very unmerry. Not only does that morning-after puffiness contribute to wrinkles, but alcohol also dehydrates you, which is anything but good for your skin, especially if you're using topical vitamin A (Retin-A), says Albert Kligman, M.D., Ph.D., professor of dermatology at the University of Pennsylvania School of Medicine and an attending physician at the Hospital of the University of Pennsylvania, both in Philadelphia, and the creator of Retin-A. "Like smoking or unprotected exposure to sunlight, too much drinking can cause skin irritation in people using Retin-A," he says.

Get plenty of water. You should drink four glasses of water a day, says Dr. Kligman, unless you are sweating heavily. If you are sweating a lot, of course, drink more water.

14 percent decrease in collagen formation among those using a cream not fortified with vitamin A.

Just don't try to get the same results by upping your dietary intake of vitamin A, warns Dr. Kligman. "When people try to get the same effects by megadosing vitamin A supplements, the results are almost the opposite," he says. "Their skin becomes dry and itchy, and their hair starts to fall out from vitamin A toxicity."

Retin-A cream comes in a variety of strengths, from 0.025 to 0.1 percent. It's available by prescription only, so your dermatologist can help determine which concentration is best for you. Generally, people beginning Retin-A treatment apply the lowest-dosage cream nightly or every other night until their dermatologists instruct them otherwise.

Because Retin-A removes the dead top layer of skin and exposes an area previously sheltered from evaporation and the elements, a common side effect is dry, sun-sensitive skin that can be irritated and scaly. Though both of these side effects typically diminish with time, if you're using Retin-A, you'll likely need a moisturizer. And you'll definitely need a sunscreen; once you start taking Retin-A, your days in the sun are over. Also, ask about Renova, an "updated" Retin-A with built-in moisturizer that has been approved by the Food and Drug Administration as a prescription cream.

C Is for Collagen

Though not as well-established in the antiwrinkle business as vitamin A, vitamin C, a nutrient known for its importance in the manufacture of collagen, is being touted by some experts as a key player in keeping the complexion smooth.

"Vitamin C is essential for connective tissue in the body, particularly for the layer where the collagen that maintains the integrity of your skin is made," explains Lorraine Meisner, Ph.D., professor of preventive medicine at the University of Wisconsin Medical School in Madison. "That's why people who eat adequate diets look younger than people who don't."

Dr. Meisner is quick to add that "adequate" vitamin C is not enough to prevent wrinkles. "The Daily Values are set incredibly low," she says. "They are enough to keep you from getting deficiency diseases but not enough to repair and maintain aging skin." Dr. Meisner generally recommends a daily vitamin C dosage of 300 to 500 milligrams. And if you smoke, you really need to boost your vitamin C intake, she says, because smoking appears to deplete vitamin C levels as well as promote wrinkles.

She also recommends topical use of high-concentration vitamin C preparation for people who are concerned about getting enough vitamin C into their skin through diet alone. "That's especially true for older people and for those who have a lot of sun exposure," says Dr. Meisner. "Their circulation tends to be impaired at the periphery, so it's harder for dietary vitamin C to get into the skin."

Topical vitamin C has also been shown to prevent the free radical skin damage that occurs following exposure to ultraviolet rays from the sun. Free radicals are unstable molecules that steal electrons from your body's healthy molecules to balance themselves. Unchecked, free radicals can cause significant tissue damage and contribute to premature wrinkling.

"It's possible that topical vitamin C, when used in conjunction with sunscreen, could prevent a significant amount of the wrinkling caused by sun exposure," says Douglas Darr, Ph.D., director of technology development at the North Carolina Biotechnology Center in Research Triangle Park.

A 10 percent vitamin C lotion called Cellex-C is available without a prescription from dermatologists, plastic surgeons and licensed aestheticians

Prescriptions for Healing

Doctors agree that certain nutrients can not only diminish some of our fine lines but also provide a touch of "permanent press" to slow the formation of new ones. Here's what some doctors recommend.

Nutrient	Daily Amount/Application
Oral	
Selenium	50–200 micrograms (l-selenomethionine)
Vitamin C	300–500 milligrams
Vitamin E	400 international units (d-alpha-tocopherol)
Topical	
Vitamin A	0.025%–0.1% cream (Retin-A), depending on skin type
Vitamin C	10% lotion (Cellex-C)
Vitamin E	5%–100% ointment or oil, applied after sun exposure

MEDICAL ALERT: *Selenium can be toxic in doses exceeding 100 micrograms daily. High amounts should be taken only under medical supervision.*

If you are taking anticoagulant drugs, you should not take oral vitamin E supplements.

(full-service beauty salon operators) and by mail order from Cellex-C Distribution, 2631 Commerce Street, Suite C, Dallas, TX 75226 (1-800-423-5592). It should be applied 15 to 30 minutes prior to sun exposure, along with sunscreen, for best results, says Dr. Meisner, one of the developers of Cellex-C.

For a burst of vitamin C in your diet, you can go the traditional orange juice and citrus route, or you can create a vegetable medley of broccoli, brussels sprouts and red bell peppers. But take note: If you want sun damage protection, don't count on being able to eat enough vitamin C, says Dr. Darr. "You can't get enough into your skin without applying it topically," he says.

Stopping Wrinkles with Vitamin E

Vitamin E, another free radical–fighting antioxidant, can also prevent skin damage from sun exposure when used topically, say researchers. But they recommend it for post-sun use rather than pre-sun use.

Vitamin E oil, applied up to eight hours after sun exposure, can prevent inflammation and skin damage, says John R. Trevithick, Ph.D., professor in the Department of Biochemistry at the University of Western Ontario in London, Ontario. But save it for after you come inside, as vitamin E itself can produce free radicals when exposed to ultraviolet light. Vitamin E oil can be bought over the counter in drugstores.

For additional sun damage protection, try taking vitamin E supplements, adds Karen E. Burke, M.D., Ph.D., a dermatologic surgeon and dermatologist in private practice in New York City. Dr. Burke recommends 400 international units daily in the form of d-alpha-tocopherol. "Although studies of oral vitamin E and wrinkles still need to be done, the supplements can help reduce photodamage and keep skin healthier," says Dr. Burke.

Vitamin E–rich foods include wheat germ, spinach and sunflower seeds.

Selenium Wrinkle Prevention

Like vitamin E, the mineral selenium quenches free radicals caused by sun exposure and prevents skin damage, says Dr. Burke. But because selenium is found in the soil and its concentrations vary nationwide, some people may get adequate amounts, while others are deficient, she says. People in the Southeast in particular tend to have low selenium levels, she notes.

For optimum skin protection, Dr. Burke recommends daily supplements of 50 to 200 micrograms of selenium (preferably the l-selenomethionine form), depending on where you live and your family history of skin cancer. Because selenium can be toxic in doses of more than 100 micrograms daily, it's best to supplement high amounts only under medical supervision.

For a big dietary boost of selenium, reach for tuna, as one three-ounce can packs 99 micrograms. Other good sources include garlic, onions and broccoli.

Dr. Burke is developing a selenium cream that she says will "work even better than Retin-A in reversing photoaging." (For more details on using nutrients to protect yourself from sun damage, see page 521.)

Yeast Infections

Ditching the Itch

Have itchy palms? Some would say that money is coming your way. A seven-year itch? Better have a heartfelt chat with your mate. An itch where . . . well, you'd rather not discuss it? Welcome to one of the most common of feminine struggles: woman versus the beast called yeast.

In fact, at some point during their childbearing years, three in four women will wonder what they did to deserve the itching, burning, odor and unpleasant discharge that accompany vaginal yeast infections. They'll also want to know exactly what they can do to stop it from ever happening again.

The Nature of the Yeast

Fortunately, there are steps women can take to prevent these itchy episodes. But first, it helps to understand why a yeast infection happens at all.

The most likely culprit behind this maddening malady is a generally mild-mannered fungus known as *Candida albicans* that lives in the vagina, mouth and intestines. Normally, candida is kept to its small, harmless colonies by the immune system and by *Lactobacillus acidophilus*, bacteria commonly found in the vagina that create an acidic environment that candida doesn't like. When something throws this ecosystem off balance, however, candida runs rampant, and yeast infections can result.

The most common offenders, things that upset this delicate ecosystem, include wet bathing suits, panty hose, skintight jeans and leotards. All of these things foster a warm, moist environment that candida loves. Women are also prone to yeast infections during pregnancy, just before they get their periods and during menopause. Candida also multiplies when women are taking antibiotics, because such medications often kill too many good bacteria, such as lactobacillus, along with the bad, leaving candida unchecked.

Be a Bad Host with Good Nutrition

Once candida has become a flaming yeast infection, doctors commonly recommend over-the-counter medications such as miconazole (Monistat)

Food Factors

You probably already know that shedding a wet bathing suit or sweaty underclothes is a good preventive against moisture-loving yeast infections. But you may not know that doctors have found that adding certain foods to your diet, or removing others, might help fight these itchy occurrences as well. Here are their dietary recommendations for staying yeast-free.

Say yes to yogurt. Whoever developed the old home remedy of douching with yogurt to stop a yeast infection was close to being right. She was just putting it in the wrong place! You have to eat a cup of it a day, and it has to contain active *Lactobacillus acidophilus* cultures. (If the yogurt contains live cultures, it will say so on the label.)

In a study of 33 women at the Long Island Jewish Medical Center in Hyde Park, New York, researchers found that women with histories of yeast infection recurrence could decrease the incidence of recurrence threefold just by eating eight ounces of yogurt a day.

Say no to sweets. *Candida albicans* (the medical term for the kind of yeast that causes vaginal infections) is a fungus with a real sweet tooth. Indulging in too many sweet, sugary foods can raise your blood sugar level and create the perfect candida breeding ground, according to William Crook, M.D., author of *The Yeast Connection and the Woman* and a physician in Jackson, Tennessee.

Skip yeasty foods. Though there hasn't been any research to confirm this, some doctors report that women prone to yeast infections can experience outbreaks from eating yeasty foods. Dr. Crook suggests avoiding foods such as pizza and beer as well as aged foods such as wine, cheeses and smoked meats.

Ward off vampires. Garlic contains an antimicrobial agent known as allicin. There is some evidence that candida simply hates garlic. Some women have found that eating a clove of garlic a day helps prevent yeast infections, says Tori Hudson, M.D., professor at the National College of Naturopathic Medicine in Portland, Oregon.

and clotrimazole (Gyne-Lotrimin) or the new one-dose, prescription-only fluconazole (Diflucan), all of which can have you sitting comfortably again in less than a week. But since these medications won't kick candida out for good, and since yeast infection recurrence is common, doctors say you have to be a bad host if you want to stay yeast-free.

"Treating the vagina alone is often a waste of time and money," says William Crook, M.D., author of *The Yeast Connection and the Woman* and a physician in Jackson, Tennessee. "Although vaginal suppositories may help, we also need to concentrate on putting the right things in your body to take care of the source of the problem."

According to the experts, that means boosting your immunity through good diet and nutritional supplements such as vitamins A, C and E and the mineral zinc. Here's what they recommend.

Note: Although *Candida albicans* is the most common cause of vaginal infections, it isn't the only cause. So if you've never had a yeast infection before, see your doctor for a proper diagnosis before starting any treatment on your own.

Keep Yeast from Rising with Zinc

When it comes to fighting disease, the mineral zinc is often a heavyweight contender. It stimulates the production of T lymphocytes, the cells in your immune system that are responsible for cleaning up cells that have been invaded by infection. According to medical research, this makes zinc a prizefighter against *Candida albicans*.

In fact, zinc supplements are likely beneficial even if your body's zinc levels are normal, according to a study done in India. Researchers there worked with laboratory animals that were not deficient in zinc. They gave these animals high-dose zinc supplements and found that they were significantly more resistant to infection from *Candida albicans* than those not supplemented with zinc.

"Zinc is essential in preventing infection," agrees Dr. Crook. "And though it's best to get your vitamins and minerals through a healthy diet, supplementation is probably a good idea, given how many essential nutrients our food loses by the time it's processed, packaged, shipped and bought."

To fight candida, Tori Hudson, M.D., professor at the National College of Naturopathic Medicine in Portland, Oregon, suggests taking the Daily Value of zinc, which is 15 milligrams. And to get more zinc through your diet, try cooked oysters. They contain about 76 milligrams of zinc per half-dozen.

Prescriptions for Healing

While medicated creams can give your most tender areas the quickest relief from an annoying yeast infection, you'll need some nutritional immunity builders if you want to prevent a recurrence. Here's what many experts suggest.

Nutrient	Daily Amount/Application
Oral	
Vitamin A	25,000 international units
Vitamin C	4,000 milligrams, taken as 2 divided doses
Vitamin E	400 international units
Zinc	15 milligrams
Topical	
Vitamin A	Gelatin capsule, used as a suppository

MEDICAL ALERT: *If you've never had a yeast infection before, be sure to see a doctor for proper diagnosis before starting treatment on your own.*

Vitamin A can be toxic in doses exceeding 15,000 international units daily and has been found to cause birth defects in doses of 10,000 international units daily when taken in early pregnancy. For this reason, the amount recommended here should be taken only under medical supervision, especially if you are a woman of childbearing age. Do not use this therapy if you are pregnant.

Some people experience diarrhea from taking more than 1,200 milligrams of vitamin C daily. So check with your doctor before trying this higher dose.

If you are taking anticoagulants, you should not take vitamin E supplements.

Acidify with Vitamin C

When it comes to fighting *Candida albicans*, vitamin C does double duty.

First, research has shown that vitamin C boosts immunity by keeping disease-fighting white blood cells up and running, so the body is better able to stave off infections, especially opportunistic ones such as candida that take advantage of a weak immune system. As a bonus, vitamin C adds acidic zip to your vaginal environment. "Candida-fighting lactobacillus grows in acid," explains Roy M. Pitkin, M.D., professor of obstetrics and gynecology at the University of California, Los Angeles. "So taking vitamin C may help, though it isn't likely to be completely effective by itself."

For optimum results, Dr. Hudson recommends 4,000 milligrams of vitamin C a day, divided into two 2,000-milligram doses and taken once in the morning and once in the evening for better absorption. This amount is considerably higher than the Daily Value, which is only 60 milligrams. Although such high amounts of vitamin C are considered safe, some people experience diarrhea from taking just 1,200 milligrams daily. If you want to try this higher dose to prevent yeast infections, discuss it with your doctor.

Think fruits and vegetables to boost the vitamin C in your diet. One cup of broccoli, orange juice or brussels sprouts provides about 100 milligrams.

Build Immunity with A and E

For women who are having ongoing battles with candida, Dr. Hudson recommends adding two more immunity-boosting nutrients to the mix: vitamins A and E.

"Vitamin A can be used either of two ways," says Dr. Hudson. Women can take vitamin A supplements of 25,000 international units a day, an amount that is five times the Daily Value and that should be taken only under medical supervision. This is especially important for women of childbearing age, since daily doses of 10,000 international units of vitamin A during early pregnancy have been linked to birth defects. It's for this reason that women who are pregnant should not use this therapy. If a woman prefers not to take such a high amount orally, she can insert the vitamin into the vagina instead.

"Inserting vitamin A stimulates the immune system right in the vagina," says Dr. Hudson. "You can simply insert a vitamin A gelatin capsule, although they are less potent than the vitamin A suppositories made by several companies."

As a final precautionary measure, she recommends taking 400 international units of vitamin E.

If you are a frequent victim of the yeast beast and would like to increase these nutrients in your diet, try cooking with vegetable oils and eating whole-grain cereals for more vitamin E, drinking fortified skim milk for a burst of vitamin A and upping your intake of bright orange and yellow vegetables to increase beta-carotene (a substance that turns to vitamin A in the body).

Index

Underlined page references indicate boxed text. Prescription drugs are denoted by the symbol Rx.

A

B

D

E

F

G

H

I

J

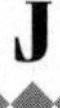

K

L

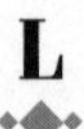

M

P

Q

R

T

W

Y

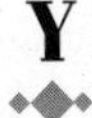

Z

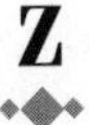